50.00

RADIATION ONCOLOGY
SELF-ASSESSMENT GUIDE

RADIATION ONCOLOGY
SELF-ASSESSMENT GUIDE

John Suh, MD
Professor and Chairman
Department of Radiation Oncology
Taussig Cancer Institute
Cleveland Clinic
Cleveland, Ohio

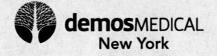

demosMEDICAL
New York

Visit our website at www.demosmedpub.com

ISBN: 9781936287536
e-book ISBN: 9781617050985

Acquisitions Editor: Rich Winters
Compositor: diacriTech

Medicine is an ever-changing science. Research and clinical experience are continually expanding our knowledge, in particular our understanding of proper treatment and drug therapy. The authors, editors, and publisher have made every effort to ensure that all information in this book is in accordance with the state of knowledge at the time of production of the book. Nevertheless, the authors, editors, and publisher are not responsible for errors or omissions or for any consequences from application of the information in this book and make no warranty, express or implied, with respect to the contents of the publication. Every reader should examine carefully the package inserts accompanying each drug and should carefully check whether the dosage schedules mentioned therein or the contraindications stated by the manufacturer differ from the statements made in this book. Such examination is particularly important with drugs that are either rarely used or have been newly released on the market.

Library of Congress Cataloging-in-Publication Data

Radiation oncology : self-assessment guide.
    p. cm.
 Includes index.
 ISBN 978-1-936287-53-6
 1. Cancer--Radiotherapy--Examinations, questions, etc.
 RC271.R3R33194 2013
 616.99'40642--dc23

                    2012026307

Special discounts on bulk quantities of Demos Medical Publishing books are available to corporations, professional associations, pharmaceutical companies, health care organizations, and other qualifying groups. For details, please contact:

Special Sales Department
Demos Medical Publishing, LLC
11 West 42nd Street, 15th Floor
New York, NY 10036
Phone: 800-532-8663 or 212-683-0072
Fax: 212-941-7842
E-mail: rsantana@demosmedpub.com

Printed in the United States of America by Gasch.
12 13 14 15 / 5 4 3 2 1

CONTENTS

Contents

PREFACE

It is with great pleasure and excitement that I introduce the first edition of *Radiation Oncology Self-Assessment Guide*. This handbook was specifically designed to help facilitate one's understanding and knowledge of the natural history, epidemiology, diagnosis, staging, treatment options, and treatment-related side effects of the various diseases encountered in radiation oncology practice by using a "flash card" format. The contributors to this guide are faculty and residents of the Department of Radiation Oncology at the Cleveland Clinic Taussig Cancer Institute. To help reinforce the reader's knowledge of each area, including key studies and treatment recommendations, each answer has key reference(s) that can be reviewed.

This handbook covers the various disease sites, including head and neck cancers, central nervous system tumors, breast cancers, thoracic cancers, gastrointestinal cancers, genitourinary cancers, gyencologic cancers, lymphomas, and pediatric cancers. Each disease site is further subdivided into specific diseases or tumor types to help facilitate further self-assessment and reinforce one's knowledge. This *Guide* uses an evidence-based approach when discussing treatment recommendations.

My sincere hope is that this self-assessment guide will provide a convenient and efficient method to enhance the understanding of radiation oncology, which is a dynamic and evolving medical specialty. By providing this unique "flash card" approach with citations of key references, I believe that *Radiation Oncology Self-Assessment Guide* will provide educational, actionable, and practical information that will enhance one's ability to provide evidence-based, high-quality patient care.
I wish to thank my many colleagues in the Department of Radiation Oncology at the Cleveland Clinic Taussig Cancer Institute whose valuable contributions made this learning resource possible and the many patients who inspire me to do better each day.

John Suh, MD

1

HEAD AND NECK CANCERS

SHLOMO KOYFMAN AND MONICA SHUKLA

Question 1

Is there a benefit to radiation intensification with altered fractionation when treating locally advanced squamous cell cancer of the head and neck (LA-HNSCC) with radiation alone?

Question 2

Is there a benefit to altered fractionation in the setting of concurrent chemotherapy?

Question 3

Is there a benefit to treating locally advanced squamous cell cancer of the head and neck (LA-HNSCC) with 6 fractions weekly rather than 5?

Answer 1

A significant benefit in local control (LC) for hyperfractionated radiotherapy (HRT) or accelerated concomitant boost (ACB) radiotherapy was shown in RTOG 90-03, a 4 arm phase III randomized trial that demonstrated ~10% improvement for either HRT (81.6 Gy/68 fx at 1.2 Gy BID) or ACB (72 Gy/42 fx at 1.8 Gy QD with an additional 1.5 Gy fx in the PM for the last 12 treatment days) compared to either standard RT (70 Gy/35 fx) or split course accelerated hyperfractionated radiotherapy (AHF-RT 67.2 Gy/42 fx at 1.6 Gy BID with a 2-week break after 38.4 Gy). Locoregional control (LRC) was ~55% in the former two groups compared to ~45% in the latter two groups. The MARCH meta-analysis also demonstrated a significant LRC advantage (7%) to both hyperfractionation and concomitant boost RT. While there was a modest survival advantage overall, hyperfractionated regimens produced an 8% OS advantage and outperformed other altered fractionation regimens (2%).

Bourhis J, Overgaard J, Audry H, et al. Hyperfractionated or accelerated radiotherapy in head and neck cancer: a meta-analysis. *Lancet.* 2006;368:843–854.

Fu KK, Pajak TF, Trotti A, et al. A Radiation Therapy Oncology Group (RTOG) phase III randomized study to compare hyperfractionation and two variants of accelerated fractionation to standard fractionation radiotherapy for head and neck squamous cell carcinomas: first report of RTOG 9003. *Int J Radiat Oncol Biol Phys.* 2000;48:7–16.

Answer 2

No. The RTOG 0129 protocol randomized patients with locally advanced HNC to standard fractionation (70 Gy/35 fx) with 3 cycles of cisplatin (d 1, 22, 43) vs ACB-RT (72 Gy in 42 fx) with 2 cycles of cisplatin (d 1, 22). There were no significant differences between the arms in terms of LRC or OS. Some hypothesize that a 3rd cycle of cisplatin offers similar benefit to hyperfractionation in this setting.

Ang KK, Harris J, Wheeler R, et al. Human papillomavirus and survival of patients with oropharyngeal cancer. *N Engl J Med.* 2010;363:24–35.

Answer 3

Yes. The phase III DAHANCA-6/7 trial randomized patients to 6 fractions a week (either an extra fraction on Saturday/Sunday, or a BID fraction given on Thursday or Friday of weeks 2–6) vs 5 fractions weekly, and demonstrated a LRC (70% vs 60%) and DFS advantage to this regimen. This forms the basis for the current RTOG standard accelerated regimen of 70 Gy in 35 fx/6 weeks with a BID fraction delivered on Thurs/Fri of weeks 2–6 being used in the RTOG 1016 trial. Of note, the DAHANCA-6/7 trial treated to 66–68 Gy with concurrent Nimorazole, and did not use concurrent chemotherapy.

Overgaard J, Hansen HS, Specht L, et al. Five compared with six fractions per week of conventional radiotherapy of squamous-cell carcinoma of head and neck: DAHANCA 6 and 7 randomised controlled trial. *Lancet.* 2003;362:933–940.

http://www.rtog.org/ClinicalTrials/ProtocolTable/StudyDetails.aspx?study=1016. Accessed October 25, 2011.

Question 4

What are the indications to add systemic chemotherapy to definitive radiotherapy in head and neck cancer?

Question 5

What induction chemotherapy regimen produces superior results to conventional cisplatin and 5-fluorouracil (PF) chemotherapy?

Question 6

How is cetuximab dosed when used concurrently with radiotherapy, and what is the evidence supporting its use?

Question 7

What structures are removed in a radical neck dissection?

Modified radical neck dissection?

Selective neck dissection?

Answer 4

Chemotherapy is indicated in stage III/IV disease based on several prospective randomized trials that demonstrated LRC, DFS and OS advantages with the addition of concurrent chemotherapy. This benefit was seen compared to standard fractionated RT (Adelstein) as well as hyperfractionated RT (Brizel). The MACH-NC meta-analysis also demonstrated a 4% 5-yr OS advantage overall, with the highest advantage seen in the setting of concurrent chemotherapy (35% vs 27%).

Adelstein DJ, Li Y, Adams GL, et al. An intergroup phase III comparison of standard radiation therapy and two schedules of concurrent chemoradiotherapy in patients with unresectable squamous cell head and neck cancer. *J Clin Oncol.* 2003;21:92–98.

Brizel DM, Albers ME, Fisher SR, et al. Hyperfractionated irradiation with or without concurrent chemotherapy for locally advanced head and neck cancer. *N Engl J Med.* 1998;338:1798–1804.

Pignon JP, le Maître A, Maillard E, et al. Meta-analysis of chemotherapy in head and neck cancer (MACH-NC): an update on 93 randomised trials and 17,346 patients. *Radiother Oncol.* 2009;2:4–14.

Answer 5

The addition of docetaxel (T) to the PF backbone was investigated in two phase III randomized studies and demonstrated improved LRC and OS (not DM), compared to PF alone. In the Vermorken study, pts were treated with TPF X 4 cycles followed by RT alone. In the Posner trial, pts were treated with similar induction chemotherapy (3 cycles) followed by RT + concurrent weekly carboplatin.

Posner MR, Hershock DM, Blajman CR, et al. Cisplatin and fluorouracil alone or with docetaxel in head and neck cancer. *N Engl J Med.* 2007;357:1705–1715.

Vermorken JB, Remenar E, van Herpen C, et al. Cisplatin, fluorouracil, and docetaxel in unresectable head and neck cancer. *N Engl J Med.* 2007;357:1695–1704.

Answer 6

400 mg/m^2 loading dose 1 week prior to RT and 250 mg/m^2 weekly during RT. It was tested in a phase III study compared to RT alone and demonstrated superior outcomes, including 2-yr LRC (50% vs 41%) and 3-yr OS (55% vs 45%). There was no difference in rates of DM (16% vs 17%). 5-yr results confirmed these findings.

Bonner JA, Harari PM, Giralt J, et al. Radiotherapy plus cetuximab for squamous-cell carcinoma of the head and neck. *N Engl J Med.* 2006;354:567–578.

Answer 7

In these procedures the following is removed:

Radical neck dissection (RND) – removes levels I–V, sternocleidomastoid muscle (SCM), omohyoid muscle, IJV, EJV, CN XI, submandibular gland.

Modified RND – removes levels I–V, but does not remove at least one of the following structures: SCM, IJV or CN XI.

Selective neck dissection – does not remove all of levels I–V. There are several named subtypes of selective neck dissections, including:

supraomohyoid neck dissection – removes levels I–III.

lateral neck dissection – removes levels II–IV.

Frank, DK, Sessions RB. Management of the neck – surgery. In: Harrison LB, Sessions RB, Hong WK, eds. *Head and Neck Cancer: A Multidisciplinary Approach.* 3rd ed. Philadelphia, PA: Lippincott Williams & Wilkins; 2008:185–189.

Question 8

In non-nasopharyngeal head and neck IMRT planning, what is the most important planning organ at risk (OAR)?

Question 9

In IMRT planning, what are the PTV coverage constraints generally mandated in RTOG studies?

Question 10

In IMRT planning, what are the three different target constraints for the parotid glands?

Question 11

What is the main benefit to IMRT planning seen in randomized studies compared to 2D/3D-CRT?

Answer 8

No more than 0.03 cc of the spinal cord planning risk volume (PRV) can receive > 50 Gy. No more than 0.03 cc of the brainstem PRV can receive > 52 Gy. The PRV cord = cord + 5 mm in each dimension. The PRV brainstem = brainstem + 3 mm in each dimension. These supercede PTV coverage.

http://www.rtog.org/ClinicalTrials/ProtocolTable/StudyDetails.aspx?study=1016. Accessed October 25, 2011.

Answer 9

> 95% of the PTV should receive prescription dose; no more than 20% of PTV will receive ≥ 110% of prescription dose (V110 ≤ 20%); no more than 5% of PTV will receive ≥ 115% of prescription dose (V115 ≤ 5%)

http://www.rtog.org/ClinicalTrials/ProtocolTable/StudyDetails.aspx?study=1016. Accessed October 25, 2011.

Answer 10

Mean dose to at least one gland (contralateral to disease) ≤ 26 Gy; or at least 50% of one gland to < 30 Gy; or at least 20 cc of the combined volume of both parotid glands to < 20 Gy.

http://www.rtog.org/ClinicalTrials/ProtocolTable/StudyDetails.aspx?study=1016. Accessed October 25, 2011.

Answer 11

IMRT has been studied in several phase III randomized trials and has been associated with reduced late grade ≥ 2 xerostomia (29%–40% for IMRT vs 80%–83% for 2/3D).

Kam MK, Leung SF, Zee B, et al. Prospective randomized study of intensity-modulated radiotherapy on salivary gland function in early-stage nasopharyngeal carcinoma patients. *J Clin Oncol.* 2007;25:4873–4879.
Nutting CM, Morden JP, Harrington KJ, et al. Parotid-sparing intensity modulated versus conventional radiotherapy in head and neck cancer (PARSPORT): a phase 3 multicentre randomised controlled trial. *Lancet Oncol.* 2011;12:127–136.

Question 12

What is the mechanism of action for amifostine and its primary side effects?

Is it beneficial in preventing xerostomia in patients treated with RT for H&N cancer?

Question 13   **OROPHARYNGEAL CANCER**

What is the risk of ipsilateral and bilateral nodal disease for a base of tongue (BOT) cancer?

Question 14

What is the risk of contralateral nodal involvement for a T1-2N0-1 well lateralized tonsil cancer?

Question 15

What are the most common assays to stain for HPV and p16?

Answer 12

Amifostine is a free radical scavenger. It can cause nausea, vomiting, hypotension and allergic reactions. The subcutaneous administration helps reduce these toxicities. It was tested in two phase III studies as an IV formulation. In the Brizel trial (RT vs RT + amifostine at 200 mg/m^2 15–30 minutes prior to RT), it significantly reduced the rate of acute (78% vs 51%) and chronic (58% vs 34%) grade $\geq$ 2 xerostomia. In the Beuntzel trial (RT + carboplatin + placebo vs RT + carboplatin + amifostine), there was no advantage to its use. It is FDA approved as a radioprotectant, but is not routinely used in many centers.

Brizel DM, Wasserman TH, Henke M, et al. Phase III randomized trial of amifostine as a radioprotector in head and neck cancer. *J Clin Oncol.* 2000;18:3339–3345.
Buentzel J, Micke O, Adamietz IA, et al. Intravenous amifostine during chemoradiotherapy for head-and-neck cancer: a randomized placebo-controlled phase III study. *Int J Radiat Oncol Biol Phys.* 2006;64:684–691.

Answer 13

About 70% of patients with BOT cancer have ipsilateral LN disease and 20% have contralateral nodal involvement at presentation.

Hu KS, Choi WH, Culliney B, et al. Cancer of the oropharynx. In: Phillips TL, Hoppe R, Leibel SA, eds. *Textbook of Radiation Oncology.* 3rd ed. Philadelphia, PA: Elsevier/Saunders; 2010:549–550.

Answer 14

The risk is below 5%. In a retrospective series from PMH in which patients with T1-2N0 tonsil cancers were treated with unilateral irradiation, the incidence of contralateral neck failure was 3.5%

O'Sullivan B, Warde P, Grice B, et al. The benefits and pitfalls of ipsilateral radiotherapy in carcinoma of the tonsillar region. *Int J Radiat Oncol Biol Phys.* 2001;51:332–343.

Answer 15

HPV is most often assessed using in situ hybridization techniques, which identifies the HPV DNA, while the p16 protein is most reliably identified through immunohistochemistry. About 20% of tumors that are p16+ are high risk HPV negative, making p16 a more sensitive assay.

Adelstein DJ, Ridge JA, Gillison ML, et al. Head and neck squamous cell cancer and the human papillomavirus. Summary of a National Cancer Institute State of the Science Meeting; November 9–10, 2008; Washington, DC. *Head Neck.* 2009;31:1393–1422.
Allen CT, Lewis JS Jr, El-Mofty SK, et al. Human papillomavirus and oropharynx cancer: biology, detection and clinical implications. *Laryngoscope.* 2010;120:1756–1772.

Question 16

Which subsite of the H&N is most associated with HPV/p16-related SCC, and what is its prognostic significance?

Question 17

What are some of the epidemiological and tumor related differences between HPV + and HPV – disease?

Question 18

What is the risk of microscopic involvement of level IB and level V in patients with T1/T2, node + SCC-OP with a negative staging CT in these levels?

Question 19

What are the early oncologic and functional results of transoral robotic surgery (TORS) for oropharyngeal cancers?

Answer 16

Oropharyngeal cancers are most heavily associated with HPV/p16+, with 60–70% of these tumors being HPV + and/or p16+. Both HPV + and p16+ status is a powerful prognostic marker, and has been shown on subset analysis of the RTOG 0129 trial to demonstrate the following improved outcomes:

	3-yr OS	3-yr PFS	3-yr LRF	3-yr DM	2nd Primary
HPV +	82%	74%	14%	9%	6%
HPV −	57%	43%	35%	15%	15%
p-value	< .001	< .001	< .001	.23	.02

Ang KK, Harris J, Wheeler R, et al. Human papillomavirus and survival of patients with oropharyngeal cancer. *N Engl J Med.* 2010;363:24–35.

Answer 17

HPV + disease tends to occur in younger, Caucasian men with limited smoking histories. It has been associated with higher number of (oral) sexual partners and marijuana use. It more frequently also presents with smaller primaries (T1/2), more advanced nodal disease (N2/3) that are often cystic appearing. HPV − disease tends to occur in patients with heavier smoking and alcohol histories, and more commonly affects older, non-Caucasian men. It is more often presents as T3/4 disease.

Gillison ML, D'Souza G, Westra W, et al. Distinct risk factor profiles for human papillomavirus type 16-positive and human papillomavirus type 16-negative head and neck cancers. *J Natl Cancer Inst.* 2008;100:407–420.

Answer 18

Less than 5% overall. In one study of patients who underwent up-front bilateral neck dissections and had negative CT necks in levels IB and V, the rates of pathologically positivity were 3% and 1%, respectively. Based on this data, some are not routinely covering these nodal stations in patients who fit these criteria.

Sanguineti G, Califano J, Stafford E, et al. Defining the risk of involvement for each neck nodal level in patients with early T-stage node-positive oropharyngeal carcinoma. *Int J Radiat Oncol Biol Phys.* 2009;74:1356–1364.

Answer 19

Early reports suggest excellent local control and functional outcomes. Results from the Univ. of Pennsylvania group suggest 98% local-regional control, with overall function returning to near baseline 1-year post treatment. About 80% of patients will require adjuvant RT with or without chemotherapy.

Cohen MA, Weinstein GS, O'Malley BW Jr, et al. Transoral robotic surgery and human papillomavirus status: Oncologic results. *Head Neck.* 2011;33:573–580.

Leonhardt FD, Quon H, Abrahão M, et al. Transoral robotic surgery for oropharyngeal carcinoma and its impact on patient-reported quality of life and function. *Head Neck.* 2012;34:146–154.

Question 20
What are the subsites of the oral cavity?

Question 21
What defines an oral cavity lesion as T4?

Question 22
What factor is an independent prognostic factor predictive of local and regional recurrence in oral tongue cancer treated primarily with surgery?

Question 23
For early stage tumors of oral tongue/floor of mouth being treated with definitive RT, what is the recommended treatment approach?

Answer 20

Mucosal lip, buccal mucosa, gingival (upper and lower), retromolar trigone, floor of mouth, mobile tongue (anterior to circumvallate papillae), hard palate.

Gomez DR, Kaplan MJ, Colevas AD, et al. Cancer of the oral cavity. In: Phillips TL, Hoppe R, Leibel SA, eds. *Textbook of Radiation Oncology.* 3rd ed. Philadelphia, PA: Elsevier Saunders; 2010:588–589.

Answer 21

T4 (Lip) – Invades through cortical bone, inferior alveolar nerve, floor of mouth, or skin of face (i.e., chin or nose).
T4a (Oral cavity) – Invades through cortical bone, into deep (extrinsic) muscle of tongue, maxillary sinus, or skin of face.
T4b (all) – Involves masticator space, pterygoid plates, or skull base, or encases internal carotid artery.

Part II, Section 3: Lip and oral cavity. In: Edge SB, Byrd DR, Compton, CC, et al., eds. *AJCC Cancer Staging Manual.* 7th ed. New York, NY: Springer; 2010:33.

Answer 22

Depth of invasion of the index lesion is prognostic. A depth of invasion of ≥ 5 mm has been shown to be prognostic for increased risk of regional failures.

I-Charoenrat P, Pillai G, Patel S, et al. Tumour thickness predicts cervical nodal metastases and survival in early oral tongue cancer. *Oral Oncol.* 2003;39:386–390.

Answer 23

A combination of EBRT and interstitial implant yields the best results. One large review demonstrated 33–60% failure with treatment with either EBRT or brachytherapy alone. EBRT dose of < 40 Gy with high proportion of brachytherapy (30–40 Gy lDR equivalent) yielded highest LC (92%). There was also a 44% neck recurrence rate when only the primary was treated.

Wendt CD, Peters L, Delclos L, et al. Primary radiotherapy in the treatment of stage I and II oral tongue cancers: importance of the proportion of therapy delivered with interstitial therapy. *Int J Radiat Oncol Biol Phys.* 1990;18:1287–1292.

Question 24

What is the significance of Ohngren's line and the Vidian canal in paranasal sinus tumors?

Question 25

What is the rate of subclinical nodal involvement for patients with maxillary sinus and nasal cavity tumors?

Question 26

How does orbital involvement affect the T stage of a maxillary sinus tumor?

Question 27

What is the anticipated 5-yr LRC and OS for patients with paranasal sinus tumors treated with surgical resection and postop RT?

Answer 24

Ohngren's line is a theoretical diagonal plane extending from the medial canthus to the angle of the mandible. Tumors arising above this line (suprastructure) have a worse prognosis than those that arise from below this line (infrastructure). The pterygoid/vidian canal is a passage in the skull leading from just anterior to the foramen lacerum in the middle cranial fossa to the pterygopalatine fossa and is a potential route of spread from the maxillary sinus to the middle cranial fossa.

Chen AM, Ryu J, Donald PJ, et al. Cancer of the nasal cavity and paranasal sinuses. In: Phillips TL, Hoppe R, Leibel SA, eds. *Textbook of Radiation Oncology*. 3rd ed. Philadelphia, PA: Elsevier Saunders; 2010:700–703.

Answer 25

The overall rate for subclinical nodal involvement is about 15%, making elective nodal radiotherapy controversial. Some report significantly distinct rates of nodal involvement based on histology. While it approaches 30–40% for poorly differentiated squamous carcinomas, it is only 10% for mucoepidermoid and adenocarcinomas.

Chen AM, Ryu J, Donald PJ, et al. Cancer of the nasal cavity and paranasal sinuses. In: Phillips TL, Hoppe R, Leibel SA, eds. *Textbook of Radiation Oncology*. 3rd ed. Philadelphia, PA: Elsevier Saunders; 2010:705.

Answer 26

Involvement of the floor or medial wall of the orbit is a T3, of the anterior orbital contents is a T4a and of the orbital apex is a T4b.

Part II, Section 6: Nasal cavity and paranasal sinuses. In: Edge SB, Byrd DR, Compton, CC, et al., eds. *AJCC Cancer Staging Manual*. 7th ed. New York, NY: Springer; 2010:71–72.

Answer 27

5-yr LRC ranges from 70–90% for T1/2 tumors and 50–60% for T3/4 tumors. 5-yr DFS is 40–50% overall. Unresectable tumors portend significantly worse prognosis.

Hoppe BS, Nelson CJ, Gomez DR, et al. Unresectable carcinoma of the paranasal sinuses: outcomes and toxicities. *Int J Radiat Oncol Biol Phys*. 2008;72:763–769.

Hoppe BS, Stegman LD, Zelefsky MJ, et al. Treatment of nasal cavity and paranasal sinus cancer with modern radiotherapy techniques in the postoperative setting--the MSKCC experience. *Int J Radiat Oncol Biol Phys*. 2007;67:691–702.

Question 28

What is the staging system for esthesioneuroblastoma, and how is it generally treated?

What are expected outcomes?

Question 29

What is the continuum of histologies of neuroendocrine differentiation that occur in the paranasal sinus/base of skull region, and their respective outcomes?

Question 30   **NASOPHARYNX**

What structures are encountered, and in what sequence, during endoscopic examination of the nasopharynx?

Answer 28

The Kadish system is most commonly used: Kadish A is limited to the nasal cavity, Kadish B extends to the paranasal sinuses, and Kadish C extends outside of the sinuses. Generally, these patients should be managed by aggressive surgical resection and postoperative radiotherapy, with expected 5-year DFS of 80–90%. Recent reports suggest a high rate of nodal failure (27%) when not electively treated.

Demiroz C, Gutfeld O, Aboziada M, et al. Esthesioneuroblastoma: is there a need for elective neck treatment? *Int J Radiat Oncol Biol Phys*. 2011;81:e255–e261.

Answer 29

There are at least four distinct histologies with variable outcomes as illustrated by one of the larger series in this disease from MD Anderson Cancer Center with median f/u of almost 7 years. The data is summarized in tabular form:

Histology	# of Pts	Treatment*	5-yr LC	5-yr RC	5-yr DMFS	5-yr OS
Esthesioneuroblastoma	31	Local only − 81%	96%	92%	100%	93%
Sinonasal undifferentiated carcinoma	16	Local + CTX − 63%	79%	84%	75%	63%
Neuroendocrine carcinoma	18	Local + CTX − 67%	72%	87%	86%	64%
Small cell carcinoma	7	Local + CTX − 71%	67%	56%	25%	29%

*Local treatment consisted of surgery, or RT, or both; CTX = chemotherapy; DMFS = distant metastasis free survival; LC = local control; RC = regional control

Rosenthal DI, Barker JL Jr, El-Naggar AK, et al. Sinonasal malignancies with neuroendocrine differentiation: patterns of failure according to histologic phenotype. *Cancer*. 2004;101:2567–2573.

Answer 30

Upon entering the nasopharynx, the lateral walls first reveal the torus tubarius, a prominence in the cartilaginous portion of the eustachian tube, followed by the eustachian tube orifice, which the torus surrounds. Posterolateral to these structures is Rosenmuller's fossa (i.e., pharyngeal recess), the most common site of origin for NPC.

Lee N, Colevas AD, Fu KK. Cancer of the nasopharynx. In: Phillips TL, Hoppe R, Leibel SA, eds. *Textbook of Radiation Oncology*. 3rd ed. Philadelphia, PA: Elsevier Saunders; 2010:523–524.

Question 31

What is the TNM staging for NPC according to the AJCC 7th edition?

Question 32

What are the different histologic subtypes of NPC?

What risk factors are associated with each?

Answer 31

Several changes were made to the staging system for NPC in the revised 7th edition of the staging manual. Note than N staging for NPC is unique. An alternative staging system used in Asia is the Ho staging system.

T1	Confined to the nasopharynx or extends to oropharynx and/or nasal cavity w/o parapharyngeal extension	**N1**	≤ 6 cm: unilateral cervical above the SCV fossa, or unilat/bilat RP nodes	**I**	T1	N0	M0
				II	T2T1-2	N0N1	M0M0
T2	Tumor with parapharyngeal extension	**N2**	≤ 6 cm: bilateral cervical LNs, above SCV fossa	**III**	T3T1-3	N0-2N2	M0M0
T3	Tumor involves bony structures of skull base and/or paranasal sinuses.	**N3a**	> 6 cm in dimension	**IVA**	T4	N0-2	M0
T4	Intracranial extension and/or involvement of cranial nerves, infratemporal fossa, masticator space, hypopharynx, or orbit	**N3b**	Supraclavicular fossa	**IVB**	Any T	N3	M0
		M1	Distant metastases	**IVC**	Any T	Any N	M1

Part II, Section 4: Pharynx. In: Edge SB, Byrd DR, Compton CC, et al., eds. *AJCC Cancer Staging Manual*. 7th ed. New York, NY: Springer; 2010:41–42.

Answer 32

Type 1 (*sporadic form*): keratinizing squamous cell carcinoma—these are histologically similar to other head and neck SCC and accounts for 20% in North America and is associated with alcohol and tobacco use. Presence of keratin has been associated with reduced local control and survival.

Type 2: Non-keratinizing carcinoma (associated with Epstein Barr Virus)

· Type 2a: differentiated – formerly WHO Type II – 30–40% in North America
· Type 2b: undifferentiated – formerly WHO Type III (lymphoepithelial carcinoma—endemic form) – 40–50% in North America.

Part II, Section 4: Pharynx. In: Edge SB, Byrd DR, Compton CC, et al., eds. *AJCC Cancer Staging Manual*. 7th ed. New York, NY: Springer; 2010:48.

Question 33

What are common clinical presentations for NPC?

What percentage of patients have associated lymphadenopathy?

Question 34

What is the general treatment paradigm for early stage nasopharyngeal lesions?

What are the approximate numbers for LRC and OS?

Answer 33

The most common presenting feature is a painless neck mass. 85–90% present with cervical lymphadenopathy with 50% having bilateral involvement. Other presentations can be refractory otitis media, decreased hearing, nasal obstruction (causing altered voice), epixtaxis, referred ear pain, and cranial neuropathies. Multiple cranial nerves can be affected in NPC, and some are associated with the following clinical syndromes:

Syndrome	Cranial Nerves	Symptoms
Jacod's (petrosphenoid)	Superior Orbital Fissure (III, IV, V1, VI) Foramen Rotundum (V2) Foramen Ovale (V3) Foramen Lacerum – pathway to these CN	Unilateral trigeminal neuralgia, ptosis, ophthalmoplegia, blindness
St. Villaret's (retroparotid)	Compression of CN IX–XII via retropharyngeal nodes	Dysphagia, abnl taste post 1/3 tongue, hoarseness, anesthesia of mucous membranes, hemiparesis of soft palate, Horner's syndrome, and atrophy of SCM, trapezius & tongue
Vernet's (jugular foramen)	CN IX–XI via invasion of jugular foramen	Paralysis of soft palate, tonsils, pharynx, and hoarseness

Lee N, Colevas AD, Fu KK. Cancer of the nasopharynx. In: Phillips TL, Hoppe R, Leibel SA, eds. *Textbook of Radiation Oncology*. 3rd ed. Philadelphia, PA: Elsevier Saunders; 2010:525–526.

Answer 34

Surgery is generally not part of the treatment strategy of NPC aside from diagnosis, biopsy, and neck dissection for residual disease. For T1N0 disease, RT alone results in excellent LC (75–90%) and OS (70–80%). The RT target includes bilateral elective nodes (levels IB-V, RP) with a nasopharyngeal boost, delivered with conformal EBRT or brachytherapy. More recently, IMRT has been used with superior ability to spare critical intracranial structures. The management of T2N0 patients is controversial as some advocate RT alone. NCCN guidelines recommend CRT.

Lee N, Colevas AD, Fu KK. Cancer of the nasopharynx. In: Phillips TL, Hoppe R, Leibel SA, eds. *Textbook of Radiation Oncology*. 3rd ed. Philadelphia, PA: Elsevier Saunders; 2010:533–534.

Question 35

What is the recommended treatment strategy for locally-advanced NPC?

What evidence supports this approach?

Question 36

What is the role of induction or adjuvant chemotherapy following definitive chemoradiotherapy or radiotherapy for advanced stage NPC?

Question 37

What are the recommended dose constraints for the optic nerves/chiasm and brainstem when treating a NPC with IMRT?

Answer 35

Chemoradiotherapy is the mainstay of treatment for locally advanced disease. Several Phase III studies confirmed a LC and OS advantage with the addition of chemotherapy. The Intergroup 00-99 Al-Sarraf study randomized patients with Stage III or IV NPC to RT (70 Gy in 2 Gy/fx) vs chemoRT (70 Gy + concurrent cisplatin (100 mg/m^2 on days 1, 22, 43) × 3 + adjuvant cisplatin/5-FU × 3 cycles). The trial closed prematurely due to the highly significant advantage to chemotherapy for both 5-yr PFS (58% vs 29%) and OS (67% vs 37%). A duplicative study from Singapore confirmed this finding, as did phase III studies from Hong Kong, and Taiwan, although these latter 2 trials did not use adjuvant chemotherapy.

Al-Sarraf M, LeBlanc M, Giri PG, et al. Chemoradiotherapy versus radiotherapy in patients with advanced nasopharyngeal cancer: Phase III randomized Intergroup study 0099. *J Clin Oncol*. 1998;16:1310–1317.
Lee AW, Lau WH, Tung SY, et al. Preliminary results of a randomized study on therapeutic gain by concurrent chemotherapy for regionally-advanced nasopharyngeal carcinoma: NPC-9901 trial by the Hong Kong Nasopharyngeal Cancer Study Group. *J Clin Oncol*. 2005;23:6966–6975.
Lin JC, Jan JS, Hsu CY, et al. Phase III study of concurrent chemoradiotherapy versus radiotherapy alone for advanced nasopharyngeal carcinoma: positive effect on overall and progression-free survival. *J Clin Oncol*. 2003;21:631–637.
Wee J, Tab EH, Tai BC, et al. Randomized trial of radiotherapy versus concurrent chemoradiotherapy followed by adjuvant chemotherapy in patients with American Joint Committee on Cancer/International Union against cancer stage III and IV nasopharyngeal cancer of the endemic variety. *J Clin Oncol*. 2005;23:6730–6738.

Answer 36

The use of induction chemotherapy prior to definitive RT has been tested in several trials in advanced stage NPC and has failed to demonstrate a survival benefit. There are no trials that have compared standard concurrent chemoradiotherapy +/− adjuvant chemotherapy. Although adjuvant chemotherapy was given on the experimental arm of the INT-0099 trial, only 55% of patients were able to complete this portion of their therapy. Other studies that did not use adjuvant chemotherapy appear to produce similar results achieved in the INT-0099 trial as well. This question is currently being studied by the Hong Kong Nasopharyngeal Cancer Study group, in which high risk patients (residual EBV DNA following the completion of CRT) are being randomized to adjuvant chemotherapy vs observation.

Hareyama M, Sakata K, Shirato H, et al. A prospective, randomized trial comparing neoadjuvant chemotherapy with radiotherapy alone in patients with advanced nasopharyngeal carcinoma. *Cancer*. 2002;94:2217–2223.
Ma J, Mai HQ, Hong MH, et al. Results of a prospective randomized trial comparing neoadjuvant chemotherapy plus radiotherapy with radiotherapy alone in patients with locoregionally advanced nasopharyngeal carcinoma. *J Clin Oncol*. 2001;19:1350–1357.
National Institutes of Health Clinical Trials Database. http://www.clinicaltrials.gov/. Accessed November 13, 2011.

Answer 37

RTOG 0615 recommends restricting the dose to the actual optic nerve/chiasm to a maximum dose of 50 Gy, and the planning risk volume (PRV) to a maximum dose of 54 Gy. The actual brainstem should be restricted to a maximum dose of 54 Gy, while 1% for the PRV brainstem can receive 60 Gy. PRVcord = cord + 5 mm in each direction. PRVoptic nerves/chiasm = optic nerves/chiasm + at least 1 mm in each direction. Of note, CTV expansions can be as little as 1 mm when disease abuts but does not invade the brainstem.

http://www.rtog.org/ClinicalTrials/ProtocolTable/StudyDetails.aspx?study=0615. Accessed November 13, 2011.

Question 38

What radiation related factor other than total dose significantly influences the risk of optic neuropathy?

Question 39   LARYNX/HYPOPHARYNX

What is the incidence of LN metastases in glottic cancer, stratified by T stage?

Question 40

Is there any randomized evidence supporting altered fractionation in T1 SCC of the glottis?

Question 41

What is the anticipated local control for a T2N0 glottic tumor?

Is there any role for altered fractionation in this disease?

Answer 38

A study from the University of Florida found that dose per fraction has been shown to significantly correlate with rates of optic neuropathy. The rate of symptomatic optic neuropathy (20/100 visual acuity or worse) was 0% for doses of < 59 Gy. For doses of ≥ 60 Gy, the rate of optic neuropathy was 11% when the dose per fraction was kept below 1.9 Gy vs 47% with dose per fraction of ≥ 1.9 Gy.

Parsons JT, Bova FJ, Fitzgerald CR, et al. Radiation optic neuropathy after megavoltage external-beam irradiation: analysis of time-dose factors. *Int J Radiat Oncol Biol Phys*. 1994;30:755–763.

Answer 39

T1: 1%; T2: 3%; T3: 15–20%; T4: 20–30%

Kaplan MJ, Johns ME, Clark DA, et al. Glottic carcinoma. The roles of surgery and irradiation. *Cancer*. 1984;53:2641–2648.

Answer 40

Yes. A single institution Japanese randomized trial examined 180 patients with T1N0 glottic cancer and found that 2.25 Gy/fx (to total dose of 56.25–63 Gy) improved 5-year LRC from 77% to 92%, compared to conventional fractionation of 2 Gy/fx (to total dose of 60 or 66 Gy). Other outcomes were similar.

Yamazaki H, Nishiyama K, Tanaka E, et al. Radiotherapy for early glottic carcinoma (T1N0M0): results of prospective randomized study of radiation fraction size and overall treatment time. *Int J Radiat Oncol Biol Phys*. 2006;64:77–82.

Answer 41

In general T2N0 tumors that exhibit impaired mobility and/or subglottic extension have inferior outcomes that those with only supraglottic extension. A large retrospective study by Le, et al found 5-yr local control of 79% vs 45% for patients without and with impaired mobility, respectively, and 77% vs 58% for those without and with subglottic extension, respectively. That same study also found patient treated with ≥ 65 Gy, ≥ 2.25 Gy/day and in ≤ 43 days had improved local control. As such, RTOG 95–12 was a randomized phase III trial in T2N0 glottic tumors comparing 70 Gy/35 fx to 79.2 Gy at 1.2 Gy BID as a means of dose escalating RT to improve LC. The study was slightly underpowered, but the results demonstrated trends towards benefit in 5-yr LC (79% vs 70%, $p = .11$) and 5-yr DFS (51% vs 37%, $p = .07$). As such, many advocate either an accelerated schedule, or the addition of chemotherapy for poor risk T2N0 tumors.

Le QT, Fu KK, Kroll S, et al: Influence of fraction size, total dose, and overall time on local control of T1-T2 glottic carcinoma. *Int J Radiat Oncol Biol Phys*. 1997;39:115–126.

Trotti A, Pajak T, Emami B, et al. A randomized trial of hyperfractionation versus standard fractionation in T2 squamous cell carcinoma of the vocal cord. *Int J Radiat Oncol Biol Phys*. 2006;66:S15.

Question 42

What are the classic field borders for T1N0 glottic tumors?

T2N0?

Question 43

What was the schema of the phase III VA larynx trial and what was its clinical significance?

Question 44

In RTOG 91–11, a three arm randomized trial between different larynx preservation regimens, what were the treatment arms?

What regimen achieved the best results?

Question 45

For patients who fail organ preservation, what is the rate of successful salvage laryngectomy?

What is the most common postoperative complication?

Answer 42

For T1 tumors, use opposed laterals with $5 \times 5 - 6 \times 6$ cm field. Upper border 0.5–1 cm above thyroid notch, posterior border 1 cm behind thyroid cartilage, inferior border at the bottom of the cricoid cartilage, and 1 cm fall off anteriorly. For T2 tumors, elective nodal irradiation is controversial but generally not used unless there is significant supra/subglottic extension or bulky T2b disease. Per RTOG 95–12, no elective nodal irradiation for T2 tumors; may cone down posteriorly off the arytenoids if the posterior 1/3 of the vocal cord is not involved by tumor. Bolus (2–5 mm) may be used over the anterior neck skin to ensure complete coverage of lesions involving the anterior 1/3 of the vocal cords or the commissure.

Trotti A, Pajak T, Emami B, et al. A randomized trial of hyperfractionation versus standard fractionation in T2 squamous cell carcinoma of the vocal cord. *Int J Radiat Oncol Biol Phys.* 2006;66:S15.

Answer 43

It was a phase III trial that randomized patients with operable stage III/IV larynx cancer to total laryngectomy + postop RT vs induction cisplatin and 5-FU with evaluation after 2 cycles. Patients with a partial response (54%) or a complete response (31%) went on to receive one more cycle of chemotherapy followed by RT alone (66–76 Gy). Patients who failed to responds were treated with TL + postop RT. Of note, 57% of pts had vocal cord fixation. OS were equivalent (68%); LRC (92% vs 80%) was better in the surgical arm; DM was lower in the conservation arm (11% vs 17%). Laryngectomy free survival was 64% in the conservation arm.

The Department of Veterans Affairs Laryngeal Cancer Study Group. Induction chemotherapy plus radiation compared with surgery plus radiation in patients with advanced laryngeal cancer. *N Eng J Med.* 1991;324:1685–1690.

Answer 44

The three arms were RT alone (70 Gy) vs induction cisplatin 100 mg/m^2 + 5-FU C.I. 1000 mg/m^2 q3 weeks × 3 cycles. Followed by RT (if CR or PR) or laryngectomy if poor response vs concurrent cisplatin 100 mg/m^2 q3 weeks + RT. Results shown in the table. Concurrent CRT achieved the best results.

Arm	5-yr LFS	5-yr LP	5-yr LRC	DM	5-yr DFS	5-yr OS	5-yr CSD
1: I + RT	44.6%	70.5%	54.9%	14.3%	38.6%	59.2%	43.8%
2: CRT	46.6%	83.6%	68.8%	13.2%	39%	54.6%	34%
3: RT	33.9%	65.7%	51%	22.3%	27.3%	53.5%	58.3%
p-value	0.011	0.0029 (2 vs 1), 0.00017 (2 vs 3)	0.0018 (2 vs 1), 0.0005 (2 vs 3)	0.06	0.016 (1 vs 3), 0.0058(2 vs 3)	NS	0.0007 (2 vs 3)

Forastiere AA, Goepfert H, Maor M, et al. Concurrent chemotherapy and radiotherapy for organ preservation in advanced laryngeal cancer. *N Engl J Med.* 2003;349:2091–2098.

Answer 45

A subset analysis of RTOG 91–11 revealed that while more patients in the RT alone arm required salvage laryngectomy as compared to the induction + RT and the CRT arms, their survival after salvage laryngectomy were similar. LRC was achieved in 75–90% of patients with 2-yr OS about 70%. Most common complication was pharyngocutaneous fistula (15–30%).

Weber RS, Berkey BA, Forastiere A, et al. Outcome of salvage total laryngectomy following organ preservation therapy: the Radiation Therapy Oncology Group trial 91–11. *Arch Otolaryngol Head Neck Surg.* 2003;129:44–49.

Question 46

What are classic contraindications to larynx preservation with definitive chemoradiotherapy?

Question 47

What are indications to boost the tracheal stoma after a total laryngectomy?

Question 48

Have organ preservation strategies been studied in hypopharyngeal cancer?

Question 49   **POSTOPERATIVE RADIOTHERAPY**

Is there evidence that supports the use of 60 Gy as the routine postoperative dose in head and neck cancer?

Answer 46

Patients with bulky T4 tumors had poor response rates to induction chemotherapy on the VA larynx cancer study, and over half of them required salvage laryngectomy. Based on this finding, patients with bulky T4 tumors (i.e., invaded cartilage and/or > 1 cm of the tongue) were excluded from RTOG 91–11 trials and are traditionally treated with TL + postop (C)RT. There are some published experiences with reasonably good outcomes for these patients with conservation approaches, but NCCN guidelines and ASCO consensus statement still recommend surgery as the primary mode of therapy.

Forastiere AA, Goepfert H, Maor M, et al. Concurrent chemotherapy and radiotherapy for organ preservation in advanced laryngeal cancer. *N Engl J Med*. 2003;349:2091–2098.

Answer 47

The tracheal stoma should be boosted to 60 Gy if there is evidence of subglottic extension, tumor invasion into the soft tissues of the neck, positive tracheal margin, or an emergency tracheostomy through tumor.

Cahlon O, Lee N, Le Q, et al. Cancer of the larynx. In: Phillips TL, Hoppe R, Leibel SA, eds. *Textbook of Radiation Oncology*. 3rd ed. Philadelphia, PA: Elsevier Saunders; 2010:658.

Answer 48

Yes. A prospective randomized trial following the same schema as the VA larynx trial was tested by the EORTC for stage II–IVB cancers of the pyriform sinus or AE fold. LRC and OS were similar between the two groups of patients. The organ preservation arm demonstrated significantly lower rates of distant failure (25% vs 36%). The rate of functional larynx preservation at 5 yrs was 35%.

Lefebvre JL, Chevalier D, Luboinski B, et al. Larynx preservation in pyriform sinus cancer: preliminary results of a European Organization for Research and Treatment of Cancer phase III trial. EORTC Head and Neck Cancer Cooperative Group. *J Natl Cancer Inst*. 1996;88:890–899.

Answer 49

Yes. A phase III PRT (RTOG 73–03) compared 50 Gy preop RT to 60 Gy postop RT. This demonstrated a LRC advantage to the postop arm (58% vs 70%) without impacting survival. There is also prospective data that confirmed that a dose of > 57.6 Gy correlated to improved local control compared to lower doses.

Peters LJ, Goepfert H, Ang KK, et al. Evaluation of the dose for postoperative radiation therapy of head and neck cancer: first report of a prospective randomized trial. *Int J Radiat Oncol Biol Phys*. 1993;26:3–11.

Tupchong L, Scott CB, Blitzer PH, et al. Randomized study of preoperative versus postoperative radiation therapy in advanced head and neck carcinoma: long-term follow-up of RTOG study 73-03. *Int J Radiat Oncol Biol Phys*. 1991;20:21–28.

Question 50

What minimum postoperative dose is recommended for dissected LN with + ECE?

Based on what evidence?

Question 51

Is there a benefit to altered fractionation in the postoperative setting?

Question 52

What are the indications and evidence for the addition of concurrent chemotherapy to postoperative radiotherapy in head and neck cancer?

Answer 50

A randomized trial was conducted in the 1980s that randomized low risk patients (1 risk factor) to 57.6 Gy (1.7 Gy/fx) vs 63 Gy and high risk patients (> 1 risk factor and/or ECE) to 63 Gy vs 68 Gy. There was no statistically significant improvement to dose escalation in general. However, patients with ECE that were treated with ≤ 57.6 Gy had inferior LC than those treated with ≥ 63 Gy (2-yr LRC 52% vs 74%, respectively).

Peters LJ, Goepfert H, Ang KK, et al. Evaluation of the dose for postoperative radiation therapy of head and neck cancer: first report of a prospective randomized trial. *Int J Radiat Oncol Biol Phys*. 1993;26:3–11.

Answer 51

A multi-institutional randomized trial that compared 63 Gy in 7 weeks vs 63 Gy in 5 weeks using a concomitant boost RT technique did not show a significant LRC or DFS benefit to altered fractionation in the postoperative setting for patient with high risk disease.

Ang KK, Trotti A, Brown BW, et al. Randomized trial addressing risk features and time factors of surgery plus radiotherapy in advanced head-and-neck cancer. *Int J Radiat Oncol Biol Phys*. 2001;51:571–578.

Answer 52

Two phase III trials were conducted comparing postop RT vs postop CRT. Chemotherapy was cisplatin 100mg/m^2 q3wk × 3. The EORTC 22931 trial demonstrated significantly improved LC (82% vs 69%), PFS (47% vs 36%) and OS (53% vs 40%) at 5 yrs with CRT. RTOG 95–01 demonstrated a LC (82% vs 72%) and DFS advantage with no OS advantage at 2 yrs. Eligibility criteria differed between studies. While the RTOG study included only those patients with + ECE, + margins, or ≥ 2 LN+, the EORTC trial also included patients with other factors including T3/4, +PNI, +LVSI or level IV/V nodes for oral cavity/ oropharynx tumors. A pooled analysis of these two trials that compared RT alone to RT + cisplatin demonstrated that ECE and positive margins were the only two scenarios in which the addition of concurrent chemotherapy improved LC and OS.

Bernier J, Cooper JS, Pajak TF, et al. Defining risk levels in locally advanced head and neck cancers: a comparative analysis of concurrent postoperative radiation plus chemotherapy trials of the EORTC (#22931) and RTOG (# 9501). *Head Neck*. 2005;27:843–850.

Bernier J, Domenge C, Ozsahin M, et al. Postoperative irradiation with or without concomitant chemotherapy for locally advanced head and neck cancer. *N Engl J Med*. 2004;350:1945–1952.

Cooper JS, Pajak TF, Forastiere AA, et al. Postoperative concurrent radiotherapy and chemotherapy for high-risk squamous-cell carcinoma of the head and neck. *N Engl J Med*. 2004;350:1937–1944.

Question 53

What is the most common type of benign salivary gland tumor?

Where is it usually found?

Question 54

What are the common malignant salivary gland tumor histologies?

Question 55

What is the most common histologic subtype of cancer in the submandibular or minor salivary glands?

What is unique about its pattern of spread and natural history?

Question 56

What is the proportion of benign and malignant lesions found in parotid glands?

Submandibular glands?

Minor salivary glands?

Answer 53

Pleomorphic adenoma is the most common benign salivary gland tumor and comprises 75% of parotid tumors. Other benign tumors include Warthin's tumor (papillary cystadenoma lymphomatosum), Godwin's tumor (benign lymphoepithelial lesions associated with Sjogren's syndrome) and oncocytomas.

Chong LM, Armstrong JG. Tumors of the salivary glands. In: Phillips TL, Hoppe R, Leibel SA, eds. *Textbook of Radiation Oncology*. 3rd ed. Philadelphia, PA: Elsevier Saunders; 2010:670.

Answer 54

Mucoepidermoid carcinoma is the most common malignant histology. It most commonly presents in the parotid gland. Other common malignant histologies include adenoid cystic carcinoma and adenocarcinoma. Acinic cell carcinoma is a common low grade malignant histology. Salivary gland tumors can be either low or high grade, which is a factor that significantly influences treatment approaches. While squamous cell carcinomas of the parotid is a recognized entity, these are more commonly found to be metastases from cutaneous SCC of the skin.

Chong LM, Armstrong JG. Tumors of the salivary glands. In: Phillips TL, Hoppe R, Leibel SA, eds. *Textbook of Radiation Oncology*. 3rd ed. Philadelphia, PA: Elsevier Saunders; 2010:670–673.

Answer 55

Adenoid cystic carcinoma. It tends to infiltrate and spread along nerves. Perineural invasion is common, especially for higher grade tumors, and is an indication to electively target the facial nerve up to the base of skull, including its origin from the stylomastoid foramen. These tumors tend not to spread to lymph nodes, and do not require elective nodal irradiation. They are also notorious for late relapses (> 10–20 yrs), most often in the form of lung metastases (40% lifetime risk).

Chong LM, Armstrong JG. Tumors of the salivary glands. In: Phillips TL, Hoppe R, Leibel SA, eds. *Textbook of Radiation Oncology*. 3rd ed. Philadelphia, PA: Elsevier Saunders; 2010:671–672.

Answer 56

In general, the smaller the gland, the more likely a tumor it is to be malignant. While only 25% of parotid lesions are malignant, about 50% of submandibular gland lesions, 75% of minor salivary gland lesions, and nearly all sublingual gland lesions are malignant.

Chong LM, Armstrong JG. Tumors of the salivary glands. In: Phillips TL, Hoppe R, Leibel SA, eds. *Textbook of Radiation Oncology*. 3rd ed. Philadelphia, PA: Elsevier Saunders; 2010:670–671.

Question 57

When is sacrifice of the facial nerve indicated in resection of a malignant parotid gland cancer?

Question 58

What are the indications for post operative radiotherapy in resected salivary gland tumors?

Question 59

What is the evidence for benefit to adjuvant radiotherapy in salivary gland cancer?

Question 60

Is there any advantage to the use of fast neutron therapy in locally advanced/unresectable salivary gland tumors?

Answer 57

Preoperative weakness or paralysis of the facial nerve usually indicates tumor involvement, and in these instances, the main trunk or the involved nerve branches may have to be sacrificed. The nerve or its involved branches should also be sacrificed if there is intra-operative evidence of gross invasion or microscopic infiltration of the nerve by tumor, even in the presence of normal preoperative facial nerve function. If the nerve appears both clinically and intraoperatively uninvolved, it should be preserved even for tumors involving the deep lobe of the gland requiring a total parotidectomy.

Adelstein DJ, Koyfman SA, El-Naggar AK, et al. The Biology and Management of Salivary Gland Cancer: Seminars in Radiation Oncology; 2012; 22(3):245–53.

Answer 58

In general, postoperative RT is indicated for close or positive margins, lymph node metastases, locally advanced disease, bone or nerve involvement, recurrent disease, or a combination of other adverse features, such as high nuclear grade, perineural invasion, and lymphovascular space invasion.

Chong LM, Armstrong JG. Tumors of the salivary glands. In: Phillips TL, Hoppe R, Leibel SA, eds. *Textbook of Radiation Oncology*. 3rd ed. Philadelphia, PA: Elsevier Saunders; 2010:683.

Answer 59

While there are no randomized data, several large institutional series have demonstrated 20–40% improvements in local control and DFS with the addition of RT to surgery alone. A match-pair analysis from MSKCC, for example, found that patients with stage III/IV disease, positive lymph nodes, or high grade tumors had improved local control and, in some instances, improved survival with the addition of adjuvant radiotherapy, while those with low grade, or early stage (I/II) disease did not appear to benefit.

Armstrong JG, Harrison LB, Thaler HT, et al. The indications for elective treatment of the neck in cancer of the major salivary glands. *Cancer*. 1992;69:615–619.

Answer 60

A randomized trial by the RTOG/MRC that compared photon/electron therapy vs fast neutron therapy demonstrated significantly improved local control (56% vs. 17%) in the fast neutron therapy arm, but distant metastases and overall survival in this arm had inferior outcomes. Severe late side effects were noted in long-term survivors. As such, it has fallen out of favor. However, dose escalation with proton and carbon ion therapies are still being investigated.

Laramore GE, Krall JM, Griffin TW, et al. Neutron versus photon irradiation for unresectable salivary gland tumors: final report of an RTOG-MRC randomized clinical trial. Radiation Therapy Oncology Group. Medical Research Council. *Int J Radiat Oncol Biol Phys*. 1993;27:235–240.

Question 61

Are there discrete molecular phenotypes that are histology specific in salivary gland tumors?

Does this impact treatment options?

Question 62   **MELANOMA**

Is there an advantage to hypofractionation in treating melanoma with radiotherapy?

Question 63

Is there randomized evidence supporting the use of adjuvant RT after resection of melanoma?

What is the benefit of RT in this setting?

Answer 61

Yes. The following table summarizes the molecular profiles of several common malignant histologies:

Histology	EGFR	HER2	c-kit	VEGF	Androgen
Mucoepidermoid	40%	25–35%	Rare	50%	rare
Adenoca/Salivary Duct Carcinoma	30–40%	20–30%	Rare	65%	15–40%
Adenoid Cystic	20%	rare	80–90%	85%	rare

Inhibitors of these various targets are currently being investigated in the metastatic setting, and some early reports suggest efficacy in a significant proportion of patients.

Adelstein DJ, Koyfman SA, El-Naggar AK, et al. The Biology and Management of Salivary Gland Cancer: Seminars in Radiation Oncology; 2012; 22(3):245–53.

Answer 62

It is unclear. In the definitive setting, large older retrospective series suggested doses of > 4 Gy per fraction significantly improved complete response rates (59% vs 33%). RTOG 8305 randomized patients with measurable melanoma to 50 Gy in 20 fx daily, vs 32 Gy in 4 weekly fractions of 8 Gy. Overall, there was no difference in response rates between the two regimens. In the postoperative setting, MDACC pioneered a regimen of 30 Gy in 5 fractions given twice weekly, which yielded 5-yr LRC of 88%. However, other retrospective series report equivalent efficacy with hypofractionated and conventionally fractionated regimens.

Ang KK, Peters LJ, Weber RS, et al. Postoperative radiotherapy for cutaneous melanoma of the head and neck region. *Int J Radiat Oncol Biol Phys*. 1994;30:795–798.
Chang DT, Amdur RJ, Morris CG, et al. Adjuvant radiotherapy for cutaneous melanoma: comparing hypofractionation to conventional fractionation. *Int J Radiat Oncol Biol Phys*. 2006;66:1051–1055.
Overgaard J. The role of radiotherapy in recurrent and metastatic malignant melanoma: a clinical radiobiological study. *Int J Radiat Oncol Biol Phys*. 1986;12:867–872.
Sause WT, Cooper JS, Rush S, et al. Fraction size in external beam radiation therapy in the treatment of melanoma. *Int J Radiat Oncol Biol Phys*. 1991;20:429–432.

Answer 63

Based on a previous phase II study, the Trans-Tasman Radiation Oncology Group (TROG) performed a phase III randomized study comparing adjuvant nodal RT (48 Gy in 20 fx) vs observation in patients who had recurrent melanoma with ≥ 1 parotid, ≥ 2 cervical or axillary or ≥ 3 groin positive nodes; or extra nodal spread of tumour; or minimum metastatic node diameter of 3 cm (neck or axilla) or 4 cm (groin). There was a significant reduction in regional failure from 31% to 18%. OS were similar between arms.

Burmeister B, Henderson M, Thompson J, et al. Adjuvant radiotherapy improves regional (lymph node field) control in melanoma patients after lymphadenectomy: Results of an intergroup randomised trial. *Int J Radiat Oncol Biol Phys*. 2009;66:S15.
Burmeister BH, Mark Smithers B, Burmeister E, et al. A prospective phase II study of adjuvant postoperative radiation therapy following nodal surgery in malignant melanoma-Trans Tasman Radiation Oncology Group (TROG) Study 96.06. *Radiother Oncol*. 2006;81:136–142.

Question 64

What is the rate of grade 3 lymphedema when radiating the axilla postoperatively for melanoma?

What is the risk for the groin?

Question 65

What is the role of sentinel lymph node biopsy (SLNB) in intermediate thickness melanoma?

Question 66   **MERKEL CELL CARCINOMA**

What margin of resection is recommended for Merkel cell carcinoma (MCC)?

What is the role of sentinel LN biopsy (SLNB)?

Question 67

What are the indications for adjuvant radiotherapy in Merkel cell carcinoma (MCC)?

What benefit does RT offer?

Answer 64

In the phase II TROG series, the risk of grade 3 lymphedema was 9% for the axilla and 19% for the groin.

Burmeister BH, Mark Smithers B, Burmeister E, et al. A prospective phase II study of adjuvant postoperative radiation therapy following nodal surgery in malignant melanoma-Trans Tasman Radiation Oncology Group (TROG) Study 96.06. *Radiother Oncol.* 2006;81:136–142.

Answer 65

A phase III randomized controlled study compared SLNB + completion LND if SLN+ for intermediate thickness melanoma vs observation + complete LND at nodal relapse. 5-yr DFS was significantly better with SLNB (78% vs 73%), but no difference in OS. SLN+ was powerful predictor of outcome and its removal slowed progression of disease, but did not affect overall survival.

Morton DL, Thompson JF, Cochran AJ, et al. Sentinel-node biopsy or nodal observation in melanoma. *N Engl J Med.* 2006;355:1307–1317.

Answer 66

Wide margins of 2 cm is generally recommended as these tumors have a high rate of recurrence. A recent study found that SLNB was feasible and the rate of sentinel lymph node positivity was at least 15–20% in all groups of patients. SLN positivity was significantly associated with the clinical size of the lesion, greatest horizontal histologic dimension, tumor thickness, mitotic rate, and histologic growth pattern. SLNB is considered standard in MCC.

Schwartz JL, Griffith KA, Lowe L, et al. Features predicting sentinel lymph node positivity in Merkel cell carcinoma. *J Clin Oncol.* 2011;29:1036–1041.

Answer 67

Indications for adjuvant RT include size > 2 cm, close/positive margins, LVSI, LN+ disease, LN not stages by SLNB or LND. A large review found that nodal recurrence rates range between 40–50% in the unsampled primary echelon nodal basin. A recent SEER analysis demonstrated an overall survival advantage for adjuvant RT. For unresectable tumors, definitive RT is appropriate, as MCC is a radiosensitive tumor.

Allen PJ, Bowne WB, Jaques DP, et al. Merkel cell carcinoma: prognosis and treatment of patients from a single institution. *J Clin Oncol.* 2005;23:2300–2309.

Mojica P, Smith D, Ellenhorn JD, et al. Adjuvant radiation therapy is associated with improved survival in Merkel cell carcinoma of the skin. *J Clin Oncol.* 2007;25:1043–1047.

National Comprehensive Cancer Network Clinical Practice Guidelines: Merkel Cell Carcinoma. Version 2.2011. http://www.nccn.org/professionals/physician_gls/pdf/head-and-neck.pdf. Accessed November 14, 2011.

Question 68

What dose of RT is used for adjuvant radiotherapy to the tumor bed?

To lymphatic region?

For unresectable disease?

Question 69

Has adjuvant chemotherapy been investigated for Merkel cell carcinoma (MCC)?

Question 70

UNKNOWN PRIMARY

What is the workup for a patient that presents with a squamous cell carcinoma metastatic to a cervical lymph node, without evidence of an obvious primary?

Answer 68

For the primary tumor bed, NCCN guidelines recommend a dose of 50–56 Gy for negative margins, 56–60 Gy for close/microscopically positive margins, and 60–66 Gy for grossly positive margins or unresectable disease. For uninvolved nodal basin, a dose of 46–50 Gy is recommended with higher doses used for gross nodal disease, or ECE.

National Comprehensive Cancer Network Clinical Practice Guidelines: Merkel Cell Carcinoma. Version 2.2011. http://www.nccn.org/professionals/physician_gls/pdf/head-and-neck.pdf. Accessed November 14, 2011.

Answer 69

Yes. A phase II study (TROG 96–07) investigated adjuvant RT (50 Gy/25 fx) with concurrent carboplatin/etoposide for patients with 1 high risk feature (recurrence after initial therapy, involved nodes, size > 1 cm, gross residual disease, or occult primary with nodes). 3-yr LF, DM, OS were 25%, 24%, and 76%, respectively, and compared favorably to historical controls.

Poulsen M, Rischin D, Walpole E, et al. High-risk Merkel cell carcinoma of the skin treated with synchronous carboplatin/etoposide and radiation: a Trans-Tasman Radiation Oncology Group Study—TROG 96:07. *J Clin Oncol.* 2003;21:4371–4376.

Answer 70

First, an FNA of the cervical LN should be performed to confirm the diagnosis of SCC. Then either a CT neck with contrast, or a PET/CT should be done. While not universally accepted, PET/CT is commonly used in this situation. One study found that it detected a primary site in 25% of patients in whom a primary had not been identified. If imaging studies are unrevealing, an EUA with direct nasopharyngolaryngoscopy and directed biopsies are then performed. In the absence of any putative primary site, biopsies are taken of the nasopharynx, BOT, and pyriform sinuses. Generally, bilateral tonsillectomies are also performed. Importantly, an isolated SCV node most likely points to a primary originating below the clavicles (e.g., esophagus, lung) rather than a true head and neck primary and should be worked up as such including bronchoscopy, esophagoscopy and CT chest, abdomen and pelvis.

Rusthoven KE, Koshy M, Paulino AC, et al. The role of fluorodeoxyglucose positron emission tomography in cervical lymph node metastases from an unknown primary tumor. *Cancer.* 2004;101:2641–2649.
Strojan P, Ferlito A, Medina JE, et al. Contemporary management of lymph node metastases from an unknown primary to the neck: I. A review of diagnostic approaches. *Head Neck.* 2011. Epub 2011 Oct 27 ahead of print.

Question 71

In what percentage of unknown primary H&N SCC is a primary site found?

What is the most common site?

Question 72

What pathologic stains can be done to help identify a primary tumor site?

Question 73

What is the recommended adjuvant therapy for a patient with an unknown primary with a single 2.5-cm level II node, found to have no additional LNs on comprehensive neck dissection and no ECE?

Question 74

What areas are targeted in definitive radiation for an unknown primary with multiple left-sided level II and III lymph nodes, the largest measuring 4.5 cm?

Answer 71

In about 50–60% of cases, a primary site will be identified after full work-up. The base of tongue and tonsils account for ~80% of primary sites of unknown primary origin.

Strojan P, Ferlito A, Medina JE, et al. Contemporary management of lymph node metastases from an unknown primary to the neck: I. A review of diagnostic approaches. *Head Neck.* 2011. Epub 2011 Oct 27 ahead of print.

Answer 72

For squamous histology, a positive EBV stain is highly suggestive of a NPC, while a positive HPV or p16 stain is highly suggestive of an oropharyngeal primary. With this information, fields can be modified to exclude the larynx/hypopharynx from the potential primary mucosal site targets, allowing for greater normal tissue sparing. For adenocarcinoma histology, calcitonin and thyroglobulin stains can be used to help identify a thyroid primary site.

National Comprehensive Cancer Network Clinical Practice Guidelines: Head and Neck Cancer. Version 2.2011. http://www.nccn.org/professionals/physician_gls/pdf/head-and-neck.pdf. Accessed November 14, 2011.

Answer 73

Observation is generally recommended in such a situation. This situation accounts for about 25% of unknown primary cases. The rate of expected failure in the neck is < 10%, with a 5% rate of a primary tumor manifestation in the future. For "all comers' with unknown primary SCC-HN, the mucosal emergence rate is closer to 15%.

Coster JR, Foote RL, Olsen KD, et al. Cervical nodal metastasis of squamous cell carcinoma of unknown origin: indications for withholding radiation therapy. *Int J Radiat Oncol Biol Phys.* 1992;23:743–749.
Grau C, Johansen LV, Jakobsen J, et al. Cervical lymph node metastases from unknown primary tumours. Results from a national survey by the Danish Society for head and neck oncology. *Radiother Oncol.* 2000;55:121–129.

Answer 74

Management options include ipsilateral neck dissection, followed by comprehensive radiation vs definitive chemoRT. Typically, comprehensive radiation is used which includes bilateral cervical nodes, as well as putative primary sites (nasopharynx, oropharynx, hypopharynx, larynx). However, with a patient presenting with level II LN, there is mature data from the University of Florida in which the larynx/hypopharynx are not targeted, and spared with a traditional larynx block in an AP SCV field. With this approach, there are virtually no failures in either of those potential primary sites. Importantly, this data applies to a cohort of patients where HPV/p16 status was unknown. For patients presenting primarily with level III and/or IV LN, then the larynx and hypopharynx would be targeted as a putative mucosal site.

Wallace A, Richards GM, Harari PM, et al. Head and neck squamous cell carcinoma from an unknown primary site. *Am J Otolaryngol.* 2011;32:286–290.

Question 75

Does unilateral radiation (for < N2c disease) offer the same benefit as bilateral radiotherapy for patients with unknown primary?

Question 76

In addition to the location of the + LNs as a guide to help tailor radiotherapy decision making, what other tumor related factor is crucial in formulating a treatment plan for an unknown primary of the head and neck?

Question 77   NON-MELANOMATOUS SKIN CANCER

What are recommended dosing regimens for definitive radiation for cutaneous BCC or SCC?

Question 78

What radiation delivery techniques are commonly used for superficial skin cancer?

What are their respective advantages/disadvantages?

Answer 75

While somewhat controversial, several studies have shown that unilateral RT results in inferior outcomes. One study showed that rates of contralateral neck failure (44% vs 14%) and mucosal primary site failure (44% vs 8%) were significantly higher for patients treated with unilateral RT.

Reddy SP, Marks JE. Metastatic carcinoma in the cervical lymph nodes from an unknown primary site: results of bilateral neck plus mucosal irradiation vs. ipsilateral neck irradiation. *Int J Radiat Oncol Biol Phys*. 1997;37:797–802.

Answer 76

Histology. Metastatic adenocarcinoma to cervical LN without a clear primary site is managed differently than a squamous cell carcinoma. Firstly, up-front neck dissection is favored over definitive (chemo) radiotherapy. Also, parotidectomy is advised as part of a comprehensive neck dissection for these patients. There are also additional putative primary sites to consider (e.g., salivary gland, paranasal sinuses) which can alter the radiation plan and argue against comprehensive radiation including potential mucosal sites.

Mendenhall WM, Amdur RJ, Hinerman RW, et al. Management of the neck including unknown primary. In: Halperin EC, Perez CA, Brady LW, eds. *Principles and Practice of Radiation Oncology*. 5th ed. Philadelphia, PA: Lippincott Williams and Wilkins; 2008:1048–1053.

Answer 77

Choice of dose/fractionation regimen depends on size and location of tumor as well and desired cosmetic outcome. Typically, the more protracted regimens yield improved long term cosmesis. NCCN recommended regimens include 64 Gy/32 fx, 55 Gy/20 fx, 50 Gy/15 fx and 35 Gy/5 fx. Other hypofractionated regimens include 40 Gy/10 fx and 20 Gy/2 fx.

National Comprehensive Cancer Network Clinical Practice Guidelines: Basal and Squamous Cell Cancer. Version 2.2011. http://www.nccn.org/professionals/physician_gls/pdf/head-and-neck.pdf. Accessed November 14, 2011.

Answer 78

Often superficial/orthovoltage therapy or electron beam therapy is used. Superficial (50–150 kv) and orthovoltage (150–500 kv) have D90 at 5 mm and 2 cm, respectively. Advantages over electrons include maximum dose at skin surface, ability to use smaller fields as there is less beam constriction at depth, and less penetration through eye shield. Electrons are typically prescribed to ensure the 90% IDL covers the deepest extent of the tumor. Wider margins (1–2 cm) are typically needed as high isodose lines constrict at depth. Advantages of electrons are widespread availability and sharper dose fall off. To minimize scatter into adjacent structures, a lead shield can be placed on patient's skin.

Question 79

Is there any evidence that higher dose/fraction is associated with improved control rates?

Question 80

When is adjuvant RT indicated after MOHS resection of a BCC/SCC?

Question 81

What factors predict for LN involvement in cutaneous SCC of the H&N?

Question 82   THYROID CANCER

What are the primary thyroid cancer histologies and their respective incidence?

Answer 79

Yes. Some retrospective series indicate that doses of > 2 Gy per fraction are associated with improved outcomes for definitive RT, even with doses above 60 Gy. This does not apply to adjuvant RT.

Locke J, Karimpour S, Young G, et al. Radiotherapy for epithelial skin cancer. *Int J Radiat Oncol Biol Phys.* 2001;51:748–755.

Answer 80

NCCN guidelines recommend adjuvant EBRT in cases with positive margins, extensive perineural or large nerve involvement, or recurrent disease. One large retrospective study showed that failure rates were significantly higher for patients treated with surgery and postop RT when there was clinical nerve involvement (symptomatic/radiographic) as opposed to only pathologic perineural involvement (5-yr LC 57% vs 90%). For the latter category, BCC seemed to do better than SCC (5-yr OC 97% vs 84%). As such, some advocate for adjuvant RT for pathologic PNI of SCC, while BCC with pathologic PNI only can be observed. Similarly, some argue that microscopic positive margins can be observed for BCC as the recurrence rate is only ~30% and usually highly salvageable with repeat surgery.

National Comprehensive Cancer Network Clinical Practice Guidelines: Basal and Squamous Cell Cancer. Version 2.2011. http://www.nccn.org/professionals/physician_gls/pdf/head-and-neck.pdf. Accessed November 14, 2011.
Jackson JE, Dickie GJ, Wiltshire KL, et al. Radiotherapy for perineural invasion in cutaneous head and neck carcinomas: Toward a risk-adapted treatment approach. *Head Neck.* 2009;31:604–610.

Answer 81

Higher grade lesions, those with LVSI, those with invasion beyond the subcutaneous fat, larger lesions and recurrent lesions are associated with significant risks of nodal metastases. In one study, 37% of lesions > 4 cm and 31% of lesions invading more than 8 mm were LN +. Consider superficial parotidectomy +/– LN dissection in patients with these high risk features undergoing surgical management.

Moore BA, Weber RS, Prieto V, et al. Lymph node metastases from cutaneous squamous cell carcinoma of the head and neck. *Laryngoscope.* 2005;115:1561–1567.

Answer 82

The most common histology is papillary (60%), followed by follicular (25%), medullary (5%), anaplastic (2%). Hurthle cell carcinoma (2%) is a rare form morphologically similar to follicular but with marked (> 75%) hypercellularity.

Swift PS, Larson S, Clark O, et al. Cancer of the thyroid. In: Phillips TL, Hoppe R, Leibel SA, eds. *Textbook of Radiation Oncology.* 3rd ed. Philadelphia, PA: Elsevier Saunders; 2010:726–727.

Question 83

What is the incidence of LN + disease in the various histologies?

What is their respective expected 10-yr OS?

Question 84

What stage is a 42 yo woman with a 3-cm thyroid tumor with metastasis to a level VI (Delphian) LN?

Question 85

What are the indications for post-thyroidectomy I-131 ablation?

Answer 83

Papillary cancer has a 30% risk of LN + and a 10-yr OS of 90–95%. Follicular cancer has a 10% risk of LN + disease and a slightly lower 10-yr OS of 85–90%. Medullary thyroid cancer has a worse survival of 80%, while anaplastic cancer is almost uniformly fatal.

Swift PS, Larson S, Clark O, et al. Cancer of the thyroid. In: Phillips TL, Hoppe R, Leibel SA, eds. *Textbook of Radiation Oncology*. 3rd ed. Philadelphia, PA: Elsevier Saunders; 2010:726–727.

Answer 84

It depends on histology. For a papillary or follicular tumor, this would be T3N1M0, stage I disease. For a medullary thyroid cancer, it would be T3N1M0, stage III, and for anaplastic thyroid cancer, it would be T4aN0M0, stage IVa. The staging scheme is as follows.

Papillary or follicular (< 45 years)
- Stage I – Any T, Any N, M0
- Stage II – Any T, Any N, M1

Papillary or follicular (≥ 45 yo) or medullary (any age)
- Stage I – T1 N0 M0
- Stage II – T2 N0 M0
- Stage III – T3 or N1a
- Stage IVA – T4a or N1b
- Stage IVB – T4b, Any N, M0
- Stage IVC – M1

Anaplastic carcinomas are considered stage IV
- Stage IVA – T4a, Any N, M0
- Stage IVB – T4b, Any N, M0
- Stage IVC – M1

Part II, Section 8:Thyroid. In: Edge SB, Byrd DR, Compton CC, et al., eds. *AJCC Cancer Staging Manual*. 7th ed. New York, NY: Springer; 2010:87.

Answer 85

In addition to TSH suppression, I-131 ablation is indicated for the following: a tumor > 1 cm, + margin, multifocal disease, LN + disease, aggressive histology (tall cell, columnar cell, poorly differentiated), gross soft tissue involvement.

National Comprehensive Cancer Network Clinical Practice Guidelines: Thyroid Cancer. Version 2.2011. http://www.nccn.org/professionals/physician_gls/pdf/head-and-neck.pdf. Accessed November 14, 2011.

Question 86

What is the procedure for postop I-131 imaging and ablation?

Question 87

What are some acute and long-term side effects of I-131 ablation?

Question 88

What are the indications for adjuvant external beam radiation therapy (EBRT) for resected thyroid cancer?

Answer 86

The procedure is as follows:

- Only applicable for patients with papillary and follicular histology.
- Withhold Synthroid (T4; levothyroxine) for 4–6 weeks. Cytomel (T3; liothyronine) can be substituted for 3–4 weeks, but discontinued at least 2 weeks before radioiodine studies. Iodine restrict diet for 2 wks prior to scan. Alternatively, rhTSH (Thyrogen) can be used to stimulate TSH without taking patients off of their synthroid.
- TSH should be 25–30 mU/L at the time of the radioiodine study
- Pregnancy test for females on day of test
- Administer 2–5 mCi I-131 tracer dose
- If high post-op uptake (> 10%), should have completion surgery.
- All others with uptake can have treatment dose of I-131.
- Dose is 30–100 mCi for patients with residual normal thyroid tissue
- Dose is 150–200 mCi for residual malignant thyroid tissue
- Perform total body scan 4–7 days after treatment dose to confirm ablation. Dose can be repeated if indicated.
- Administer levothyroxine suppressive therapy
- Repeat total body scan in 6 months, and then at q2–3 yr intervals.

National Comprehensive Cancer Network Clinical Practice Guidelines: Head and Neck Cancer. Version 2.2011. http://www.nccn.org/professionals/physician_gls/pdf/head-and-neck.pdf. Accessed November 14, 2011.

Answer 87

Acute side effects include sialadenitis, cystitis and GI irritation. Patients are also instructed to use their own toilet, flush twice, wash hands well after urination, avoid close contacts for several days after ablation, especially with children, to avoid unnecessary exposure to others. Long term toxicities may rarely include pulmonary fibrosis, oligospermia, and leukemias.

Swift PS, Larson S, Clark O, et al. Cancer of the thyroid. In: Phillips TL, Hoppe R, Leibel SA, eds. *Textbook of Radiation Oncology*. 3rd ed. Philadelphia, PA: Elsevier Saunders; 2010:732–733.

Answer 88

For papillary and follicular histologies, indications for adjuvant EBRT include age > 45 and pT4 tumor; gross disease in neck despite I-131 therapy, gross residual disease with inadequate iodine uptake. EBRT is indicated in medullary cancers for patients with T4 disease and positive margins, or bulky nodal disease, or with gross ECE. All patients with anaplastic cancer should be treated with adjuvant (chemo)radiotherapy.

Swift PS, Larson S, Clark O, et al. Cancer of the thyroid. In: Phillips TL, Hoppe R, Leibel SA, eds. *Textbook of Radiation Oncology*. 3rd ed. Philadelphia, PA: Elsevier Saunders; 2010:733.

2

CENTRAL NERVOUS SYSTEM

SAMUEL T. CHAO AND GAURAV MARWAHA

Question 1

What are the recommended doses for cranial radiosurgery for brain metastases as determined by the dose escalation study performed by Radiation Therapy Oncology Group?

Question 2

What are the three prognostic groups for brain metastases based on the recursive partitioning analysis (RPA) from Radiation Therapy Oncology Group (RTOG) studies?

Question 3

For single brain metastasis, is there benefit to surgical resection?

Question 4

Is there benefit to whole brain radiation in addition to surgical resection of single brain metastases?

Answer 1

The Radiation Therapy Oncology Group performed a dose escalation study (RTOG 9005) to determine the maximum tolerated dose (MTD) for each given size of tumor based on maximum diameter. For tumors 2 cm or less, the study did not meet MTD and the recommended dose was 24 Gy. For tumors 2.1 cm to 3.0 cm, the MTD was 18 Gy. For tumors 3.1 cm to 4 cm, the MTD was 15 Gy.

Shaw E, Scott C, Souhami L, et al. Single dose radiosurgical treatment of recurrent previously irradiated primary brain tumors and brain metastases: final report of RTOG protocol 90-05. *Int J Radiat Oncol Biol Phys*. 2000;47:291–298.

Answer 2

Gaspar et al. did an analysis of three consecutive RTOG brain metastases studies (1200 patients) to group prognostic factors to predict survival. These phase III studies compared different dosing schemes and radiation sensitizers for patients undergoing whole brain radiation therapy.

RPA Class	Characteristics	Median Survival (mo)
I	KPS ≥ 70, age < 65, primary controlled, no extracranial metastases	7.1
II	All others	4.2
III	KPS < 70	2.3

Gaspar L, Scott C, Rotman M, et al. Recursive partitioning analysis (RPA) of prognostic factors in three Radiation Therapy Oncology Group (RTOG) brain metastases trials. *Int J Radiat Oncol Biol Phys*. 1997;37:745–751.

Answer 3

Based on a prospective study of 48 patients with single brain metastasis comparing resection with whole brain radiation vs biopsy followed by whole brain radiation therapy, there was a significant improvement in survival, functional independence and local recurrence. Median survival was 40 weeks in the resection arm vs 15 weeks in the biopsy arm ($p < .01$). Functional independence was longer in the resection arm, 38 weeks vs 8 weeks ($p < .005$). Local recurrence was 18% in the resection arm vs 52% in the biopsy arm ($p < .02$).

Patchell RA, Tibbs PA, Walsh JW, et al. A randomized trial of surgery in the treatment of single metastases to the brain. *N Engl J Med*. 1990;322:494–500.

Answer 4

Yes. Based on a prospective phase III study of adjuvant whole brain radiation therapy (50.4 Gy/28 fx) vs no whole brain radiation therapy after resection for single brain metastasis, local recurrence decreased from 46% to 10% with the addition of whole brain radiation ($p < .001$). Intracranial failure also decreased from 70% to 18% with the addition of WBRT ($p < .001$). Neurologic death was decreased from 44% to 14% ($p = .003$). There was no difference in overall survival, however, the study was not powered for survival.

	Resection Alone	Resection + WBRT	*p* Value
Local recurrence	46%	10%	< .001
Distant recurrence	37%	14%	< .01
Intracranial failure	70%	18%	< .001
Neurologic death	44%	14%	.003

Patchell RA, Tibbs PA, Regine WF, et al. Postoperative radiotherapy in the treatment of single metastases to the brain: a randomized trial. *JAMA*. 1998;280:1485–1489.

Question 5

According to RTOG 95-08 which was a phase III study comparing WBRT alone vs WBRT + SRS for patients with 1–3 brain metastases, which subgroups showed an improvement in overall survival?

Question 6

Based on a phase III Japanese study for patients with 1–4 brain metastases randomizing patients to stereotactic radiosurgery (SRS) alone vs whole brain radiation therapy with SRS, did WBRT provide benefit?

Question 7

According to a phase III study of SRS vs SRS + WBRT for patients with brain metastases performed at MD Anderson, which arm had worse neurocognitive outcomes?

Answer 5

Overall, the study did not demonstrate a survival advantage. For patient with a single brain metastasis, the addition of SRS significantly improved survival from 4.9 months to 6.5 months ($p = .0393$). Patients undergoing SRS were more likely to have stable or improved KPS (43% vs 27%, $p = .03$). Local control was also significantly better (82% vs 71%).

On subset analysis, patients with a single brain metastasis, RPA Class I patients, and those with squamous/NSCLC histology showed an improvement in overall survival. For RPA Class I, the addition of SRS improved survival from 9.6 months to 11.6 months. For NSCLC patients, the addition of SRS improved survival from 3.9 months to 5.9 months.

Andrews DW, Scott CB, Sperduto PW, et al. Whole brain radiation therapy with or without stereotactic radiosurgery boost for patients with one to three brain metastases: phase III results of the RTOG 9508 randomised trial. *Lancet*. 2004;363:1665–1672.

Answer 6

This study enrolled 132 patients with 1–4 brain metastases, randomizing patients to SRS alone vs SRS + WBRT. WBRT decreased any brain recurrence from 76% to 47% ($p < .001$). WBRT decreased 1-year local recurrence from 27.5% to 11% ($p = .002$). WBRT also decreased 1-year distant brain recurrence from 64% to 42% ($p = .003$). Median survival was the same, but the study was underpowered for overall survival.

Aoyama H, Shirato H, Tago M, et al. Stereotactic radiosurgery plus whole-brain radiation therapy vs stereotactic radiosurgery alone for treatment of brain metastases: a randomized controlled trial. *JAMA*. 2006;295:2483–2491.

Answer 7

This study reported by Chang et al. randomized 58 patients with 1 to 3 brain metastases to SRS vs SRS + WBRT. Primary endpoint of the study was neurocognitive function as measured by the Hopkins Verbal Learning Test – Revised (HVLT-R) total recall at 4 months. There was significantly worse neurocognitive function in the whole brain radiation arm with a mean posterior probability of decline of 52% vs 24% for SRS alone. There was decreased CNS recurrence in the WBRT arm (73% were free from CNS recurrence with WBRT vs 27%) at 1 year ($p = .0003$).

Chang EL, Wefel JS, Hess KR, et al. Neurocognition in patients with brain metastases treated with radiosurgery or radiosurgery plus whole-brain irradiation: a randomised controlled trial. *Lancet Oncol*. 2009;10:1037–1044.

Question 8

What is the Graded Prognostic Assessment (GPA) for brain metastases?

Question 9

In a phase III study evaluating the role of motexafin gadolinium with whole brain radiation therapy for brain metastases, what factor is a major predictor of neurocognitive outcome?

Question 10

What are the most common cancers that metastasize to the brain?

Answer 8

The Graded Prognostic Assessment (GPA) is a prognostic index incorporating data from RTOG 95-08 and four additional phase III brain metastases trials. Unlike RPA, the GPA is less subjective and more quantitative compared to recursive partitioning analysis. A score is given based on age, KPS, number of CNS metastases, and the presence of extracranial metastases.

	0	0.5	1
Age	> 60	50–59	< 50
KPS	< 70	70–80	90–100
Number of CNS metastases	> 3	2–3	1
Extracranial metastases	Present		None

Median survival were: GPA 0–1, 2.6 months; GPA 1.5–2.5, 3.8 months; GPA 3, 6.9 months; GPA 3.5–4, 11 months.

A diagnosis specific GPA has also been developed.

Sperduto PW, Berkey B, Gaspar LE, et al. A new prognostic index and comparison to three other indices for patients with brain metastases: an analysis of 1,960 patients in the RTOG database. *Int J Radiat Oncol Biol Phys.* 2008;70:510–514.

Sperduto PW, Chao ST, Sneed PK, et al. Diagnosis-specific prognostic factors, indexes, and treatment outcomes for patients with newly diagnosed brain metastases: a multi-institutional analysis of 4,259 patients. *Int J Radiat Oncol Biol Phys.* 2010;77:655–661.

Answer 9

401 patients were randomized to receiving whole brain radiation vs whole brain radiation with motexafin gadolinium in this phase III study, which tested neurocognitive outcomes. Disease progression was found to be a major predictor of neurocognitive outcomes. In addition, neurocognitive function tests are predictors of overall survival.

Meyers CA, Smith JA, Bezjak A, et al. Neurocognitive function and progression in patients with brain metastases treated with whole-brain radiation and motexafin gadolinium: results of a randomized phase III trial. *J Clin Oncol.* 2004;22:157–165.

Answer 10

The most common cancers that metastasize to the brain are lung at 16–20% incidence, breast at 5% incidence, renal at 6–10% incidence, melanoma at 7% incidence, and colorectal at 1–2% incidence. Due to difficulties in ascertainment, these numbers probably underestimate the true incidence.

Kamar FG, Posner JB. Brain metastases. *Semin Neurol.* 2010;30:217–235.

Question 11

Is there a difference in response for whole-brain radiation for brain metastases for doses of 40 Gy in 4 weeks, 40 Gy in 3 weeks, 30 Gy in 3 weeks, 30 Gy in 2 weeks, 10 Gy in 1 fraction or 12 Gy in 2 fractions?

Question 12

Is there a role for accelerated hyperfractionated radiation in the treatment of brain metastases?

Question 13

What other phase III studies aside from the University of Kentucky (Patchell) evaluated the role of surgery + whole brain radiation vs whole brain radiation alone?

Question 14

According to an EORTC phase III trial assessing surgical resection or SRS +/− WBRT, what benefit does WBRT provide?

Answer 11

No. There were 2 prospective randomized trials by the RTOG evaluating different accelerated fractionation regimens. There was no difference in overall response. The duration of neurologic improvement was shorter for patients treated with 10 Gy in 1 fraction or 12 Gy in 2 fractions.

Borgelt B, Gelber R, Kramer S, et al. The palliation of brain metastases: final results of the first two studies by the Radiation Therapy Oncology Group. *Int J Radiat Oncol Biol Phys*. 1980;6:1–9.

Answer 12

RTOG 91-04 compared accelerated hyperfractionation (32 Gy in 20 fractions delivered at 1.6 Gy BID to the whole brain followed by 22.4 Gy in 14 fractions to visible lesions + 2 cm margin for a total dose of 54.4 Gy) vs whole brain to 30 Gy in 10 fractions. Median survival was the same at 4.5 months. There is no benefit to accelerated hyperfractionation.

Murray KJ, Scott C, Greenberg HM, et al. A randomized phase III study of accelerated hyperfractionation versus standard in patients with unresected brain metastases: a report of the Radiation Therapy Oncology Group (RTOG) 9104. *Int J Radiat Oncol Biol Phys*. 1997;39:571–574.

Answer 13

Noordijk et al., a Dutch trial, was a prospective randomized trial showing significantly better overall survival (43 weeks vs 26 weeks) with the addition of surgery. Mintz et al., a Canadian trial, did not show a benefit to surgery (6.3 mo with WBRT alone vs 5.6 mo for WBRT + surgery, $p = .24$), but this study included more patients with poor KPS and extracranial metastases.

Noordijk EM, Vecht CJ, Haaxma-Reiche H, et al. The choice of treatment of single brain metastasis should be based on extracranial tumor activity and age. *Int J Radiat Oncol Biol Phys*. 1994;29:711–717.

Mintz AH, Kestle J, Rathbone MP, et al. A randomized trial to assess the efficacy of surgery in addition to radiotherapy in patients with a single cerebral metastasis. *Cancer*. 1996;78:1470–1476.

Answer 14

This trial, EORTC 22952-26001, enrolled 359 patients. Functional independence and overall survival were the same in both arms. WBRT decreased the 2-year relapse rate at initial sites (surgery: 59% to 27%, $p < .001$; SRS: 31% to 19%, $p = .040$) and at new sites (surgery: 42% to 23%, $p = .008$; SRS: 48% to 33%, $p = .023$).

Kocher M, Soffietti R, Abacioglu U, et al. Adjuvant whole-brain radiotherapy versus observation after radiosurgery or surgical resection of one to three cerebral metastases: results of the EORTC 22952-26001 study. *J Clin Oncol*. 2011;29:134–141.

Question 15

What is the role of re-irradiation for progressive brain metastases?

Question 16

Is there any role for stereotactic radiosurgery to the resection bed following resection or brain metastases?

Question 17

What type of local control rates are seen with stereotactic radiosurgery in the management of brain metastases, and how does this compare to surgical resection?

Answer 15

Wong et al. performed a retrospective reivew of 86 patients who underwent re-irradiation for progressive brain metastases. Median dose for the second course was 20 Gy. 27% had resolution of neurologic symptoms and 43% had partial resolution. Median survival was 4 months. One patient developed dementia. There was one long-term survivor at 72 months. Lack of extracranial metastasis was a significant predictor of survival.

Wong WW, Schild SE, Sawyer TE, et al. Analysis of outcome in patients reirradiated for brain metastases. *Int J Radiat Oncol Biol Phys*. 1996;34:585–590.

Answer 16

SRS to the resection bed may be used to defer whole-brain radiation by providing local control to the resection bed. Acturarial local control at 6 and 12 months was 88% and 79%, respectively. Higher conformality index correlated to better local control. The authors recommend a 2-mm margin around the resection cavity.

North Central Cancer Treatment Group (NCCTG) N107C is a phase III trial of SRS to the resection bed compared to WBRT. The primary endpoints are overall survival and neurocognitive progression at 6 months postradiation. This study is currently open with a planned accrual of 192.

Soltys SG, Adler JR, Lipani JD, et al. Stereotactic radiosurgery of the postoperative resection cavity for brain metastases. *Int J Radiat Oncol Biol Phys*. 2008;70:187–193.

Answer 17

Local control rates with SRS range from 73–98%. SRS in the treatment for single brain appears to be roughly equivalent to local control rates seen with surgery followed by WBRT.

Shrieve DC, Loeffler JS, McDermott MW, et al. Radiosurgery. In: Hoppe R, Phillips TL, Roach M, eds. *Leibel and Phillips Textbook of Radiation Oncology*. 3rd ed. Philadelphia, PA: Elsevier Saunders; 2010:487–508.
Suh JH. Stereotactic radiosurgery for the management of brain metastases. *N Engl J Med*. 2010;362:1119–1127.

Question 18

What is the role of temozolomide in the management of glioblastoma?

Question 19

What extent of resection was determined to be prognostic for glioblastoma?

Question 20

What is the role of methylation of the MGMT promoter in glioblastoma?

Answer 18

Based on the EORTC-NCIC study, temozolomide improved median survival from 12.1 months to 14.6 months ($p < .001$). For this study, temozolomide was given daily 7 days per week at a dose of 75 mg per meter squared during the radiation, followed by six cycles of adjuvant temozolomide (started at 150 mg per meter squared for the first cycle, then 200 mg per meter squared for subsequent cycles). This trial enrolled patients between ages of 18 to 70 years of age. The update to this study showed an improvement in 5-year survival from 1.9% to 9.8% ($p < .0001$) with the addition of temozolomide. As such, temozolomide is considered standard of care for newly diagnosed glioblastoma.

Stupp R, Hegi ME, Mason WP, et al; European Organisation for Research and Treatment of Cancer Brain Tumour and Radiation Oncology Groups; National Cancer Institute of Canada Clinical Trials Group. Effects of radiotherapy with concomitant and adjuvant temozolomide versus radiotherapy alone on survival in glioblastoma in a randomised phase III study: 5-year analysis of the EORTC-NCIC trial. *Lancet Oncol.* 2009;10:459–466.

Stupp R, Mason WP, van den Bent MJ, et al; European Organisation for Research and Treatment of Cancer Brain Tumor and Radiotherapy Groups; National Cancer Institute of Canada Clinical Trials Group. Radiotherapy plus concomitant and adjuvant temozolomide for glioblastoma. *N Engl J Med.* 2005;352:987–996.

Answer 19

From a multivariate analysis of 416 patients treated at MD Anderson from 6/93 to 6/99, those with a resection of 98% or greater had a median survival of 13 months vs 8.8 months for those less than 98% ($p < .0001$). Another study shows benefit to gross total resection over incomplete resections with a survival advantage of 16.8 months vs 11.8 months ($p < .0001$).

Lacroix M, Abi-Said D, Fourney DR, et al. A multivariate analysis of 416 patients with glioblastoma multiforme: prognosis, extent of resection, and survival. *J Neurosurg.* 2001;95:190–198.

Stummer W, Reulen HJ, Meinel T, et al; ALA-Glioma Study Group. Extent of resection and survival in glioblastoma multiforme: identification of and adjustment for bias. *Neurosurgery.* 2008;62:564–576.

Answer 20

Hegi et al. tested the relationship of MGMT (O6-methylguanine-DNA methyltransferase – repair enzyme) silencing by methylation and survival from Stupp study. Methylation of MGMT promoter: 2-year OS = 46% in temozolomide arm vs 22.7% in RT alone arm ($p = .007$ by the log-rank test). Unmethylated MGMT promoter: 2-year OS = 13.8% in temozolomide arm vs < 2% in RT alone arm. Based on the results of this study, RTOG 0525 randomized patients with GBM to conventional adjuvant temozolomide dosing per EORTC-NCIC trial vs a dose dense regimen of 100 mg per meter squared days 1–21 per 28 day cycle.

Hegi ME, Diserens AC, Gorlia T, et al. MGMT gene silencing and benefit from temozolomide in glioblastoma. *N Engl J Med.* 2005;352:997–1003.

Question 21
Is there any benefit to doses higher than 60 Gy for treatment of glioblastoma?

Question 22
For elderly patients (70 years old or greater), is there a benefit to radiation over supportive care for patients with glioblastoma based on phase III data?

Question 23
Regarding recursive partitioning analysis (RPA) for malignant gliomas, which is the best group for patients with glioblastoma?

Answer 21

There was no benefit shown to 90 Gy of radiation using IMRT. There was also no benefit to brachytherapy in addition to conventional RT and no benefit to stereotactic radiosurgery boost (RTOG 9305).

Chan JL, Lee SW, Fraass BA, et al. Survival and failure patterns of high-grade gliomas after three-dimensional conformal radiotherapy. *J Clin Oncol*. 2002;20:1635–1642.

Laperriere NJ, Leung PM, McKenzie S, et al. Randomized study of brachytherapy in the initial management of patients with malignant astrocytoma. *Int J Radiat Oncol Biol Phys*. 1998;41:1005–1011.

Selker RG, Shapiro WR, Burger P, et al; Brain Tumor Cooperative Group. The Brain Tumor Cooperative Group NIH Trial 87-01: a randomized comparison of surgery, external radiotherapy, and carmustine versus surgery, interstitial radiotherapy boost, external radiation therapy, and carmustine. *Neurosurgery*. 2002;51:343–355; discussion 355–357.

Souhami L, Seiferheld W, Brachman D, et al. Randomized comparison of stereotactic radiosurgery followed by conventional radiotherapy with carmustine to conventional radiotherapy with carmustine for patients with glioblastoma multiforme: report of Radiation Therapy Oncology Group 93-05 protocol. *Int J Radiat Oncol Biol Phys*. 2004;60:853–860.

Answer 22

Keime-Guilbert et al. reported on 85 patients enrolled in a study comparing supportive care alone vs radiation to 50.4 Gy at 1.8 Gy per fraction. Radiation improved overall survival from 16.9 weeks to 29.1 weeks ($p = .002$). Quality of life and cognitive evaluation did not differ between the groups.

Keime-Guibert F, Chinot O, Taillandier L, et al. Radiotherapy for glioblastoma in the elderly. *N Engl J Med*. 2007;356:1527–1535.

Answer 23

RPA for malignant gliomas were recently redefined by Li, et al. The best group is RPA Class III. For GBM patients, the defining variables are:

RPA Class	Defining Variables	Median Survival Time (mo)	Overall Survival Rates: 1-yr, 3-yr, and 5-yr
III	< 50 y and KPS ≥ 90	17.1	70%, 20%, 14%
IV	< 50 y and KPS < 90; ≥ 50 y, KPS ≥ 70, resection, and working;	11.2	46%, 7%, 4%
V + VI	≥ 50 y, KPS ≥ 70, resection, and not working ≥ 50 y, KPS ≥ 70, biopsy only ≥ 50 y, KPS < 70	7.5	28%, 1%, 0%

Li J, Wang M, Won M, et al. Validation and simplification of the Radiation Therapy Oncology Group recursive partitioning analysis classification for glioblastoma. *Int J Radiat Oncol Phys*. 2011;81:623–630.

Question 24

For elderly patients with glioblastoma, is there a benefit to a higher, more protracted course of radiation?

Question 25

In the adjuvant setting, is there a benefit to standard temozolomide dose regimen vs dose-dense temozolomide regimen?

Question 26

Are imaging changes (increase in lesion size) one month post radiation with concurrent temozolomide sufficient to diagnose progression?

Question 27

Is there any benefit to whole brain radiation vs partial brain radiation in the management of malignant gliomas?

Answer 24

There was no difference between a conventional course of radiation (60 Gy in 30 fractions) vs an abbreviated course of radiation (40 Gy in 15 fractions) according to a phase III study reported by Roa et al. Median overall survival for standard RT was 5.1 months for standard fractionation vs 5.6 months for the shorter course.

Roa W, Brasher PM, Bauman G, et al. Abbreviated course of radiation therapy in older patients with glioblastoma multiforme: a prospective randomized clinical trial. *J Clin Oncol.* 2004;22:1583–1588.

Answer 25

RTOG 0525 compared two dosing scheme. The standard regimen based on the Stupp regimen was compared to a dose-dense regimen. *Standard arm:* 60 Gy XRT + TMZ 75 mg/m^2 qd -> TMZ 150 mg × 1 w/ dose escalation to 200 mg/m^2 d1-5 q4w × 6. *Experimental arm:* 60 Gy XRT + 75 mg/m^2 × 1 w/dose escalation to 100 mg/m^2 d1-21 of 28 day cycle × 7. No survival benefit was seen.

Gilbert MR, Wang M, Aldape K, et al. RTOG 0525: a randomized phase III trial comparing standard adjuvant temozolomide (TMZ) with a dose-dense (dd) schedule in newly diagnosed glioblastoma (GBM). *ASCO Proc.* 2011;15(suppl):2006.

Answer 26

No. Pseudoprogression may be seen and in fact, may predict for improved survival. Pseudoprogression is difficult to distinguish from progression radiographically. Overall survival in patients with properly defined pseudoprogression is 38 months per Brandes et al.

Brandes AA, Franceschi E, Tosoni A, et al. MGMT promoter methylation status can predict the incidence and outcome of pseudoprogression after concomitant radiochemotherapy in newly diagnosed glioblastoma patients. *J Clin Oncol.* 2008;26:2192–2197.

Answer 27

There is no difference between whole brain radiation and partial field radiation in terms of survival or local control. According to Shibamoto et al., median overall survival was 12 months for GBM patients treated with a local field covering tumor plus less than 2 cm margin, 12 months for those treated with a generous field (2 cm or more margin), and 13 months for those treated to whole brain. 80% of the recurrences occurred within 2 cm of the primary. 50% recur within 1 cm based on some older series.

Hochberg FH, Pruitt A. Assumptions in the radiotherapy of glioblastoma. *Neurology.* 1980;30:907–911.

Shibamoto Y, Yamashita J, Takahashi M, et al. Supratentorial malignant glioma: an analysis of radiation therapy in 178 cases. *Radiother Oncol.* 1990;18:9–17.

Wallner KE, Galicich JH, Krol G, et al. Patterns of failure following treatment for glioblastoma multiforme and anaplastic astrocytoma. *Int J Radiat Oncol Biol Phys.* 1989;16:1405–1409.

Question 28

Is there any benefit to hyperfractionation in the treatment of high-grade gliomas?

Question 29

According to the Stupp regimen for GBM, what is the dose of temozolomide concurrent with the radiation and adjuvant after the radiation?

Question 30

In the treatment of malignant gliomas, how common is it to see pseudoprogression after treatment with concurrent radiation therapy and temozolomide?

Question 31

Is there a benefit to higher doses of radiation up to 60 Gy in the treatment of malignant gliomas?

Answer 28

RTOG 83-02 was a phase I/II trial of hyperfractionation of 1.2 Gy BID or accelerated hyperfractionation of 1.6 Gy BID (interfraction interval 4–8 hr). 72 Gy at 1.2 Gy BID was found to have the best median survival with the least toxicity. RTOG 90-06 and other studies failed to show a benefit to altered fractionation.

Nieder C, Andratschke N, Wiedenmann N, et al. Radiotherapy for high-grade gliomas. Does altered fractionation improve the outcome? *Strahlenther Onkol.* 2004;180:401–407.
Werner-Wasik M, Scott CB, Nelson DF, et al. Final report of a phase I/II trial of hyperfractionated and accelerated hyperfractionated radiation therapy with carmustine for adults with supratentorial malignant gliomas. Radiation Therapy Oncology Group Study 83-02. *Cancer.* 1996;77:1535–1543.

Answer 29

The dose of temozolomide given concurrently with radiation is 75 mg per square meter of body-surface area per day, 7 days per week from the first to the last day of radiotherapy. This is followed by six cycles of adjuvant temozolomide at 150 to 200 mg per square meter for 5 days during each 28-day cycle.

Stupp R, Mason WP, van den Bent MJ, et al. Radiotherapy plus concomitant and adjuvant temozolomide for glioblastoma. *N Engl J Med.* 2005;352:987–996.

Answer 30

In a retrospective review of malignant glioma patients who were identified on imaging 4 weeks after therapy to have progression of disease, 50% developed pseudoprogression. The authors recommended continuation of adjuvant temozolomide in these cases.

Taal W, Brandsma D, deBruin HG, et al. Incidence of early pseudo-progression in a cohort of malignant glioma patients treated with chemoirradiation with temozolomide. *Cancer.* 2008;113:405–410.

Answer 31

Walker et al. performed a retrospective review of three Brain Tumor Study Group trials and found that a dose of 60 Gy had the best median survival.

	No RT	≤ 45 Gy	50 Gy	55 Gy	60 Gy
MS (weeks)	18	13.5	28	36	42
p-value		.346	< .001	< .001	< .001

Walker MD, Strike TA, Sheline GE. An analysis of dose-effect relationship in the radiotherapy of malignant gliomas. *Int J Radiat Oncol Biol Phys.* 1979;5:1725–1731.

Question 32

Aside from MGMT methylation, what is another strong molecular predictor of overall survival in patients with glioblastoma?

Question 33

Is there a role for radiosurgery (SRS) in the management of recurrent glioblastoma?

Question 34   LOW-GRADE GLIOMAS

Is there a benefit to higher doses vs lower doses of radiation in the management of low-grade gliomas?

Answer 32

IDH1 mutation is associated with prolonged PFS and OS. These mutations occurred in 16/286 patients in a recent study by Weller M et al. In the study, patients with IDH1 mutation had improved PFS (16.2 mo vs 6.5 mo, $p < .001$) and improved OS (30.2 mo vs 11.2 mo, $p = .002$). There is a greater difference in survival seen with IDH1 mutations than with MGMT promotor methylation.

Weller M, Felsberg J, Hartmann C, et al. Molecular predictors of progression-free and overall survival in patients with newly diagnosed glioblastoma: a prospective translational study of the German Glioma Network. *J Clin Oncol.* 2009;27:5743–5750.

Answer 33

SRS may be a viable treatment option in the recurrent setting following standard therapy. With radiosurgery in the recurrent setting, studies have shown a median survival time of 8–10.2 months.

Shrieve DC, Loeffler JS, McDermott MW, et al. Radiosurgery. In: Hoppe R, Phillips TL, Roach M, eds. *Leibel and Phillips Textbook of Radiation Oncology*. 3rd ed. Philadelphia, PA: Elsevier Saunders; 2010:487–508.

Answer 34

Per RTOG and EORTC studies, there is no benefit in terms of progression free survival or overall survival for higher doses of radiation vs lower doses of radiation. In the EORTC study, 5-year OS was 58% in the 45 Gy arm and 59% in the 59.4 Gy arm. 5 year PFS was also the same, 47% in the 45 Gy arm and 50% in the 59.4 Gy arm. In the RTOG study, 5-year OS was 72% in the 50.4 Gy arm and 65% in the 64.8 Gy arm. As a result, 50.4 to 54 Gy in 1.8 Gy per fraction is typically used, with a 2 cm margin.

Karim AB, Maat B, Hatlevoll R, et al. A randomized trial on dose-response in radiation therapy of low-grade cerebral glioma: European Organization for Research and Treatment of Cancer (EORTC) Study 22844. *Int J Radiat Oncol Biol Phys.* 1996;36:549–556.

Shaw E, Arusell R, Scheithauer B, et al. Prospective randomized trial of low- versus high-dose radiation therapy in adults with supratentorial low-grade glioma: initial report of a North Central Cancer Treatment Group/Radiation Therapy Oncology Group/Eastern Cooperative Oncology Group study. *J Clin Oncol.* 2002;20:2267–2276.

Question 35

What is the role of radiation in low-grade gliomas?

Question 36

From the Intergroup (NCCTG/RTOG 91-10) study randomizing patients with low-grade gliomas to 50.4 Gy of radiation vs 64.8 Gy of radiation, was there a significant difference in overall survival?

Question 37

What are the unfavorable risk factors for patients with low-grade gliomas used for the RTOG 0424 trial?

Answer 35

Per EORTC study, radiation improves progression free survival. EORTC 22845 was a prospective study of 314 patients, which randomized patients to observation vs upfront RT to 54 Gy/30 fx. No difference in 5-year OS: 65.7% in observation arm vs 68.7% in immediate post-op RT arm. 5-year PFS (34.6% in observation arm vs 55.0% in immediate postop RT arm) and decrease in seizures at 1 year (41% in the observation arm vs 25.0% in the immediate postop RT arm) were significantly improved.

	Observation Arm	Immediate Post-operative Radiation	*p* Value
5-year overall survival	65.7%	68.7%	.872
5-year progression free survival	34.6%	55.0%	< .0001
Seizures at 1 year	41%	25%	.0329

van den Bent MJ, Afra D, de Witte O, et al. EORTC Radiotherapy and Brain Tumor Groups and the UK Medical Research Council. Long-term efficacy of early versus delayed radiotherapy for low-grade astrocytoma and oligodendroglioma in adults: the EORTC 22845 randomised trial. *Lancet.* 2005;366:985–990.

Answer 36

No overall survival difference was seen for the two arms for this trial, which enrolled 203 patients from 1986 to 1994. On subset analysis, patients less than 40 years old (5-year OS of 77% vs 60%), oligodendroglioma predominance (5-year OS of 74% vs 56%), tumor less than 5 cm (5-year OS of 81% vs 61%), and gross total resection (5-year OS of 88% vs 56% for subtotal resection vs 71% for biopsy alone) showed improved survival. There was a higher incidence of radiation necrosis in the higher dose arm (5% vs 2.5%).

Shaw E, Arusell R, Scheithauer B, et al. Prospective randomized trial of low- versus high-dose radiation therapy in adults with supratentorial low-grade glioma: initial report of a North Central Cancer Treatment Group/Radiation Therapy Oncology Group/Eastern Cooperative Oncology Group study. *J Clin Oncol.* 2002;20:2267–2276.

Answer 37

The EORTC identified 5 unfavorable prognostic factors from two large randomized trials: age ≥ 40 years, largest tumor diameter ≥ 6 cm, tumor crossing midline, astrocytoma dominant histology, and neurologic symptoms (Pignatti et al). RTOG 04-24 was a phase II study of concurrent and adjuvant temozolomide for patients with 3 or greater risk factors. Those risk factors include: age ≥ 40, largest preoperative diameter of tumor ≥ 6 cm, tumor crosses midline, tumor subtype of astrocytoma (astrocytoma dominant), and preoperative Neurological Function Status > 1.

Pignatti F, van den Bent M, Curran D, et al; European Organization for Research and Treatment of Cancer Brain Tumor Cooperative Group; European Organization for Research and Treatment of Cancer Radiotherapy Cooperative Group. Prognostic factors for survival in adult patients with cerebral low grade glioma. *J Clin Oncol.* 2002;20:2076–2084.

Shaw E, Arusell R, Scheithauer B, et al. Prospective randomized trial of low- versus high-dose radiation therapy in adults with supratentorial low-grade glioma: initial report of a North Central Cancer Treatment Group/Radiation Therapy Oncology Group/Eastern Cooperative Oncology Group study. *J Clin Oncol.* 2002;20:2267–2276.

Question 38

Is there a benefit to PCV (procarbazine, CCNU, and vincristine) chemotherapy in the management of higher risk low-grade gliomas (patients 40 years or older without a gross total resection)?

Question 39

What are the three major types of low-grade gliomas seen in adults, and how common are each of them?

Collectively, in what age groups are they most commonly seen?

Question 40

What is the hallmark histopathologic feature for pilocytic astrocytomas?

Question 41

What is the relevance of Ki-67 labeling index in the evaluation of low-grade gliomas?

Answer 38

RTOG 98-02 randomized these patients to receive no chemotherapy vs 6 cycles of chemotherapy following radiation. There was no overall survival advantage to the addition of PCV. There was a progression-free survival advantage to PCV. Median PFS and 5-yr PFS favored RT + PCV (not reached vs 4.4 yrs, and 63% vs 46%; $p = .005$).

Shaw EG, Wang M, Coons SW, et al. Final report of Radiation Therapy Oncology Group (RTOG) protocol 9802: radiation therapy (RT) versus RT + procarbazine, CCNU, and vincristine (PCV) chemotherapy for adult low-grade glioma (LGG). *J Clin Oncol.* 2008;26(May 20 suppl):90s. Abstract 2006.

Answer 39

Low-grade astrocytoma: 67%

Mixed oligoastrocytomas: 19%

Oligodendrogliomas: 13%

These low-grade gliomas are most common between ages 20–40 years, rarely occurring after age 50.

Narayana A, Recht L, Gutin PH. Central nervous system tumors. In: Hoppe R, Phillips TL, Roach M, eds. *Leibel and Phillips Textbook of Radiation Oncology.* 3rd ed. Philadelphia, PA: Elsevier Saunders; 2010:421–425.

Answer 40

They are made up of fusiform cells with very long, wavy processes known as "Rosenthal fibers." Mitosis is rarely observed in these tumors.

Narayana A, Recht L, Gutin PH. Central nervous system tumors. In: Hoppe R, Phillips TL, Roach M, eds. *Leibel and Phillips Textbook of Radiation Oncology.* 3rd ed. Philadelphia, PA: Elsevier Saunders; 2010:421–425.

Answer 41

Even though low-grade gliomas are similar in histologic appearance, varying levels of proliferative markers like Ki-67 labeling index (LI) can affect prognosis. In one particular study, Ki-67 LI of > 10% was associated with higher grade and worse survival – this index proved to be more significant than histologic grading. Thus patients with a high LI can possibly benefit from more aggressive treatment.

Calvar JA, Meli FJ, Romero C, et al. Characterization of brain tumors by MRS, DWI and Ki-67 labeling index. *J Neurooncol.* 2005;72:273–280.

Question 42

What is unique about the growth behavior of pilocytic astrocytomas vs non-pilocytic tumors?

Question 43

How do WHO grade I astrocytomas appear on imaging, and how does this differ from other astrocytomas?

Question 44

What is the role of surgery and radiation in the management of pilocytic astrocytomas?

What kind of outcomes can be achieved?

Question 45

Is there increased toxicity with higher doses of radiation for low-grade gliomas?

Answer 42

Pilocytic astrocytomas tend to grow by expansion, and do not diffusely infiltrate adjacent tissue like non-pilocytic tumors.

Narayana A, Recht L, Gutin PH. Central nervous system tumors. In: Hoppe R, Phillips TL, Roach M, eds. *Leibel and Phillips Textbook of Radiation Oncology*. 3rd ed. Philadelphia, PA: Elsevier Saunders; 2010:421–425.

Answer 43

On imaging, the classic appearance of pilocytic astrocytomas (WHO grade 1) is a large cyst with an enhancing mural nodule. MRI generally reveals non-enhancing lesions for ordinary astrocytomas, however around 40% of ordinary astrocytomas may enhance and 10% may have calcifications.

Narayana A, Recht L, Gutin PH. Central nervous system tumors. In: Hoppe R, Phillips TL, Roach M, eds. *Leibel and Phillips Textbook of Radiation Oncology*. 3rd ed. Philadelphia, PA: Elsevier Saunders; 2010:421–425.

Answer 44

60–80% of pilocytic astrocytomas are amenable to GTR. Long-term survival is nearly 100% after GTR, and 5-year OS of 80–90% after STR. Postoperative radiation is generally not indicated in completely resected pilocytic astrocytomas. However, in the STR/biopsy setting, close follow-up is indicated, because in the event of disease progression, radiation may be an option.

Narayana A, Recht L, Gutin PH. Central nervous system tumors. In: Hoppe R, Phillips TL, Roach M, eds. *Leibel and Phillips Textbook of Radiation Oncology*. 3rd ed. Philadelphia, PA: Elsevier Saunders; 2010:421–425.

Answer 45

The NCCTG/RTOG performed a prospective, randomized study of low-dose vs high-dose radiation for low-grade gliomas. The 2-year actuarial incidence of grade 3 to 5 radiation necrosis was 2.5% with low-dose RT (50.4 Gy) and 5% with high-dose RT (64.8 Gy), which was statistically significant ($p = .04$).

Shaw E, Arusell R, Scheithauer B, et al. Prospective randomized trial of low- versus high-dose radiation therapy in adults with supratentorial low-grade glioma: initial report of a North Central Cancer Treatment Group/Radiation Therapy Oncology Group/Eastern Cooperative Oncology Group study. *J Clin Oncol*. 2002;20:2267–2276.

Question 46

What is the progression-free survival rate at 5 years following neurosurgeon-determined gross total resection for low-grade gliomas?

Question 47   **CRANIOPHARYNGIOMA**

Should gross total resection be the goal when resecting a craniopharyngioma?

Question 48

How common are craniopharyngiomas?

Question 49

What is the role of radiation therapy in the management of craniopharyngiomas?

What are the doses?

Answer 46

Using data from RTOG 9802, phase II component which was observation following gross-total resection of grade II gliomas for patients younger than 40 years old, the 5-year PFS was 48%. The 5-year OS was 93%. Preoperative tumor size of 4 cm or greater, astrocytoma/oligoastrocytoma, and imaging residual disease of 1 cm or greater predicted for poorer PFS.

Shaw EG, Berkey B, Coons SW, et al. Recurrence following neurosurgeon-determined gross-total resection of adult supratentorial low-grade glioma: results of a prospective clinical trial. *J Neurosurg*. 2008;109:835–841.

Answer 47

Limited surgery followed by radiation leads to excellent outcomes and good local control. In a study by Merchant et al., the surgery only group had more frequent neurologic, ophthalmic, and endocrine complications. Also, the combined modality group had less of a decline in IQ compared to surgery only group (1.25 vs 9.8 points, $p < .063$). Limited resection followed by radiation is a good treatment option for most patients.

Merchant TE, Kiehna EN, Sanford RA, et al. Craniopharyngioma: the St. Jude Children's Research Hospital experience 1984-2001. *Int J Radiat Oncol Biol Phys*. 2002;53:533–542.

Answer 48

The U.S. incidence of craniopharyngioma is 350 cases per year. They constitute 1–3% of all brain tumor diagnoses, and 3–5% of brain tumors diagnosed in children.

Jane JA Jr, Laws ER. Craniopharyngioma. *Pituitary*. 2006;9:323–326.

Answer 49

Radiation therapy can be used in the treatment of residual disease post-operatively, and/or in the setting of recurrent disease. Typically, 54 Gy is used because this has been shown to have significantly better local control in various retrospective series. In a recent retrospective review, for example, among patients managed with partial resection, the 10-year recurrence-free rates were 77% and 38%, with and without postoperative RT.

Karavitaki N, Brufani C, Warner JT, et al. Craniopharyngiomas in children and adults: systematic analysis of 121 cases with long-term follow-up. *Clin Endocrinol (Oxf)*. 2005;62:397–409.
Minniti G, Esposito V, Amichetti M, et al. The role of fractionated radiotherapy and radiosurgery in the management of patients with craniopharyngioma. *Neurosurg Rev*. 2009;32:125–132; discussion 132.

Question 50

Craniopharyngiomas often present with cysts that frequently recur despite resection. What are the management options for these cysts?

Question 51

What are the long-term outcomes for patients with craniopharyngiomas?

Question 52   **ANAPLASTIC GLIOMAS**

What is the impact of 1p19q deletion in anaplastic oligodendroglioma and oligoastrocytoma?

Answer 50

Management options include percutaneous aspiration (which can be done intermittently, with an Ommaya reservoir system, as well), intracavitary irradiation with the use of beta-emitters (P32 used most commonly, with dose of 250 Gy), and intracavitary chemotherapy (bleomycin).

Kun LE, MacDonald S, Tarbell NJ. Craniopharyngioma. In: Halperin E, Constine L, Tarbell N, et al, eds. *Pediatric Radiation Oncology*. 5th ed. Philadelphia, PA: Lippincott Williams & Wilkins; 2011:40–44.

Answer 51

In general patients do well with a long-term overall survival rate of around 80–90%. In one series of 121 patients, for example, the 10-year survival rate was 90% when non-tumor related deaths were excluded. However, prognosis is not only affected by ability to control the tumor, but treatment-related complications as well.

Karavitaki N, Brufani C, Warner JT, et al. Craniopharyngiomas in children and adults: systematic analysis of 121 cases with long-term follow-up. *Clin Endocrinol (Oxf)*. 2005;62:397–409.

Answer 52

Patients with 1p19q deletion were found in RTOG 9402 (phase III study of PCV chemotherapy followed by radiation therapy vs radiation therapy alone) to have longer progression free survival and longer overall survival. The 1p19q codeleted subset had a median survival of > 7 years compared to 2.8 years. This was also shown in a similar study conducted by EORTC (phase III study of RT alone vs RT + PCV) with 74% of the 1p19q codeleted subgroup still alive after 60 months. Most recently, an update from RTOG 94-02 revealed that 1p19q status is both prognostic and predictive after PCV chemotherapy. In 126 patients with 1p19q codeletion, MS was 14.7 years versus 7.3 years in patients receiving PCV + RT vs. RT alone, respectively.

van den Bent MJ, Carpentier AF, Brandes AA, et al. Adjuvant procarbazine, lomustine, and vincristine improves progression-free survival but not overall survival in newly diagnosed anaplastic oligodendrogliomas and oligoastrocytomas: a randomized European Organisation for Research and Treatment of Cancer phase III trial. *J Clin Oncol*. 2006;24:2715–2722.

Cairncross G, Berkey B, Shaw E, et al. Phase III trial of chemotherapy plus radiotherapy compared with radiotherapy alone for pure and mixed anaplastic oligodendroglioma: Intergroup Radiation Therapy Oncology Group Trial 9402. *J Clin Oncol*. 2006;24:2707–2714.

Cairncross JG, Wang M, Shaw EG, et al. Chemotherapy plus radiotherapy (CT-RT) versus RT alone for patients with anaplastic oligodendroglioma: Long-term results of the RTOG 9402 phase III study. Abstract #2008b, Oral Abstract Session, Central Nervous System Tumors. 2012 ASCO Annual Meeting.

Question 53

For patients with anaplastic astrocytomas, does the addition of bromodeoxyuridine (BUdR) improve outcomes?

Question 54

What is the recommended treatment paradigm for anaplastic gliomas?

Question 55

What are the median and 3-year survival rates for patients with anaplastic astrocytomas?

Answer 53

No. The RTOG performed a phase III study (RTOG 9404) evaluating radiation therapy with PCV chemotherapy vs radiation therapy with PCV and BudR (which gets incorporated into the DNA of actively dividing cells and acts as a radiation sensitizer). The radiation dose was 59.4 Gy/33 fractions using 1.5 cm margin around the area of edema. The 4-year overall survival was 51% in both arms. There was one treatment related death in the BUdR arm. BUdR does not add benefit in the management of anaplastic astrocytomas.

Prados MD, Seiferheld W, Sandler HM, et al. Phase III randomized study of radiotherapy plus procarbazine, lomustine, and vincristine with or without BUdR for treatment of anaplastic astrocytoma: final report of RTOG 9404. *Int J Radiat Oncol Biol Phys*. 2004;58:1147–1152.

Answer 54

Maximal safe resection followed by radiation therapy to 50.4 Gy/28 fx (1.8 Gy/fx) to the CTV1 volume (which is defined by T2 hyperintensity + surgical bed + T1 contrast enhancement expanded volumetrically by 2 cm). An extra 9 Gy/5 fx (1.8 Gy/fx) boost field (CTV2 = MRI T1 contrast enhancement and resection bed + 1 cm margin). Alternatively, the open CATNON/RTOG study delivers 59.4 Gy/33 fx to CTV1. WBRT is recommended for multifocal tumors. The role for PCV chemotherapy, per RTOG 9402 and EORTC 26591 suggested PFS benefit but no OS benefit. However, in patients with 1p/19q codeletion, a recent update of 9402 suggests a doubling of median survival in patients treated with PCV.

Additionally, the role of temozolomide is currently being investigated. RTOG 0834 is a randomized study looking at the role of temozolomide concurrently and adjuvantly with radiation in patients with non-1p and 19q deletion. The four arms are radiation alone, radiation with concurrent temozolomide, radiation with adjuvant temozolomide, and radiation with concurrent and adjuvant temozolomide.

Cairncross G, Berkey B, Shaw E, et al. Phase III trial of chemotherapy plus radiotherapy compared with radiotherapy alone for pure and mixed anaplastic oligodendroglioma: Intergroup Radiation Therapy Oncology Group Trial 9402. *J Clin Oncol*. 2006;24:2707–2714.

Cairncross JG, Wang M, Shaw EG, et al. Chemotherapy plus radiotherapy (CT-RT) versus RT alone for patients with anaplastic oligodendroglioma: Long-term results of the RTOG 9402 phase III study. Abstract #2008b, Oral Abstract Session, Central Nervous System Tumors. 2012 ASCO Annual Meeting.

Answer 55

Median survival is 36 months, and the 3-year survival rate is approximately 50%.

Narayana A, Recht L, Gutin PH. Central nervous system tumors. In: Hoppe R, Phillips TL, Roach M, eds. *Leibel and Phillips Textbook of Radiation Oncology*. 3rd ed. Philadelphia, PA: Elsevier Saunders; 2010:421–425.

Question 56

What is the incidence for anaplastic oligodendrogliomas?

How common are they amongst gliomas?

Question 57

What is the role for chemotherapy in the management of anaplastic oligodendrogliomas?

Question 58

Is there a benefit to radiation in the treatment of anaplastic gliomas?

Answer 56

There are approximately 2000 cases/year diagnosed in the United States. They represent only 3–5% of all malignant gliomas.

Fine VH, Barker GF II, Markert JM, et al. Neoplasms of the central nervous system. In: DeVita VT Jr, Hellman S, Steven A, eds. *Cancer: Principles and Practice of Oncology.* 7th ed. Philadelphia, PA: JB Lippincott; 2005:1834–1932.

Answer 57

The role of chemotherapy has been investigated in the following 2 randomized trials:

RTOG 9402 – Patients with anaplastic oligodendroglioma or oligoastrocytma (AO/AOA) were randomized to: postoperative PCV (4 cycles every 6 weeks) followed by RT (59.4 Gy/33 fx) versus RT alone. The MS was 4.9 years for the PCV + RT arm versus 4.7 y and the 3y PFS was 2.6 years for the PCV + RT arm versus 1.7 years. 46% of pts had 1p/19q loss and demonstrated better survival regardless of tx arm (MS > 7 years with 1p/19q loss vs. 2.8 years). In update of 126 patients with 1p19q codeletion, MS was 14.7 years versus 7.3 years in patients receiving PCV+RT vs RT alone, respectively.

EORTC 26951 – AO/AOA were randomized to: postoperative RT (59.4 Gy/33 fx) followed by PCV (6 cycles q6w) versus RT alone. The PFS was 32 months in patients receiving PCV versus 13.2 months. The MS was 40.3 months in patients receiving PCV versus 30.6 months. The 5y OS was 42% with PCV versus 35%. 25% of pts had 1p/19q loss and demonstrated better survival (5y OS of 75% with 1p/19q loss versus 28%).

van den Bent MJ, Carpentier AF, Brandes AA, et al. Adjuvant procarbazine, lomustine, and vincristine improves progression-free survival but not overall survival in newly diagnosed anaplastic oligodendrogliomas and oligoastrocytomas: a randomized European Organisation for Research and Treatment of Cancer phase III trial. *J Clin Oncol.* 2006;24:2715–2722.
Cairncross G, Berkey B, Shaw E, et al. Phase III trial of chemotherapy plus radiotherapy compared with radiotherapy alone for pure and mixed anaplastic oligodendroglioma: Intergroup Radiation Therapy Oncology Group Trial 9402. *J Clin Oncol.* 2006;24:2707–2714.
Cairncross JG, Wang M, Shaw EG, et al. Chemotherapy plus radiotherapy (CT–RT) versus RT alone for patients with anaplastic oligodendroglioma: Long-term results of the RTOG 9402 phase III study. Abstract #2008b, Oral Abstract Session, Central Nervous System Tumors. 2012 ASCO Annual Meeting.

Answer 58

BTSG 6901 was a randomized trial of best supportive care, BCNU alone, radiation alone, and radiation + BCNU. Patients who received radiation (+/− BCNU) survived 35 weeks vs 18.5 weeks with BCNU alone vs 14 weeks with supportive care. This study established radiation as a standard in the treatment of anaplastic gliomas.

Walker MD, Alexander E Jr, Hunt WE, et al. Evaluation of BCNU and/or radiotherapy in the treatment of anaplastic gliomas. A cooperative clinical trial. *J Neurosurg.* 1978;49:333–343.

Question 59   PROPHYLACTIC CRANIAL IRRADIATION

Is there an overall survival advantage to prophylactic cranial irradiation (PCI) for limited stage lung cancer patients?

Question 60   SPINE METASTASES

For patients with malignant spinal cord compression, what role does decompressive surgery with spinal stabilization play based on a phase III trial?

Question 61

Is there any benefit to 100 mg IV dexamethasone compared to 10 mg IV dexamethasone initial bolus for patients with malignant spinal cord compression?

Question 62

What is the local control rate of spine radiosurgery for re-irradiation of spine metastases?

Answer 59

Auperin et al. performed a meta-analysis of 7 randomized controlled trials on PCI. There was improvement in overall survival with PCI (3 year OS improved to 15.3% to 20.7%). The incidence of brain metastases decreased from 58.6% to 33.3% at 3 years with the addition of PCI.

Aupérin A, Arriagada R, Pignon JP, et al; Prophylactic Cranial Irradiation Overview Collaborative Group. Prophylactic cranial irradiation for patients with small-cell lung cancer in complete remission. *N Engl J Med*. 1999;341:476–484.

Answer 60

Patchell et al. reported a phase III study of 101 patients who were randomized to radiation alone vs direct decompressive surgery followed by radiation (30 Gy in 10 fx). The surgical arm had a significantly higher ambulation rate (84% vs 57%), longer persistence of ambulation (122 days vs 13 days), median survival (126 days vs 100 days), and more patients becoming ambulatory if they presented non-ambulatory (62% vs 19%).

Patchell RA, Tibbs PA, Regine WF, et al. Direct decompressive surgical resection in the treatment of spinal cord compression caused by metastatic cancer: a randomised trial. *Lancet*. 2005;366:643–648.

Answer 61

There is no benefit to high dose steroids as the initial dose. There was no difference in ambulatory rate, bladder function, or pain relief. There was significant pain relief in both arms by 3 hours ($p < .001$).

Vecht CJ, Haaxma-Reiche H, van Putten WL, et al. Initial bolus of conventional versus high-dose dexamethasone in metastatic spinal cord compression. *Neurology*. 1989;39:1255–1257.

Answer 62

MD Anderson performed a prospective study using spine radiosurgery to retreat spine metastases. 59 patients with 63 metastases were reirradiated. 1-year radiographic local control and overall survival were both 76%. Of the tumors that progressed, 81% had tumors within 5 mm of the spinal cord.

Garg AK, Wang XS, Shiu AS, et al. Prospective evaluation of spinal reirradiation by using stereotactic body radiation therapy: The University of Texas MD Anderson Cancer Center experience. *Cancer*. 2011;117:3509–3516.

Question 63

What is the RPA classification scheme for patients undergoing spine radiosurgery?

Question 64

What is the role of spine radiosurgery in the treatment of spine metastases?

Question 65

How frequent is adjacent vertebral body failure in spine radiosurgery?

Answer 63

RPA analysis of patients treated with spine radiosurgery at the Cleveland Clinic resulted in 3 classes ($p < .0001$). Class 1 is defined as: Time from diagnosis of primary cancer to being seen for spine radiosurgery (TPD) > 30 months (mo) and Karnofsky Performance Status (KPS) > 70; Class 2: TPD > 30 mo and KPS < 70 (or) TPD < 30 mo and age < 70 years (yr); Class 3: TPD < 30 mo and age > 70 yr. Median OS was 21.1 mo for Class 1 (n = 59), 8.7 mo for Class 2 (n = 104), and 2.4 mo for Class 3 (n = 11). This may be used to predict which patients may benefit the most from spine radiosurgery.

Chao ST, Koyfman SA, Woody N, et al. Recursive partitioning analysis index is predictive for overall survival in patients undergoing spine stereotactic body radiation therapy for spinal metastases. *Int J Radiat Oncol Biol Phys*. 2011;82:1738–1743.

Answer 64

Spine radiosurgery is being used to retreat the spine in a previously irradiated area or to treat radioresistant histology upfront. The ideal candidates are those with 1–3 contiguous vertebral body involvement with 3 separate sites of disease. The no more than 10% of the spinal cord should receive 10 Gy or more.

The use of spine radiosurgery in an upfront setting is being investigated in RTOG 0631, which is a phase II/III study of spine stereotactic radiosurgery for localized spine metastases. This has been shown to be safe in the phase II component of the study and has moved to the phase III component, which is a randomization of spine radiosurgery to 16 Gy in 1 fraction compared to conventional radiation to 8 Gy in 1 fraction.

Dahele M, Fehlinigs MG, Sahgal A. Stereotactic radiotherapy: an emerging treatment for spinal metastases. *Can J Neurol Sci*. 2011;38:247–250.
Masucci GL, Yu E, Chang EL, et al. Stereotactic body radiotherapy is an effective treatment in reirradiating spinal metastases: current status and practical considerations for safe practice. *Expert Rev Anticancer Ther*. 2011;11:1923–1933.
Shin JH, Chao ST, Angelov L. Stereotactic radiosurgery for spinal metastases: update on treatment strategies. *J Neurosurg Sci*. 2011;55:197–209.

Answer 65

Local failure of the unirradiated adjacent vertebral body occurs in less than 5% to 8% of patients with isolated spinal metastases.

Klish DS, Grossman P, Allen PK, et al. Irradiation of spinal metastases: should we continue to include one uninvolved vertebral body above and below in the radiation field? *Int J Radiat Oncol Biol Phys*. 2011;8:1495–1499.
Koyfman SA, Djemil T, Burdick MJ, et al. Marginal recurrence requiring salvage radiotherapy after stereotactic body radiotherapy for spinal metastases. *Int J Radiat Oncol Biol Phys*. 2011;83:297–302.

Question 66

Does dose impact the control rate seen with radiosurgery?

Question 67

PRIMARY CNS LYMPHOMA

Is there any role to CHOD (cyclophosphamide, doxorubicin, vincristine, and dexamethasone) chemotherapy in the management of primary CNS lymphoma?

Question 68

Is there any role for methotrexate-based chemotherapy in the management of primary CNS lymphoma?

Question 69

According to the Prognostic Scoring System for primary CNS lymphoma, what are the risk factors?

Answer 66

Dose may play a role in control rates for radiosurgery. In a study by Memorial Sloan Kettering, 126 metastases that underwent stereotactic body radiation therapy were studied. The control rate was higher in patients receiving high dose (23–24 Gy) compared to low doses (less than or equal to 22 Gy). The local relapse free survival was 80% in the high dose level vs 37% in the low dose level ($p = .029$).

Greco C, Zelefsky MH, Lovelock M, et al. Predictors of local control after single-dose stereotactic image-guided intensity-modulated radiotherapy for extracranial metastases. *Int J Radiat Oncol Biol Phys*. 2011;79:1151–1157.

Answer 67

This was assessed in RTOG 88-06, a phase I/II study of pre radiation CHOD of 52 patients. The use of CHOD prior to radiation did not show a survival benefit when compared to historical studies. Median survival was 16.1 months.

Schultz C, Scott C, Sherman W, et al. Preirradiation chemotherapy with cyclophosphamide, doxorubicin, vincristine, and dexamethasone for primary CNS lymphomas: initial report of Radiation Therapy Oncology Group protocol 88-06. *J Clin Oncol*. 1996;14:556–564.

Answer 68

DeAngelis et al. performed a phase II study of 47 patients. 31 patients received Dexamethasone 16 mg IV → MTX 1 g/m^2 × 2 overlapping with intra-Ommaya MTX 12 mg × 6 doses → WBRT 40 Gy + 14.4 Gy boost → taper steroids → Ara-C 3 g/m^2 × 2. 16 patients received RT alone. MTX and Ara-C improved DFS to 41 months vs 10 months for WBRT ($p = .003$) and MS to 42.5 vs 21.7 months. Late neurologic toxicity, with dementia and ataxia, was seen in three of 31 (9.7%) combined modality patients.

DeAngelis LM, Yahalom J, Thaler HT, et al. Combined modality therapy for primary CNS lymphoma. *J Clin Oncol*. 1992;10:635–643.

Answer 69

The risk factors are age > 60 years old, performance status > 1, elevated LDH, elevated CSF protein, and involvement of the deep regions of the brain. Using these prognostic factors, 0–1 risk factors have an 80% 2 year overall survival, 2–3 risk factors have a 48% 2 year overall survival, and 4–5 have a 15% 2-year overall survival.

Ferreri AJ, Blay JY, Reni M, et al. Prognostic scoring system for primary CNS lymphomas: the International Extranodal Lymphoma Study Group experience. *J Clin Oncol*. 2003;21:266–272.

Question 70

What are the 3 RPA classes according to the Memorial Sloan-Kettering RPA Classification for primary CNS lymphoma?

Question 71

What is the median survival with radiation alone for primary CNS lymphoma?

Question 72

How are patients with primary CNS lymphoma and HIV treated?

Question 73   **MENINGIOMAS**

For meningiomas, how is extent of resection graded?

Answer 70

Class 1 patients are patients less than 50 years of age and have a median survival of 85 months. Class 2 patients are 50 years old and above and have a KPS of 70 or greater. These patients have a median survival of 3.2 years. Class 3 patients are patients 50 years and above and have a KPS below 70. They have a median survival of 1.1 years.

Abrey LE, Ben-Porat L, Panageas KS, et al. Primary central nervous system lymphoma: the Memorial Sloan-Kettering Cancer Center prognostic model. *J Clin Oncol.* 2006;24:5711–5715.

Answer 71

Median survival according to RTOG 83-15 (prospective phase II study) was 11.6 months. This study treated patients to 40 Gy whole brain with a boost to 60 Gy to the GTV plus 2 cm. On subset analysis, patients with KPS of 70–100 had a median survival of 21.1 months vs 5.6 months and patients < 60 years of age had a median survival of 23.1 months vs 7.6 months.

Nelson DF, Martz KL, Bonner H, et al. Non-Hodgkin's lymphoma of the brain: can high dose, large volume radiation therapy improve survival? Report on a prospective trial by the Radiation Therapy Oncology Group (RTOG): RTOG 8315. *Int J Radiat Oncol Biol Phys.* 1992;23:9–17.

Answer 72

There is no established standard regarding treating primary CNS lymphoma in a patient with HIV. Patients should be given highly active antiretroviral therapy (HAART) as a component of their management. HAART improves survival from 1 month to 4 months ($p = .007$). Whole brain radiation may also be given.

Bayrakar S, Bayrakar UD, Ramos JC, et al. Primary CNS lymphoma in HIV positive and negative patients: comparison of clinical characteristics, outcome and prognostic factors. *J Neurooncol.* 2011;101:257–265.

Answer 73

Simpson grade defines extent of resection and predicts for recurrence after surgery.

Grade	Extent of Resection	10-Year Recurrence Rate
I	GTR of tumor, dural attachments, abnormal bone	9%
II	GTR of tumor, coagulation of dural attachments	19%
III	GTR of tumor, without resection or coagulation of dural attachments	29%
IV	Partial resection of tumor	40%
V	Simple decompression (biopsy)	

Simpson D. The recurrence of intracranial meningiomas after surgical treatment. *J Neurol Neurosurg Psychiatry.* 1957;20:22–39.

Question 74

What is the control rate with radiosurgery for imaging-diagnosed meningiomas?

Question 75

Is there a dose-response relationship in treating meningiomas with fractionated radiation?

Question 76

Can stereotactic radiosurgery be used in the treatment of meningiomas, and if so, what sort of control rates can one expect?

Question 77   **TRIGEMINAL NEURALGIA**

In regards to radiosurgery, is there any benefit to higher doses for trigeminal neuralgia?

Answer 74

From the University of Pittsburgh, 219 patients treated with radiosurgery for imaging-diagnosed meningiomas were treated with SRS. The control rate with radiosurgery was 90% + at 10 years. Tumor progression developed in 7 patients, 2 of which were found to be misdiagnoses of metastatic nasopharyngeal adenoid cystic carcinoma and chondrosarcoma.

Flickinger JC, Kondziolka D, Maitz AH, et al. Gamma knife radiosurgery of imaging-diagnosed intracranial meningioma. *Int J Radiat Oncol Biol Phys*. 2003;56:801–806.

Answer 75

In a retrospective review conducted at UCSF of 140 patients receiving radiation for subtotally resected meningioma, the 5 year progression free survival was 93% for patients receiving greater than 52 Gy vs 65% for 52 Gy or less for benign meningiomas ($p = .04$). For malignant meningiomas, the 5-year progression free survival was 63% for doses greater than 53 Gy vs 17% for 53 Gy or less.

Goldsmith BJ, Wara WM, Wilson CB, et al. Postoperative irradiation for subtotally resected meningiomas. A retrospective analysis of 140 patients treated from 1967 to 1990. *J Neurosurg*. 1994;80:195–201.

Answer 76

Yes, doses typically range from 12–16 Gy. Local control rates can be > 90%, with one study illustrating a 98% control rate at 5 years.

Kollová A, Liscák R, Novotný J Jr, et al. Gamma Knife surgery for benign meningioma. *J Neurosurg*. 2007;107:325–336.
Pollock BE, Stafford SL, Link MJ, et al. Stereotactic radiosurgery of World Health Organization grade II and III intracranial meningiomas: treatment results on the basis of a 22-year experience. Cancer. 2011;118:1048–1054.

Answer 77

Initial studies did not show a benefit to higher doses, however, more recent retrospective studies do suggest improved outcomes with higher doses of radiosurgery (such as 85 Gy). Higher doses do lead to higher risk for trigeminal neuropathy.

Kim YH, Kim DG, Kim JW, et al. Is it effective to raise the irradiation dose from 80 to 85 Gy in gamma knife radiosurgery for trigeminal neuralgia? *Stereotact Funct Neurosurg*. 2010;88:169–176.
Pollock BE, Phuong LK, Foote RL, et al. High-dose trigeminal neuralgia radiosurgery associated with increased risk of trigeminal nerve dysfunction. *Neurosurgery*. 2001;49:58–62; discussion 62–64.

Question 78

What are the potential long-term side effects of SRS in the treatment of trigeminal neuralgia?

Question 79

What is the role for medical treatment of trigeminal neuralgia, and what are those treatment options?

Question 80   **VESTIBULAR SCHWANNOMAS**

What is the risk of facial weakness and trigeminal disturbance with radiosurgery compared to surgery for patients with vestibular schwannomas?

Question 81

What are the doses for radiation therapy and associated outcomes in the management of vestibular schwannomas?

Answer 78

Rates of facial dysesthesias range from 0–10% with doses < 90 Gy. Facial numbness is the most commonly observed side effect. Anesthesia dolorosa is a potential effect of GKRS though reports are scarce at best. Other side effects like dysguesia, hearing loss, and secondary malignancies are extremely rare.

Guo S, Chao ST, Reuther AM, et al. Review of the treatment of trigeminal neuralgia with gamma knife radiosurgery. *Stereotact Funct Neurosurg*. 2008;86:135–146.

Answer 79

Pharmacologic therapy is the initial recommended treatment, reserving surgery and radiation for those who fail medical management. Carbamazapine (200–2400 mg daily depending on severity of pain symptoms) is the best studied, and most efficacious medical treatment for TN. Complete or near complete control of pain was attained in 58–100% of patients in a recently reported review by the American Academy of Neurology (AAN) and European Federation of Neurological Societies (EFNS). Other pharmacologic options include oxcarbazepine, baclofen, lamotrigine, and pimozide, though these have not proven to be as effective.

Gronseth G, Cruccu G, Alksne J, et al. Practice parameter: the diagnostic evaluation and treatment of trigeminal neuralgia (an evidence-based review): report of the Quality Standards Subcommittee of the American Academy of Neurology and the European Federation of Neurological Societies. *Neurology*. 2008;71:1183–1190.

Answer 80

According to a prospective study performed in France, the risk of facial weakness with surgery was 37% compared to 0% with radiosurgery. The risk of trigeminal nerve disturbance was 29% vs 4% with radiosurgery.

Régis J, Pellet W, Delsanti C, et al. Functional outcome after gamma knife surgery or microsurgery for vestibular schwannomas. *J Neurosurg*. 2002;97:1091–1100.

Answer 81

Radiation therapy in the form of single fraction (12–13 Gy) or fractionated (20–35 Gy in 4–5 Gy fractions or 45–54 Gy in 1.8 Gy/fx) has been used. SRS provides excellent local control rates > 90%. In one series of Gamma Knife 12–13 Gy, 10-year local control rate was 98.3%.

Andrews DW, Suarez O, Goldman HW, et al. Stereotactic radiosurgery and fractionated stereotactic radiotherapy for the treatment of acoustic schwannomas: comparative observations of 125 patients treated at one institution. *Int J Radiat Oncol Biol Phys*. 2001;20:1265–1278.

Chopra R, Kondziolka D, Niranjan A. Long-term follow-up of acoustic schwannoma radiosurgery with marginal tumor doses of 12–13 Gy. *Int J Radiat Oncol Biol Phys*. 2007;68:845–851.

Murphy ES, Suh JH. Radiotherapy for vestibular schwannomas: a critical review. *Int J Radiat Oncol Biol Phys*. 2011;79:985–997.

Question 82

What are the significant morbidities associated with surgical and radiotherapeutic management of vestibular schwannomas?

Question 83

Is observation considered an acceptable approach to the management of vestibular schwannomas, and if so, when can it be employed?

Question 84   **ARTERIOVENOUS MALFORMATIONS**

Does the risk of hemorrhage increase or decrease during the latency period (between radiosurgery and angiographic obliteration) following radiosurgery for arteriovenous malformation?

Answer 82

Hearing loss and facial neuropathy (weakness and numbness) are the major concerning toxicities. A recent prospective study comparing Gamma Knife radiosurgery vs surgery illustrated better hearing preservation (68% vs 0%) and facial nerve preservation (98% vs 50%) in the Gamma Knife group.

Myrseth E, Møller P, Pedersen PH, et al. Vestibular schwannoma: surgery or gamma knife radiosurgery? A prospective, nonrandomized study. *Neurosurgery*. 2009;64:654–661; discussion 661–663.

Answer 83

Yes, observation is appropriate if the lesions are small (< 2 cm), and/or associated with no increase in size or symptoms. The majority of patients over 65 years of age do not require intervention. Reason for eventual intervention is based upon rapid tumor growth with associated onset of symptoms.

Rosenberg SI. Natural history of acoustic neuromas. *Laryngoscope*. 2000;110:497–508.

Answer 84

In a study of 500 patients treated with Gamma Knife radiosurgery in Japan, the risk of hemorrhage decreases by 54% during the latency period. The risk of hemorrhage decreases by 88% after obliteration.

Maruyama K, Kawahara N, Shin M, et al. The risk of hemorrhage after radiosurgery for cerebral arteriovenous malformations. *N Engl J Med*. 2005;352:146–153.

Question 85

What is the Spetzler-Martin grading scheme?

Question 86

How effective is stereotactic radiosurgery (SRS) in the treatment of AVMs?

Question 87

What are the implications for not treating an AVM?

Answer 85

The Spetzler-Martin grading system allocates points for certain features of intracranial AVM's. The total score correlates with operative outcome. Low scores (1–3) are typically amenable to surgery.

Size of nidus
Small (< 3 cm) = 1
Medium (3–6 cm) = 2
Large (> 6 cm) = 3
Eloquence of adjacent brain
Non-eloquent = 0
Eloquent = 1
Venous drainage
Superficial only = 0
Deep = 1

Spetzler RF, Martin NA. A proposed grading system for arteriovenous malformations. *J Neurosurg*. 1986;65:476–483.

Answer 86

Most reported angiographic obliteration rates range between 74%–92% at a time point 2–3 years post SRS. Smaller AVMs tend to have a much higher rate of obliteration (80–100%) than larger AVMs (40–70%) 2 years post SRS.

Flickinger JC, Kondziolka D, Maitz AH, Lunsford LD. An analysis of dose-response for arteriovenous malformation radiosurgery and other factors affecting obliteration. *Radiother Oncol*. 2002;63:347–354.

Miyawaki L, Dowd C, Wara W, et al. Five year results of LINAC radiosurgery for arteriovenous malformations: outcome for large AVMs. *Int J Radiat Oncol Biol Phys*. 1999;44:1089–1106.

Answer 87

The average annual rate of hemorrhage for untreated AVM ranges between 2.8% to 4.6%. Risk of hemorrhage is influenced by older age, deep brain location and exclusive deep venous drainage. The average annual mortality rate ranges from 0.7 to 1.0% in previous retrospective reviews.

da Costa L, Wallace MC, Ter Brugge KG, et al. The natural history and predictive features of hemorrhage from brain arteriovenous malformations. *Stroke*. 2009;40:100–105.

Ondra SL, Troupp H, George ED, et al. The natural history of symptomatic arteriovenous malformations of the brain: a 24-year follow-up assessment. *J Neurosurg*. 1990;73:387–391.

Question 88

What are the toxicities associated with SRS in the treatment of AVM?

Question 89   **PITUITARY TUMORS**

Which modality results in faster time to normalization of endocrinopathies from secretory pituitary adenomas, fractionated radiation or stereotactic radiosurgery?

Question 90

What is the primary treatment modality for prolactinomas?

Question 91

What is the control rate with fractionated radiation for nonfunctional pituitary adenomas?

Answer 88

Early effects include seizures, nausea/vomiting, and headache. Late effects can include radionecrosis (associated with permancent neurologic deficit in 2–3% of patients), edema, venous congestion, cyst formation, cranial nerve deficits, and bleeding risk. Larger AVMs (> 3 cm) are more likely to have significant toxicities.

Flickinger JC, Kondziolka D, Lunsford LD, et al. A multi-institutional analysis of complication outcomes after arteriovenous malformation radiosurgery. *Int J Radiat Oncol Biol Phys*. 1999;44:67–74.

Miyawaki L, Dowd C, Wara W, et al. Five year results of LINAC radiosurgery for arteriovenous malformations: outcome for large AVMs. *Int J Radiat Oncol Biol Phys*. 1999;44:1089–1106.

Answer 89

No randomized trials have compared SRS vs radiation therapy. Stereotactic radiosurgery appears to result in a faster time to normalization of endocrinopathies. In one study evaluating patients treated for acromegaly, the mean time to normalization was 1.4 years with radiosurgery vs 7.1 years in patients treated with fractionated radiation.

Landolt AM, Haller D, Lomax N, et al. Stereotactic radiosurgery for recurrent surgically treated acromegaly: comparison with fractionated radiotherapy. *J Neurosurg*. 1998;88:1002–1008.

Answer 90

Medical management is the primary treatment modality for prolactinomas. Primary therapy is bromocriptine and cabergoline. These drugs normalize prolactin levels and shrink tumors.

Melmed S, Casaneueva FF, Hoffman AR, et al. Diagnosis and treatment of hyperprolactinemia, an Endocrine Society clinical practice guidline. *J Clin Endocinol Metab*. 2011;96:273–288.

Answer 91

Many studies report excellent local control rates: > 95% at 10 years, and > 90% at 20 years, with most common doses between 45–50.4 Gy.

Suh JH, Chao ST, Weil RJ. Pituitary tumors. In: Gunderson LL, Tepper J, eds. *Clinical Radiation Oncology*. 3rd ed. Philadelphia, PA: Elsevier Saunders; 2012:493–509.

Question 92

What is the most common side effect of external-beam radiation treatment for pituitary adenomas?

Question 93

What are the various types of secretory pituitary adenomas, and how prevalent are each of them?

Question 94

What are the recommended SRS doses for pituitary tumors for both functional and nonfunctional types, and what is the most important dose constraint?

Question 95

What physical exam findings can one expect to see in patients with pituitary adenoma-induced acromegaly, and how can the condition be treated?

Answer 92

The most frequent side effect is hypopituitarism. The cumulative actuarial risk is approximately 50% at 10 to 20 years.

Littley MD, Shalet SM, Beardwell CG, et al. Hypopituitarism following external radiotherapy for pituitary tumours in adults. *Q J Med*. 1989;70:145–160.

Snyder PJ, Fowble PF, Schatz NJ, et al. Hypopituitarism following radiation therapy of pituitary adenomas. *Am J Med*. 1986;81:457–462.

Suh JH, Chao ST, Weil RJ. Pituitary tumors. In: Gunderson LL, Tepper J, eds. *Clinical Radiation Oncology*. 3rd ed. Philadelphia, PA: Elsevier Saunders; 2012:493–509.

Answer 93

Prolactinomas (most common), growth hormone (GH) releasing adenomas, adrenocorticotropic hormone (ACTH) releasing adenomas, and thyroid stimulating hormone (TSH) releasing adenomas (rare).

Suh JH, Chao ST, Weil RJ. Pituitary tumors. In: Gunderson LL, Tepper J, eds. *Clinical Radiation Oncology*. 3rd ed. Philadelphia, PA: Elsevier Saunders; 2012:493–509.

Answer 94

SRS doses range from 14–18.5 Gy for nonfunctioning adenomas, and 18–35 Gy for functioning adenomas. Reports of visual complications are extremely rare when the optic apparatus is limited to 8–9 Gy.

Suh JH, Chao ST, Weil RJ. Pituitary tumors. In: Gunderson LL, Tepper J, eds. *Clinical Radiation Oncology*. 3rd ed. Philadelphia, PA: Elsevier Saunders; 2012:493–509.

Answer 95

Acromegaly occurs when GH is oversecreted by a GH-releasing adenoma of the pituitary gland. This condition leads to multi-organ disturbances including cardiovascular, musculoskeletal (bony enlargement, of frontal bones, hands/feet, nose, spine, and mandible, in particular), respiratory, and a possible increased chance of developing colon cancer. Treatment is surgery if possible (and/or radiation), though multidisciplinary care is required as the primary goal of treatment is to normalize IGF-1 levels. Somatostatin analogues have been shown to have the greatest effect in reducing IGF-1 levels (by ~50%). Radiation and radiosurgery maybe given for incompletely resected disease or persistent IGF-1 levels.

Suh JH, Chao ST, Weil RJ. Pituitary tumors. In: Gunderson LL, Tepper J, eds. *Clinical Radiation Oncology*. 3rd ed. Philadelphia, PA: Elsevier Saunders; 2012:493–509.

Question 96   OPTIC GLIOMAS

What is the risk of second primary tumors in patients with NF1 being treated with radiation for optic glioma?

Question 97   OLIGODENDROGLIOMAS

What chromosome abnormalities are commonly observed in oligodendrogliomas?

Question 98   CNS RADIATION TOXICITIES/THERAPIES FOR TOXICITIES

What evidence is there to suggest a benefit to donepezil for patients treated with radiation for primary brain tumors?

Question 99

What is the role of bevacizumab in the treatment of radiation necrosis?

Answer 96

The relative risk of developing a second primary tumor is 3.04 in patients receiving radiation compared to patients who did not receive radiation. The median time frame to developing a secondary tumor from the time of radiation was 14 years.

Sharif S, Ferner R, Birch JM, et al. Second primary tumors in neurofibromatosis 1 patients treated for optic glioma: substantial risks after radiotherapy. *J Clin Oncol.* 2006;24:2570–2575.

Answer 97

Overall, in oligodendrogliomas, 75% have loss of genetic information from chromosome 1p, and 81% loss of genetic information from 19q. Anaplastic oligodendrogliomas additionally have losses in chromosomes 9p and 10q, and sometimes EGFR gene amplification similar to that seen in anaplastic astrocytomas.

Narayana A, Recht L, Gutin PH. Central nervous system tumors. In: Hoppe R, Phillips TL, Roach M, eds. *Leibel and Phillips Textbook of Radiation Oncology.* 3rd ed. Philadelphia, PA: Elsevier Saunders; 2010:421–425.

Answer 98

A phase II study of donepezil, an acetylcholinesterase inhibitor, was conducted at Wake Forest University. This study of 35 patient, 24 of which remained on study for 24 weeks, showed an improvement in cognitive functioning, quality of life, and mood.

Shaw EG, Rosdhal R, D'Agostino RB Jr, et al. Phase II study of donepezil in irradiated brain tumor patients: effect on cognitive function, mood, and quality of life. *J Clin Oncol.* 2006;24:1415–1420.

Answer 99

A randomized, double-blind placebo controlled trial was performed using bevacizumab to treat central nervous system radiation necrosis. Improvement was seen on MRI (T2 weighted imaging and T1 with contrast imaging) in all patients receiving bevacizumab. Clinical improvement was also seen in all patients receiving bevacizumab. This drug is a monoclonal antibody that binds VEGF. In radiation necrosis, perinecrotic astrocytes produce VEGF which acts as a vascular permeability factor and maybe responsible for late CNS injury.

Levin VA, Bidaut L, Hou P, et al. Randomized double-blind placebo-controlled trial of bevacizumab therapy for radiation necrosis of the central nervous system. *Int J Radiat Oncol Biol Phys.* 2011;79:1487–1495.
Nonoguchi N, Miyatake S, Fukumoto M, et al. The distribution of vascular endothelial growth factor-producing cells in clinical radiation necrosis of the brain: pathological consideration of their potential roles. *J Neurooncol.* 2011;105:423–431.

Question 100
What is the risk of optic neuropathy from radiosurgery?

Question 101
What is Cahan's criteria for radiation-induced neoplasm?

Question 102
How is radiation injury classified according to temporal relationship to radiation treatment?

Question 103
What are the additional risks when a patient on phenytoin starts radiation?

Answer 100

The risk of optic neuropathy is dose dependent. In a study of 50 patients, the risk of optic neuropathy was 0% for less than 10 Gy, 26.7% for 10 to < 15 Gy, and 77.8% for 15 Gy or more. In another study, the rate of optic neuropathy was 1.1% for 12 Gy or less.

Leber KA, Bergloff J, Pendl G. Dose-response tolerance of the visual pathways and cranial nerves of the cavernous sinus to stereotactic radiosurgery. *J Neurosurg.* 1998;88:43–50.

Stafford SL, Pollock BE, Leavitt JA, et al. A study on the radiation tolerance of the optic nerves and chiasm after stereotactic radiosurgery. *Int J Radiat Oncol Biol Phys.* 2003;55:1177–1181.

Answer 101

Cahan's criteria defines what can be considered a radiation-induced neoplasm. The criteria includes:

1. Tumor must originate in a previously irradiated region.
2. Must be a sufficiently long time interval from irradiation and the onset of post-radiation tumor.
3. Histology must be different than the primary tumor.
4. Patient must not have a genetic predisposition for tumor development.

Cahan WG, Woodard HQ, Higinbotham NL, et al. Sarcoma arising in irradiated bone: report of eleven cases. *Cancer.* 1948;82:8–34.

Answer 102

Acute injury occurs during or after completion of radiation. It is reversible and is characterized by edema. Early delayed injury occurs up to 12 weeks after completion of radiation. This is also reversible and is characterized by increased signal on FLAIR and T2. Late injury of radiation necrosis occurs a few months to several years after radiation. It is irreversible and can be characterized by a focal pattern (circumscribed lesion) or a diffuse pattern (wide spread periventricular white matter changes).

Sheline GE, Wara WM, Smith V. Therapeutic irradiation and brain injury. *Int J Radiat Oncol Biol Phys.* 1980;6: 1215–1228.

Answer 103

Erythema multiforme and Stevens-Johnson syndrome are associated with being on phenytoin and radiation at the same time. If anticonvulsants are necessary during radiation, it is best to avoid phenytoin.

Delattre JY, Safai B, Posner JB. Erythema multiforme and Stevens-Johnson syndrome in patients receiving cranial irradiation and phenytoin. *Neurology.* 1988;38:194–198.

Question 104

Is there any benefit to methylphenidate for primary or metastatic brain tumors?

Question 105   **SPINAL CORD TUMORS**

Is there any benefit to radiation for spinal myxopapillary ependymoma after surgery?

Question 106

How common are primary spinal canal tumors in adults and children?

Question 107

What is the anatomical distribution for primary spinal cord tumors?

Which types of tumors are most commonly found in each anatomic location?

Answer 104

No. In a double-blind trial that was terminated prematurely, 68 patients with primary or metastatic brain tumors were randomly assigned to methylphenidate or placebo. Eight weeks after completion of RT, there was no difference in fatigue or cognition compared to placebo.

Butler JM Jr, Case LD, Atkins J, et al. A phase III, double-blind, placebo-controlled prospective randomized clinical trial of d-threo-methylphenidate HCl in brain tumor patients receiving radiation therapy. *Int J Radiat Oncol Biol Phys*. 2007;69:1496–1501.

Answer 105

A retrospective study of 85 patients was performed by the Rare Cancer Network. There appears to be a benefit to high-dose radiation (50.4 Gy and above) following surgery. There is a benefit to low-dose radiation, but not as much as high dose. For patients with an upfront diagnosis, observation may be considered after surgery due to the long natural history of this tumor.

Chao ST, Kobayashi T, Benzel E, et al. The role of adjuvant radiation therapy in the treatment of spinal myxopapillary ependymomas. *J Neurosurg Spine*. 2011;14:59–64.
Pica A, Miller R, Villà S, et al. The results of surgery, with or without radiotherapy, for primary spinal myxopapillary ependymoma: a retrospective study from the rare cancer network. *Int J Radiat Oncol Biol Phys*. 2009;74:1114–1120.

Answer 106

Overall, primary spinal canal tumors are rare in adults, comprising only 2–4% of all primary CNS tumors. In adults, they are outnumbered by primary brain tumors 20:1, while in children the ratio is 5:1.

Linstadt DE, Nakamura JL. Spinal cord tumors. In: Hoppe R, Phillips TL, Roach M, eds. *Leibel and Phillips Textbook of Radiation Oncology*. 3rd ed. Philadelphia, PA: Elsevier Saunders; 2010:509–522.

Answer 107

Extradural	10%	Metastatic Lesions
Intradural, extramedullary	65%	Meningiomas and nerve sheath tumors
Intramedullary	25%	Gliomas (ependymomas and astrocytomas)

Linstadt DE, Nakamura JL. Spinal cord tumors. In: Hoppe R, Phillips TL, Roach M, eds. *Leibel and Phillips Textbook of Radiation Oncology*. 3rd ed. Philadelphia, PA: Elsevier Saunders; 2010:509–522.

Question 108

What is the role for adjuvant radiation in the treatment of spinal gliomas?

Question 109

What dose of radiation is typically used in the management of subtotally resected spinal meningiomas and ependymomas?

Question 110

What is the role for spinal radiosurgery in the management of benign intradural, extramedullary tumors?

Question 111

How do spinal cord tumors most commonly present?

Answer 108

Post-operative radiation is not indicated for low-grade gliomas that have been completely resected. For subtotally resected low-grade gliomas, focal field radiation therapy to 50.4 Gy is indicated. For high-grade gliomas, resection is difficult and focal radiation therapy to 54 Gy is recommended.

Linstadt DE, Nakamura JL. Spinal cord tumors. In: Hoppe R, Phillips TL, Roach M, eds. *Leibel and Phillips Textbook of Radiation Oncology.* 3rd ed. Philadelphia, PA: Elsevier Saunders; 2010:509–522.
Robinson CG, Prayson RA, Hahn JF, et al. Long-term survival and functional status of patients with low-grade astrocytoma of spinal cord. *Int J Radiat Oncol Biol Phys*. 2005;63:91–100.

Answer 109

With the use of standard external beam radiation, 50.4 Gy (1.8 Gy/fx or 1 Gy/bid) has been shown to be efficacious.

Bhatnagar AK, Gerszten PC, Ozhasaglu C, et al. Cyberknife frameless radiosurgery for the treatment of extracranial benign tumors. *Technol Cancer Res Treat*. 2005;4:571–576.

Answer 110

While surgical resection remains the gold standard, there is no prospective data comparing surgery to SRS. In a recent retrospective review of 32 meningiomas, 24 neurofibromas, and 47 schwannomas treated with SRS with a mean radiographic f/u of 33 months, clinically 91% of meningiomas, 67% of neurofibromas, and 86% of schwannomas were symptomatically stable to improved at time of last follow-up. The authors concluded that SRS provides safe and efficacious long-term control of benign intradural, extramedullary spinal tumors with low rates of complications.

Sachdev S, Dodd RL, Chang SD, et al. Stereotactic radiosurgery yields long-term control for benign intradural, extramedullary spinal tumors. *Neurosurg*. 2011;69:533–539.

Answer 111

75% of patients present with pain. Tumor pain is often worse at night with lying down (due to venous congestion) causing nocturnal wakening. Spinal cord tumor pain is commonly described as gnawing and unremitting.

Welch WC, Jacobs GB. Surgery for metastatic spinal disease. *J Neurooncol*. 1995;23:163–170.

Question 112

What is the most concerning toxicity with radiation of the spinal cord, and how does it typically present?

Answer 112

Radiation myelitis. It can occur 1–2 years after radiation therapy with paresthesias, weakness, sensation/autonomic loss, and loss of motor function. It may present in a transient form, within months post radiation, known as L'hermitte's sign, where upon neck flexion, shock-like sensations can be felt in the extremities.

Gemici C. Lhermitte's sign: review with special emphasis in oncology practice. *Crit Rev Oncol Hematol.* 2010;74:79–86.

3

BREAST CANCER

RAHUL TENDULKAR

Question 1   EPIDEMIOLOGY AND CANCER RISK

What is the incidence of new breast cancer diagnoses per year in the United States?

Question 2

What is the risk of being diagnosed with breast cancer for the average American female?

What is the risk for the average American male?

Question 3

What percentage of breast cancers occurs in men?

Question 4

What are risk factors for developing breast cancer?

Answer 1

In 2010, there were an estimated 207,090 cases of breast cancer in women. Breast cancer incidence rates have slightly decreased over the past decade. Potential attributing factors include decreased hormonal therapy usage and a leveling-off of increased mammography usage noted during the decade prior.

Jemal A, Siegel R, Xu J, et al. Cancer statistics, 2010. *CA Cancer J Clin*. 2010;60:277–300.

Answer 2

The lifetime risk of being diagnosed with breast cancer in a woman is 1 in 8. The lifetime risk in males is 1 in 1000. (The risk rises to 6.8 in 100 for men who carry a BRCA2 mutation and 1.2 in 100 for men with BRCA1.)

Tai YC, Domchek S, Parmigiani G, et al. Breast cancer risk among male BRCA1 and BRCA2 mutation carriers. *J Natl Cancer Inst*. 2007;99:1811–1814.

Answer 3

1% of breast cancer cases occur in men; about 90% are ER+. Men often present with more advanced disease at the time of diagnosis compared to women. However, when matched stage for stage, survival rates between male and female breast cancers are not significantly worse.

Giordano SH, Cohen DS, Buzdar AU, et al. Breast carcinoma in men: a population-based study. *Cancer*. 2004;101:51–57.

Answer 4

Female sex, older age, family history of breast cancer, early menarche, late menopause, nulliparity, later age at first pregnancy, lack of breast feeding, hormone replacement therapy, hereditary mutations, dense breast tissue, prior radiation to breast, obesity, and a prior history of breast cancer, DCIS, or LCIS. After gender, the strongest risk factor is age; the median age of diagnosis in the U.S. is 61 years old. Other strong risk factors (relative risk ratio > 3.0) include BRCA1/2 gene mutation, > 1 immediate family member with breast cancer, history of atypical ductal hyperplasia, history of LCIS, a personal history of cancer, and a history of radiation treatment during youth.

Haffty BG, Buchholz TA, Perez CA. Early stage breast cancer. In: Halperin EC, Perez CA, Brady LW, eds. *Principles and Practice of Radiation Oncology*. New York, NY: Lippincott Williams and Wilkins; 2008:1175–1291.

Question 5

What is the relative reduction in breast cancer mortality by routine screening mammography?

Question 6   **IMAGING**

What is the recommended annual mammographic screening schedule according to the American Cancer Society guidelines?

Question 7

What high risk patients are recommended for annual MRI screening according to the American Cancer Society guidelines?

Question 8

What are suspicious findings on a mammogram?

Answer 5

Screening mammograms reduce breast cancer mortality by about 20–35% in women between 50–69 years of age.

Elmore JG, Armstrong K, Lehman CD, et al. Screening for breast cancer. *JAMA*. 2005;293:1245–1256.

Answer 6

Annual mammograms starting at 40 years of age.

Smith RA, Cokkinides V, Eyre HJ. American Cancer Society guidelines for the early detection of cancer, 2003. *CA Cancer J Clin*. 2003;53:27–43.

Answer 7

Screening MRI is recommended for women with an approximately 20–25% or greater lifetime risk of breast cancer, including women with a certain hereditary mutations (BRCA, Li-Fraumeni, Cowden), a strong family history of breast or ovarian cancer, and women who were treated for Hodgkin disease before age 30. Although MRI specificity is inferior to that of mammography, the increased mortality risk from breast cancer justify its use in screening this population.

Saslow D, Boetes C, Burke W, et al. American Cancer Society guidelines for breast screening with MRI as an adjunct to mammography. *CA Cancer J Clin*. 2007;57:75–89.

Answer 8

Mammographic abnormalities which are suspicious for malignancy and would prompt for further evaluation include a spiculated soft tissue mass, architectural distortion, clustered microcalcifications, developing asymmetry, focal asymmetry, and linear branching microcalcifications.

Haffty BG, Buchholz TA, Perez CA. Early stage breast cancer. In: Halperin EC, Perez CA, Brady LW, eds. *Principles and Practice of Radiation Oncology*. 5th ed. New York, NY: Lippincott Williams and Wilkins; 2008:1175–1291.

Question 9

What is the BI-RADS lexicon?

Question 10

What is the recommended follow-up for a BI-RADS 1 lesion?

Question 11

What is the recommended follow-up for a BI-RADS 3 lesion?

Question 12

What is the recommended follow-up for a BI-RADS 5 lesion?

Answer 9

The breast imaging reporting and data system is summarized as follows: BI-RADS 0 = incomplete study, needs additional imaging. BI-RADS 1 = negative. BI-RADS 2 = benign. BI-RADS 3 = probably benign. BI-RADS 4 = suspicious abnormality. BI-RADS 5 = highly suggestive of malignancy. BI-RADS 6 = known biopsy-proven malignancy.

American College of Radiology. *Breast Imaging Reporting and Data System (BIRADS)*. Reston, VA: ACR; 2003.

Answer 10

Routine annual mammography.

American College of Radiology. *Breast Imaging Reporting and Data System (BIRADS)*. Reston, VA: ACR; 2003.

Answer 11

Short interval follow-up (e.g., 6 months).

American College of Radiology. *Breast Imaging Reporting and Data System (BIRADS)*. Reston, VA: ACR; 2003.

Answer 12

Biopsy and/or additional action should be taken.

American College of Radiology. *Breast Imaging Reporting and Data System (BIRADS)*. Reston, VA: ACR; 2003.

Question 13

What are different types of a diagnostic mammogram?

Question 14

How often does staging breast MRI change management?

Question 15

What is the role of staging MRI in early breast cancer?

Question 16

What day of the menstrual cycles should breast MRI be conducted?

Answer 13

Magnification views are conducted to examine microcalcifications, and spot compression views to examine asymmetric densities. Tangential views are helpful in confirming dermal calcifications. Rolled views help evaluate lesions by moving them away from dense breast parenchyma. A 90-degree lateral view is a direct orthogonal view to the CC projection, which can be helpful in localizing lesions.

Helvie MA. Imaging analysis: mammography. In: Harris J, Lippman ME, Morrow M, et al., eds. *Diseases of the Breast*. 4th ed. Philadelphia, PA: Lippincott Williams & Wilkins; 2010:116–130.

Answer 14

Breast MRI changes surgical management by identifying additional mammographically-occult disease in up to 16–37% of cases.

Van Goethem M, Tjalma W, Schelfout I, et al. Magnetic resonance imaging in breast cancer. *Eur J Surg Oncol*. 2006;32:901–10.

Answer 15

No prospective studies have shown that MRI in early breast cancer results in lower rates of local recurrence. A retrospective study from Solin demonstrated no differences for in-breast tumor recurrence (IBTR) after BCT in women with or without staging MRI.

Solin LJ, Orel SG, Hwang WT, et al. Relationship of breast magnetic resonance imaging to outcome after breast-conservation treatment with radiation for women with early-stage invasive breast carcinoma or ductal carcinoma in situ. *J Clin Oncol*. 2008;26:386–391.

Answer 16

Breast MRI should be performed around day 7–14 of the menstrual cycle because parenchymal enhancement at other times of the cycle reduces its sensitivity.

Roth SE. Imaging analysis: magnetic resonance imaging. In: Harris J, Lippman ME, Morrow M, et al., eds. *Diseases of the Breast*. 4th ed. Philadelphia, PA: Lippincott Williams & Wilkins; 2010:152–170.

Question 17

What anatomic landmark delineates the three levels of the axilla?

Question 18

What levels are routinely dissected in a standard axillary lymph node dissection?

Question 19

Where are the internal mammary lymph nodes located?

Question 20

What is the most common location of a primary breast tumor?

Answer 17

The pectoralis minor muscle demarcates the Level I, II, and III axillary lymph nodes. Level I nodes lie inferior and lateral; Level II is posterior, and Level III (aka infraclavicular nodes) are medial to the pectoralis minor and against the chest wall. The pectoralis minor muscle inserts onto the coracoid process of the scapula.

Haffty BG, Buchholz TA, Perez CA. Early stage breast cancer. In: Halperin EC, Perez CA, Brady LW, eds. *Principles and Practice of Radiation Oncology*. New York, NY: Lippincott Williams and Wilkins; 2008:1175–1291.

Answer 18

Levels I–II. Data have demonstrated increased rates of axillary recurrence when < 5 lymph nodes are removed; 10 or more nodes are ideally submitted for pathologic review in a standard axillary lymph node dissection.

Fowble B, Solin LJ, Schultz DJ, et al. Frequency, sites of relapse, and outcome of regional node failures following conservative surgery and radiation for early breast cancer. *Int J Radiat Oncol Biol Phys*. 1989;17:703–710.

Answer 19

Lateral to the sternum in the first three intercostal spaces. Approximately 30% of medial tumors and 15% of lateral tumors drain to the internal mammary nodes.

Chen RC, Lin NU, Golshan M, et al. Internal mammary nodes in breast cancer: diagnosis and implications for patient management – a systematic review. *J Clin Oncol*. 2008;26:4981–4989.

Answer 20

Most breast cancers arise in the upper outer quadrant of the breast (53%). The least common location is the lower inner quadrant (6%).

Darbre PD. Recorded quadrant incidence of female breast cancer in Great Britain suggests a disproportionate increase in the upper outer quadrant of the breast. *Anticancer Res*. 2005;25:2543–2550.

Question 21
GENETICS

What percentage of breast cancers is associated with hereditary mutations or syndromes?

Question 22

What are some hereditary mutations or syndromes associated with breast cancer?

Question 23

On what chromosomes are BRCA-1 and BRCA-2 located?

Question 24

What is the lifetime risk of developing a breast cancer or ovarian cancer for a BRCA-1 mutation carrier?

Answer 21

About 5–10% of new diagnoses of breast cancer are attributed to inherited genetic mutations.

Ashworth A, Weber BL, Domchek SM. Inherited genetic factors and breast cancer. In: Harris J, Lippman ME, Morrow M, et al., eds. *Diseases of the Breast*. 4th ed. Philadelphia, PA: Lippincott Williams & Wilkins; 2010:209–223.
Haffty BG, Buchholz TA, Perez CA. Early stage breast cancer. In: Halperin EC, Perez CA, Brady LW, eds. *Principles and Practice of Radiation Oncology*. 5th ed. New York, NY: Lippincott Williams and Wilkins; 2008:1175–1291.

Answer 22

BRCA-1, BRCA-2, Cowden syndrome (PTEN), Li-Fraumeni (p53), ataxia-telangiectasia (ATM), and Peutz-Jeghers syndrome.

Ashworth A, Weber BL, Domchek SM. Inherited genetic factors and breast cancer. In: Harris J, Lippman ME, Morrow M, et al., eds. *Diseases of the Breast*. 4th ed. Philadelphia, PA: Lippincott Williams & Wilkins; 2010:209–223.

Answer 23

BRCA-1 is located on 17q, and BRCA-2 is located on 13q.

Ashworth A, Weber BL, Domchek SM. Inherited genetic factors and breast cancer. In: Harris J, Lippman ME, Morrow M, et al., eds. *Diseases of the Breast*. 4th ed. Philadelphia, PA: Lippincott Williams & Wilkins; 2010:209–223.

Answer 24

Breast cancer ~60–80%, ovarian cancer ~30–50%.

Ashworth A, Weber BL, Domchek SM. Inherited genetic factors and breast cancer. In: Harris J, Lippman ME, Morrow M, et al., eds. *Diseases of the Breast*. 4th ed. Philadelphia, PA: Lippincott Williams & Wilkins; 2010:209–223.

Question 25
What is the lifetime risk of developing a breast cancer or ovarian cancer for a BRCA-2 mutation carrier?

Question 26
What hormone receptor status is associated with breast cancers occurring in BRCA-1 mutation carriers?

Question 27   GENERAL TREATMENT CONCEPTS
What is the most important prognostic factor for survival in breast cancer?

Question 28
What is the most important predictor of locoregional recurrence after mastectomy?

Answer 25

Breast cancer ~50–60%, ovarian cancer ~10–20%.

Ashworth A, Weber BL, Domchek SM. Inherited genetic factors and breast cancer. In: Harris J, Lippman ME, Morrow M, et al., eds. *Diseases of the Breast*. 4th ed. Philadelphia, PA: Lippincott Williams & Wilkins; 2010:209–223.

Answer 26

Triple negative phenotype (ER-negative, PR-negative, Her2/neu not amplified). 20% of patients with triple-negative breast cancer carry BRCA mutations.

Gonzalez-Angulo AM, Timms KM, Liu S, et al. Incidence and outcome of BRCA mutations in unselected patients with triple receptor-negative breast cancer. *Clin Cancer Res*. 2011;17:1082–1089.

Answer 27

Axillary lymph node positive breast cancer has a worse prognosis than lymph node-negative disease. Estimated 10-yr survival based upon number of involved axillary lymph nodes: 0: 75%; 1–3: 62%; 4–9: 42%; 10+: 20%.

Fisher ER, Anderson S, Redmond C, et al. Pathologic findings from the National Surgical Adjuvant Breast Project Protocol B-06: 10-year pathologic and clinical prognostic discriminants. *Cancer*. 1993;71:2507–2514.

Answer 28

The extent of axillary nodal involvement is the strongest prognostic factor. The 10-yr actuarial rates of isolated locoregional recurrence have been reported based upon number of involved nodes: 0: 4%; 1–3: 10%; 4–9: 21%; 10+: 22% ($p < .0001$). In addition, younger age, high nodal ratio, larger tumor size, ER-negative tumors, and positive margins increase the risk of recurrence.

Voogd AC, Nielsen M, Peterse JL, et al. Differences in risk factors for local and distant recurrence after breast-conserving therapy or mastectomy for stage I and II breast cancer: pooled results of two large European randomized trials. *J Clin Oncol*. 2001;19:1688–1697.

Question 29
Which patients are at highest risk of internal mammary node metastases?

Question 30
What are some differences in the Halsted and Fisher theories of breast cancer?

Question 31
What is the likelihood of lymphedema after lumpectomy and whole breast radiation therapy?

Question 32
What are the anatomic borders for a standard tangential whole breast field?

Answer 29

Patients with axillary node positive disease and medial primary tumors. In historical surgical series, these patients had a 50% risk of IM nodal metastases. 6% to 16% of patients with negative axillary nodes had positive IMNs.

Chen RC, Lin NU, Golshan M, et al. Internal mammary nodes in breast cancer: diagnosis and implications for patient management – a systematic review. *J Clin Oncol.* 2008;26:4981–4989.

Answer 30

Halsted theorized that breast cancer spreads with an orderly anatomic progression of disease, such that aggressive local treatment should improve survival. Fisher theorized that intrinsic tumor factors dictate patterns of spread, such that systemic therapy should improve survival.

Rabinovitch R, Kavanagh B. Double helix of breast cancer therapy: intertwining the Halsted and Fisher hypotheses. *J Clin Oncol.* 2009;27:2422–2423.

Answer 31

Lymphedema may occur in about 15% after BCT with a full axillary LND, and about 5% after sentinel LND. The rate of lymphedema increases with irradiation of the supraclavicular field, particularly when a posterior axillary boost field is added. Lymphedema rates due to the addition of a supraclavicular field have been reported at 29%. Another study has observed no significant increase in lymphedema with a supraclavicular field that does not extend more laterally than the coracoid process.

Graham P, Jagavkar R, Browne L, et al. Supraclavicular radiotherapy must be limited laterally by the coracoid to avoid significant adjuvant breast nodal radiotherapy lymphoedema risk. *Australas Radiol.* 2006;50:578–582.
Hinrichs CS, Watroba NL, Rezaishiraz H, et al. Lymphedema secondary to postmastectomy radiation: incidence and risk factors. *Ann Surg Oncol.* 2004;11:573–580.

Answer 32

The anatomic borders for a standard tangential whole breast field include the sternum (medially), midaxillary line (laterally), sternoclavicular junction (superiorly), and 2 cm below the inframammary fold (inferiorly).

Vassil AD, Tendulkar RD. Breast radiotherapy. In: Videtic GM, Vassil AD, eds. *Handbook of Treatment Planning in Radiation Oncology.* New York, NY: Demos Medical Publishing; 2011:67–84.

Question 33

What lung bite is acceptable for tangential whole breast irradiation?

Question 34

What are potential advantages of prone breast RT?

Question 35

What are potential limitations of prone breast RT?

Question 36

What is the role of IMRT in the adjuvant treatment of breast cancer?

Answer 33

The lung bite should be limited to less than 3 cm in order to spare the ipsilateral lung. Typically 1.5–2 cm of lung bite is sufficient. CT-based planning allows for careful dosimetry to ensure adequate coverage to the breast tissue.

Vassil AD, Tendulkar RD. Breast radiotherapy. In: Videtic GM, Vassil AD, eds. *Handbook of Treatment Planning in Radiation Oncology*. New York, NY: Demos Medical Publishing; 2011:67–84.

Answer 34

Avoidance of heart and lung, and a more homogeneous dose distribution due to decreased skin separation. Lung dose is decreased in comparison to a supine position. Additionally, there is decreased inframammary skin fold, thereby decreasing skin toxicity for women with pendulous breasts.

Vassil AD, Tendulkar RD. Breast radiotherapy. In: Videtic GM, Vassil AD, eds. *Handbook of Treatment Planning in Radiation Oncology*. New York, NY: Demos Medical Publishing; 2011:67–84.

Answer 35

Inability to adequately treat the regional lymph nodes, patient discomfort, and potentially inadequate coverage on a posteriorly located tumor bed.

Vassil AD, Tendulkar RD. Breast radiotherapy. In: Videtic GM, Vassil AD, eds. *Handbook of Treatment Planning in Radiation Oncology*. New York, NY: Demos Medical Publishing; 2011:67–84.

Answer 36

Two trials have demonstrated an improvement in desquamation, cosmetic outcomes, and fibrosis with IMRT compared to standard 2D treatment planning.

Donovan E, Bleakley N, Denholm E, et al. Randomised trial of standard 2D radiotherapy (RT) versus intensity modulated radiotherapy (IMRT) in patients prescribed breast radiotherapy. *Radiother Oncol*. 2007;82:254–264.
Pignol JP, Olivotto I, Rakovitch E, et al. A multicenter randomized trial of breast intensity-modulated radiation therapy to reduce acute radiation dermatitis. *J Clin Oncol*. 2008;26:2085–2092.

Question 37

What is the role of the 21-gene recurrence score (Oncotype DX)?

Question 38

What is the optimal sequence of adjuvant chemotherapy and radiation therapy for breast cancer?

Question 39   **DCIS / LCIS**

How does LCIS appear on imaging?

Question 40

What subtype of LCIS has the worst prognosis?

Answer 37

Patients with lymph node negative, ER+ breast cancers are stratified into a low-, intermediate-, and high-risk of recurrence in order to estimate the relative benefit of chemotherapy in addition to hormonal therapy.

Paik S, Shak S, Tang G, et al. A multigene assay to predict recurrence of tamoxifen-treated, node-negative breast cancer. *New Engl J Med*. 2004;351:2817–2826.

Answer 38

The Recht trial from Boston demonstrated reduced distant metastases in patients treated with chemotherapy then radiation, however, the survival cures converged at later follow-up.

Recht A, Come SE, Henderson IC, et al. The sequencing of chemotherapy and radiation therapy after conservative surgery for early-stage breast cancer. *N Engl J Med*. 1996;334:1356–1361.

Answer 39

LCIS does not have a physical or mammographic correlate. It is an incidental histopathologic finding on a biopsy usually done for other mammographic abnormalities. An underlying DCIS or invasive cancer must be ruled out by excisional biopsy.

Wazer DE, Arthur DW. Breast: stage tis. In: Halperin EC, Perez CA, Brady LW, eds. *Principles and Practice of Radiation Oncology*. 5th ed. New York, NY: Lippincott Williams and Wilkins; 2008:1162–1174.

Answer 40

The pleomorphic subtype has an unfavorable prognosis. It has been reported to have a more aggressive behavior than classic LCIS, and warrants consideration for primary surgical and adjuvant treatment.

Buchanan CL, Flynn LW, Murray MP, et al. Is pleomorphic lobular carcinoma really a distinct clinical entity? *J Surg Oncol*. 2008;98:314–317.

Question 41

What are treatment options for LCIS?

Question 42

Is LCIS a precursor to invasive breast cancer?

Question 43

What is the relative risk reduction by tamoxifen in developing an invasive cancer in a patient with LCIS?

Question 44

What are the five subtypes of ductal carcinoma in situ?

Answer 41

Treatment may range from observation to tamoxifen, or bilateral mastectomies. There is no role for a negative margin excision (controversial in the more aggressive pleomorphic LCIS subtype) since classic LCIS is often multifocal, multicentric, or bilateral. There is no role for radiation therapy for LCIS.

Wazer DE, Arthur DW. Breast: stage tis. In: Halperin EC, Perez CA, Brady LW, eds. *Principles and Practice of Radiation Oncology.* 5th ed. New York, NY: Lippincott Williams and Wilkins; 2008:1162–1164.

Answer 42

This is controversial. LCIS is a marker for subsequent breast cancer which may occur in either breast, but it has not been proven to be a precursor lesion. Invasive ductal carcinoma is the most common subsequent cancer in women with a prior history of LCIS.

Wazer DE, Arthur DW. Breast: stage tis. In: Halperin EC, Perez CA, Brady LW, eds. *Principles and Practice of Radiation Oncology.* 5th ed. New York, NY: Lippincott Williams and Wilkins; 2008:1162–1174.

Answer 43

The relative risk reduction is 50% per NSABP P-1. NSABP P-1 was a phase III trial which randomized women to tamoxifen 20 mg daily or placebo. Women were eligible if they were age 60 or older, between the ages of 35 and 59 years with a 5-year estimated risk for breast cancer of at least 1.66% as predicted by the Gail model, or age 35 years or older with a history of LCIS.

Fisher B, Costantino JP, Wickerham DL, et al. Tamoxifen for the prevention of breast cancer: current status of the National Surgical Adjuvant Breast and Bowel Project P-1 study. *J Natl Cancer Inst.* 2005;97:1652–1662.

Answer 44

Comedo, cribriform, papillary, micropapillary, and solid. The comedo subtype is more often associated with invasion; the presence of marked comedonecrosis is also an independent predictor for local recurrence.

Fisher ER, Costantino J, Fisher B, et al. Pathologic findings from the National Surgical Adjuvant Breast Project (NSABP) Protocol B-17. Intraductal carcinoma (ductal carcinoma in situ). The National Surgical Adjuvant Breast and Bowel Project Collaborating Investigators. *Cancer.* 1995;75:1310–1319.

Question 45

What are the components of the Van Nuys prognostic index for ductal carcinoma in situ?

Question 46

What are treatment options for DCIS?

Question 47

What is the local control for DCIS treated with mastectomy?

Question 48

What is the absolute reduction in breast tumor recurrence (IBTR) by adding radiation to lumpectomy for DCIS?

Answer 45

Size, surgical margin status, pathologic grade, and age. This index was derived from a database of 706 patients with DCIS treated with breast conservation surgery with or without RT. Patients with scores of 4–6 did not show a 12-yr local recurrence-free survival from RT; this finding was not statistically significant. Patients with scores of 7–9 had a 12–15% local recurrence-free survival benefit ($p = .03$). Patients with scores of 10–12, showed the greatest absolute benefit from radiation therapy; recurrence rates remained a significant issue even with RT in this group.

Silverstein MJ. The University of Southern California/Van Nuys prognostic index for ductal carcinoma in situ of the breast. *Am J Surg.* 2003;186:337–343.

Answer 46

DCIS may be treated with mastectomy or breast conservation therapy consisting of lumpectomy and radiation +/− tamoxifen. No randomized trials have been conducted comparing the two surgical approaches for DCIS.

Wazer DE, Arthur DW. Breast: stage tis. In: Halperin EC, Perez CA, Brady LW, eds. *Principles and Practice of Radiation Oncology.* 5th ed. New York, NY: Lippincott Williams and Wilkins; 2008:1162–1174.

Answer 47

Approximately 98%. Because sentinel lymph node biopsy is not feasible post-mastectomy, it should be considered if mastectomy is planned, especially if the patient is felt to be at high risk for occult invasive cancer. Axillary lymph node involvement is 3% in DCIS.

Intra M, Veronesi P, Mazzarol G, et al. Axillary sentinel lymph node biopsy in patients with pure ductal carcinoma in situ of the breast. *Arch Surg.* 2003;138:309–313.

Answer 48

NSABP B-17, which randomized women to observation or breast radiation (50 Gy/25 fx), demonstrated that whole breast radiotherapy after lumpectomy significantly decreased the 12-year local recurrence rate from 31% to 16%. EORTC 10853 demonstrated that whole breast radiotherapy decreased the 4-year local recurrence rate from 16% to 9%.

Fisher B, Land S, Mamounas E, et al. Prevention of invasive breast cancer in women with ductal carcinoma in situ: an update of the National Surgical Adjuvant Breast and Bowel Project experience. *Semin Oncol.* 2001;28:400–418.
Julien JP, Bijker N, Fentiman IS, et al. Radiotherapy in breast-conserving treatment for ductal carcinoma in situ: first results of the EORTC randomised phase III trial 10853. EORTC Breast Cancer Cooperative Group and EORTC Radiotherapy Group. *Lancet.* 2000;355:528–533.

Question 49

What is the relative reduction in IBTR from radiation following lumpectomy for DCIS?

Question 50

After BCT for DCIS, what percentage of recurrences are invasive cancers?

Question 51

What is benefit of tamoxifen in ductal carcinoma in situ?

Question 52

What is the role of a radiation boost in DCIS?

Answer 49

Adjuvant radiation reduced in breast tumor recurrence (IBTR) by about 50% per NSABP B-17 and the EORTC 10853 trials.

Fisher B, Land S, Mamounas E, et al. Prevention of invasive breast cancer in women with ductal carcinoma in situ: an update of the National Surgical Adjuvant Breast and Bowel Project experience. *Semin Oncol.* 2001;28:400–418.

Julien JP, Bijker N, Fentiman IS, et al. Radiotherapy in breast-conserving treatment for ductal carcinoma in situ: first results of the EORTC randomised phase III trial 10853. EORTC Breast Cancer Cooperative Group and EORTC Radiotherapy Group. *Lancet.* 2000;355:528–533.

Answer 50

Based on the NSABP and EORTC data, about 50% of recurrences after BCT for DCIS are invasive breast cancers and 50% are DCIS.

Fisher B, Land S, Mamounas E, et al. Prevention of invasive breast cancer in women with ductal carcinoma in situ: an update of the National Surgical Adjuvant Breast and Bowel Project experience. *Semin Oncol.* 2001;28:400–418.

Julien JP, Bijker N, Fentiman IS, et al. Radiotherapy in breast-conserving treatment for ductal carcinoma in situ: first results of the EORTC randomised phase III trial 10853. EORTC Breast Cancer Cooperative Group and EORTC Radiotherapy Group. *Lancet.* 2000;355:528–533.

Answer 51

NSABP B-24, a phase III trial comparing women treated with lumpectomy and RT to tamoxifen 20 mg daily for 5 years versus placebo, demonstrated that the addition of tamoxifen to partial mastectomy and radiation improved the overall breast cancer event rate from 13% to 8%. The subset of ER+ patients derives the greatest benefit.

Fisher B, Dignam J, Wolmark N, et al. Tamoxifen in treatment of intraductal breast cancer: National Surgical Adjuvant Breast and Bowel Project B-24 randomised controlled trial. *Lancet.* 1999;353:1993–2000.

Answer 52

No prospective trials have been conducted to evaluate the role of a tumor bed boost for DCIS. In retrospective series, women under 45 years of age may benefit from a boost after whole breast radiation therapy. Median boost dose in this series was 10 Gy.

Omlin A, Amichetti M, Azria D, et al. Boost radiotherapy in young women with ductal carcinoma in situ: a multicentre, retrospective study of the rare cancer network. *Lancet Oncology.* 2006;7:652–656.

Question 53
What margin is adequate for DCIS treated with BCT?

Question 54
Which subset of DCIS patients may be spared adjuvant radiotherapy?

Question 55
What is an extensive intraductal component?

Question 56   **Early Stage Breast Cancer**
What are contraindications to BCT, consisting of lumpectomy and adjuvant radiation?

Answer 53

A margin of at least 2 mm has a lower risk of local recurrence than margins < 2 mm.

Dunne C, Burke JP, Morrow M, et al. Effect of margin status on local recurrence after breast conservation and radiation therapy for ductal carcinoma in situ. *J Clin Oncol.* 2009;27:1615–1620.

Answer 54

The ECOG 5194 trial demonstrated a 5-year IBTR of 6% in patients with low-intermediate grade DCIS up to 2.5 cm in size with at least 3 mm margins. High-grade DCIS up to 1 cm in size had a higher rate of IBTR of 15% at 5 years, and adjuvant radiation is recommended in this population. Long term data are not yet available.

Hughes LL, Wang M, Page DL, et al. Local excision alone without irradiation for ductal carcinoma in situ of the breast: a trial of the Eastern Cooperative Oncology Group. *J Clin Oncol.* 2009;27:5319–5324.

Answer 55

EIC is defined as a component of DCIS comprising at least 25% of the invasive specimen and also present in surrounding tissue (beyond the border of invasive disease). Initially EIC was described as a risk factor for local recurrence, but it no longer appears to be an adverse factor as long as the tumor is resected with widely negative margins.

Gage I, Schnitt SJ, Nixon AJ, et al. Pathologic margin involvement and the risk of recurrence in patients treated with breast-conserving therapy. *Cancer.* 1996;78:1921–1928.

Answer 56

Multicentric tumors, diffuse malignant-appearing calcifications, inability to achieve negative margins, pregnancy, prior breast/chest irradiation, large tumors, active lupus or scleroderma. Other connective tissue disorders are considered a relative contraindication to radiation therapy, and should be considered on a case-by-case basis.

Haffty BG, Buchholz TA, Perez CA. Early stage breast cancer. In: Halperin EC, Perez CA, Brady LW, eds. *Principles and Practice of Radiation Oncology.* 5th ed. New York, NY: Lippincott Williams and Wilkins; 2008:1175–1291.

Question 57

Is lymph node positive disease a contraindication to BCT?

Question 58

What are common side effects of whole breast radiotherapy?

Question 59

What percentage of patients treated with BCT have a good-to-excellent cosmetic outcomes?

Question 60

What is the most common histology of a radiation-induced sarcoma after prior breast irradiation?

Answer 57

No. Patients with lymph node positive disease benefit from adjuvant whole breast radiation in a similar proportion to node-negative patients. In pooled data from European randomized trials, nodal disease did not predict a significantly increased risk of ipsilateral breast recurrence compared to node-negative disease following BCT.

Voogd AC, Nielsen M, Peterse JL, et al. Differences in risk factors for local and distant recurrence after breast-conserving therapy or mastectomy for stage I and II breast cancer: pooled results of two large European randomized trials. *J Clin Oncol.* 2001;19:1688–1697.

Answer 58

Acute side effects may include fatigue, erythema, edema, pruritis, desquamation, and pneumonitis. Late side effects may include poor cosmesis, lymphedema, rib fracture, cardiotoxicity, pulmonary fibrosis, and second malignancies. The incidence for a rib fracture has been reported to be < 3%; this is an unusual occurrence for RT doses < 50 Gy. The risk for a secondary non-breast malignancy is 1%. Inclusion of the high axillary or supraclavicular lymph nodes may result in brachial plexopathy.

Pierce SM, Recht A, Lingos TI, et al. Long-term radiation complications following conservative surgery (CS) and radiation therapy (RT) in patients with early stage breast cancer. *Int J Radiat Oncol Biol Phys.* 1992;23:915–923.

Answer 59

Per the Whelan trial, about 70% of cosmetic outcomes are rated as good or excellent following BCT. Breast cosmesis is related to radiation-induced skin telangiectasia and fibrosis of subcutaneous tissue. Cosmetic outcome is affected by older age and large tumor size.

Whelan TJ, Pignol JP, Levine MN, et al. Long-term results of hypofractionated radiation therapy for breast cancer. *N Engl J Med.* 2010;362:513–520.

Answer 60

Angiosarcoma. The magnitude of the risk of a radiation-induced sarcoma is small: 3.2 per 1,000. The same report documented the risk to be 2.3 per 1,000 for patients who did not receive radiation therapy. Of the sarcomas occurring within the field of radiation, angiosarcoma accounts for 56.8%.

Yap J, Chuba PJ, Thomas R, et al. Sarcoma as a second malignancy after treatment for breast cancer. *Int J Radiat Oncol Biol Phys.* 2002;52:1231–1237.

Question 61

What is the most common histology of an invasive breast cancer?

Question 62

What breast cancer histology is associated with lymphoplasmacytic infiltrates?

Question 63

What breast cancer histology is associated with Indian filing?

Question 64

What percentage of invasive breast cancers express the estrogen receptor and/or progesterone receptor?

Answer 61

The majority of invasive breast cancer is infiltrating ductal carcinomas (75–80%), followed by infiltrating lobular carcinomas (10%).

Haffty BG, Buchholz TA, Perez CA. Early stage breast cancer. In: Halperin EC, Perez CA, Brady LW, eds. *Principles and Practice of Radiation Oncology*. 5th ed. New York, NY: Lippincott Williams and Wilkins; 2008:1175–1291.

Answer 62

Medullary breast cancers. These often present with large lymph nodes that are histologically negative for cancer. Medullary carcinoma tends to occur more frequently in younger patients, and has a more favorable prognosis.

Vu-Nishino H, Tavassoli FA, Ahrens WA, et al. Clinicopathologic features and long-term outcome of patients with medullary breast carcinoma managed with breast-conserving therapy (BCT). *Int J Radiat Oncol Biol Phys*. 2005;62:1040–1047.

Answer 63

Infiltrating lobular carcinoma. "Indian filing" is the term given to describe the small cells that infiltrate the mammary stroma and adipose tissue in a single file pattern.

Simpson PT, Reis-Filho JS, Lakhani SR. Lobular carcinoma in situ: biology and pathology. In: Harris J, Lippman ME, Morrow M, et al., eds. *Diseases of the Breast*. 4th ed. Philadelphia, PA: Lippincott Williams & Wilkins; 2010:333–340.

Answer 64

ER and PR are positive in approximately 70–80% of invasive breast cancers.

Schiff R, Osborne CK, Fuqua SAW. Clinical aspects of estrogen and progesterone receptors. In: Harris J, Lippman ME, Morrow M, et al., eds. *Diseases of the Breast*. 4th ed. Philadelphia, PA: Lippincott Williams & Wilkins; 2010:408–430.

Question 65

What percentage of invasive breast cancers overexpresses the HER2/neu oncogene?

Question 66

What are the molecular subtypes of invasive breast cancer?

Question 67

What defines microinvasive breast cancer (T1mic)?

Question 68

What is the risk of lymph node involvement with microinvasive breast cancer?

Answer 65

HER2/neu is overexpressed in approximately 25% of invasive breast cancers. Patients with high levels of HER2 expression benefit from HER2-targeted therapies. HER2 gene overexpression is determined by 3+ staining by IHC, or FISH positivity. About 24% of IHC 2+ tumors demonstrate gene amplification when tested by FISH.

Dybdal N, Leiberman G, Anderson S, et al. Determination of HER2 gene amplification by fluorescence in situ hybridization and concordance with the clinical trials immunohistochemical assay in women with metastatic breast cancer evaluated for treatment with trastuzumab. *Breast Cancer Res Treat*. 2005;93:3–11.

Answer 66

Luminal A, luminal B, normal-like, HER2 overexpressing, and basal types. The basal type (commonly associated with triple negative receptor status) has the worst prognosis.

Perou CM, Sorlie T, Eisen MB, et al. Molecular portraits of human breast tumours. *Nature*. 2000;406:747–752.

Answer 67

Invasive tumor less than or equal to 1 mm in size.

Breast. Edge SB, Byrd DR, Compton CC, et al., eds. *AJCC Cancer Staging Manual*. 7th ed. New York, NY: Springer; 2010:347–376.

Answer 68

Less than 5%. Other estimates of lymph node involvement based on tumor diameter:

Tis – 0.8%; T1a – 5%; T1b – 16%; T1c – 28%; T2 – 47%; T3 – 68%; T4 – 86%.

Silverstein MJ, Skinner KA, Lomis TJ. Predicting axillary nodal positivity in 2282 patients with breast carcinoma. *World J Surg*. 2001;25:767–772.

Question 69

What is the difference between pN0(i+) and pN1mi?

Question 70

What is the false negative rate of sentinel lymph node (SLN) biopsy?

Question 71

What was the 20-year risk of local recurrence in patients receiving breast conservation therapy (BCT) on NSABP B-06?

Question 72

What was the 5-year risk of ipsilateral breast tumor recurrence after partial mastectomy with or without adjuvant radiation on the Early Breast Cancer Trialists' Collaborative Group meta-analysis?

Answer 69

Isolated tumor cells or foci of metastases in lymph nodes that are less than or equal to 0.2 mm are considered pN0(i+), and foci that are > 0.2 mm or > 200 cells but less than or equal to 2 mm are considered pN1mi.

Breast. Edge SB, Byrd DR, Compton CC, et al., eds. *AJCC Cancer Staging Manual.* 7th ed. New York, NY: Springer; 2010:347–376.

Answer 70

Approximately 8–10%. However, about half of patients in whom the identified sentinel lymph node proves to be falsely negative will have had clinically suspicious nodes palpable at surgery; gross tumor involvement may interfere with the uptake of both radiolabeled colloid and dye and deviate lymph flow to a node other than the true SLN.

Hill AD, Tran KN, Akhurst T, et al. Lessons learned from 500 cases of lymphatic mapping for breast cancer. *Ann Surg.* 1999;229:528–535.
Veronesi U, Paganelli G, Viale G, et al. A randomized comparison of sentinel-node biopsy with routine axillary dissection in breast cancer. *N Engl J Med.* 2003;349:546–53.

Answer 71

The local recurrence rate was 39% with lumpectomy alone, and 14% with lumpectomy and whole breast radiation (50 Gy). There was no difference in overall survival between the arms.

Fisher B, Anderson S, Bryant J, et al. Twenty-year follow-up of a randomized trial comparing total mastectomy, lumpectomy, and lumpectomy plus irradiation for the treatment of invasive breast cancer. *N Engl J Med.* 2002;347:1233–1241.

Answer 72

This meta-analysis of 42,000 women in 78 randomized treatment comparisons demonstrated a 5-yr ipsilateral breast tumor recurrence risk of 26% with partial mastectomy alone, compared to 7% with partial mastectomy and adjuvant radiation.

Clarke M, Collins R, Darby S, et al. Effects of radiotherapy and of differences in the extent of surgery for early breast cancer on local recurrence and 15-year survival: an overview of the randomised trials. *Lancet.* 2005;366: 2087–2106.

Question 73

According to the Early Breast Cancer Trialists Collaborative Group meta-analysis, how many local recurrences must be prevented to avoid one death due to breast cancer?

Question 74

What were the key findings of the NSABP B-04 trial?

Question 75

According to NSABP B-04, what percent of clinically node-negative patients harbored microscopic lymph node metastases?

Answer 73

A 19% reduction in 5-year IBTR after adjuvant radiation led to a 5% improvement in 15-year breast cancer mortality, suggesting a "4-to-1" ratio.

Clarke M, Collins R, Darby S, et al. Effects of radiotherapy and of differences in the extent of surgery for early breast cancer on local recurrence and 15-year survival: an overview of the randomised trials. *Lancet.* 2005;366:2087–2106.

Answer 74

NSABP B-04 was a phase III clinical trial, which evaluated 1765 women with operable breast cancer. Women with clinically negative nodes who underwent total mastectomy with neither axillary dissection nor irradiation and subsequently had pathologically positive axillary nodes in the absence of other manifestations of disease then underwent axillary dissection. None of the women received adjuvant systemic therapy. Women with negative nodes received 50 Gy to the chest wall; node-positive women received an additional boost of 10 to 20 Gy. 45 Gy was delivered to both the internal mammary nodes and the supraclavicular nodes. Among clinically lymph-node negative patients there was no difference in survival between radical mastectomy and total mastectomy, with or without axillary radiation. The rate of pathologic nodal involvement was 40% in patients undergoing ALND, however only 18% suffered a clinical nodal failure in the absence of ALND.

Fisher B, Jeong JH, Anderson S, et al. Twenty-five-year follow-up of a randomized trial comparing radical mastectomy, total mastectomy, and total mastectomy followed by irradiation. *N Engl J Med.* 2002;347:567–575.

Answer 75

In NSABP B-04, about 40% of patients were found to have nodal metastases on axillary dissection. As the patients in the total mastectomy arm achieved the same survival as those with radical mastectomy, this data indicated that leaving positive nodes unremoved did not significantly increase the rate of distant recurrence or breast-cancer–related mortality.

Fisher B, Redmond C, Fisher ER, et al. Ten-year results of a randomized clinical trial comparing radical mastectomy and total mastectomy with or without radiation. *N Engl J Med.* 1985;312:674–681.

Question 76

According to NSABP B-04, what percent of clinically node-negative patients not undergoing either axillary dissection or radiation suffered an axillary recurrence?

Question 77

What is the role of a tumor bed boost after whole breast radiation?

Question 78

Which population of breast cancer patients derives the greatest benefit from tumor bed boost after whole breast radiation?

Question 79

What were the eligibility criteria for the Canadian hypofractionated radiation randomized trial (Whelan trial)?

Answer 76

In NSABP B-04, about 18% of patients in the total mastectomy alone arm had an axillary recurrence (which is about half of the 40% found to have nodal metastases on axillary dissection). Patients with nodes that became positive after a distant recurrence were not included in this figure.

Fisher B, Redmond C, Fisher ER, et al. Ten-year results of a randomized clinical trial comparing radical mastectomy and total mastectomy with or without radiation. *N Engl J Med*. 1985;312:674–681.

Answer 77

Two trials (EORTC, Lyon) demonstrated an improvement in IBTR with the addition of a 10–16 Gy boost to standard whole breast radiation, with some resultant worsening of cosmesis/fibrosis.

Bartelink H, Horiot JC, Poortmans PM, et al. Impact of a higher radiation dose on local control and survival in breast-conserving therapy of early breast cancer: 10-year results of the randomized boost versus no boost EORTC 22881-10882 trial. *J Clin Oncol*. 2007;25:3259–3265.
Romestaing P, Lehingue Y, Carrie C, et al. Role of a 10-Gy boost in the conservative treatment of early breast cancer: results of a randomized clinical trial in Lyon, France. *J Clin Oncol*. 1997;15:963–968.

Answer 78

Younger women have the greatest absolute risk reduction from radiation boost because of a higher baseline risk for local recurrence, although the relative risk reduction is the same (40%) across all age groups.

Bartelink H, Horiot JC, Poortmans PM, et al. Impact of a higher radiation dose on local control and survival in breast-conserving therapy of early breast cancer: 10-year results of the randomized boost versus no boost EORTC 22881-10882 trial. *J Clin Oncol*. 2007;25:3259–3265.

Answer 79

Women had pathologic stage T1-T2 N0 invasive breast cancer s/p partial mastectomy with negative margins. DCIS was not included on the trial.

Whelan TJ, Pignol JP, Levine MN, et al. Long-term results of hypofractionated radiation therapy for breast cancer. *N Engl J Med*. 2010;362:513–20.

Question 80

What were the arms of the Canadian hypofractionation phase III trial?

Question 81

What was the size limitation of the Canadian hypofractionation phase III trial?

Question 82

What were the results of the Canadian hypofractionated radiation randomized trial?

Question 83

Which patients are eligible for the RTOG 0413/NSABP B-39 trial of accelerated partial breast irradiation (APBI) vs. whole breast radiation?

Answer 80

Both arms received whole breast radiation without a boost, using two-dimensional planning. The doses were 50 Gy in 25 fractions versus 42.5 Gy in 16 fractions. No boost was given.

Whelan TJ, Pignol JP, Levine MN, et al. Long-term results of hypofractionated radiation therapy for breast cancer. *N Engl J Med*. 2010;362:513–520.

Answer 81

Patients with a breast width of more than 25 cm at the posterior border of the medial and lateral tangential beams were excluded from the trial because of concerns about the potential for excess toxicity from hotspots in the hypofractionated arm, as two-dimensional treatment planning was used.

Whelan TJ, Pignol JP, Levine MN, et al. Long-term results of hypofractionated radiation therapy for breast cancer. *N Engl J Med*. 2010;362:513–520.

Answer 82

There was no difference in overall survival, ipsilateral breast tumor recurrence, cosmesis, or toxicity between the two dose fractionation schedules at 10 years of follow-up. The subset of women with high-grade disease had a higher rate of IBTR in the hypofractionated arm.

Whelan TJ, Pignol JP, Levine MN, et al. Long-term results of hypofractionated radiation therapy for breast cancer. *N Engl J Med*. 2010;362:513–520.

Answer 83

Stage Tis-T2, N0-N1, with a unifocal tumor < 3 cm in size, and negative margins after lumpectomy. The primary endpoint for analysis is in-breast tumor recurrence as a first event; secondary endpoints are distant disease-free survival, recurrence-free survival, overall survival, quality of life, and treatment toxicities.

NSABP B-39. Rockville, MD: Cancer trials support unit, 2011. https://www.ctsu.org/public/data/protocols/NSABP/NSABP-B-39/ec.pdf. Accessed November 22, 2011.

Question 84

What are the doses for accelerated partial breast irradiation on the RTOG 0413/NSABP B-39 trial?

Question 85

According to the ASTRO consensus statement, which patients may be considered suitable for APBI off trial?

Question 86

What is the role of completion axillary dissection in patients with limited volume metastatic disease in a sentinel lymph node?

Question 87

Can radiation be omitted in elderly patients with ER+ early stage breast cancer?

Answer 84

3D-conformal EBRT 38.5 Gy in 10 BID fractions, or brachytherapy 34 Gy in 10 BID fractions by either interstitial or MammoSite balloon-catheter based intracavitary brachytherapy.

NSABP B-39. Rockville, MD: Cancer trials support unit, 2011. https://www.ctsu.org/public/data/protocols/NSABP/NSABP-B-39/ec.pdf. Accessed November 22, 2011.

Answer 85

Patients with age > 60, unifocal invasive tumor less than or equal to 2 cm, LN-negative, ER+, margin of at least 2 mm, and without LVI, EIC, or BRCA mutations have acceptable rates of IBTR in several non-randomized studies. Definitive results are awaited from the NSABP B-39 study.

Smith BD, Arthur DW, Buchholz TA, et al. Accelerated partial breast irradiation consensus statement from the American Society for Radiation Oncology (ASTRO). *Int J Radiat Oncol Biol Phys*. 2009;74:987–1001.

Answer 86

Controversial. The ACOSOG Z0011 trial included 891 women with clinical stage T1-T2 N0 breast cancer and 1–2 SLNs positive, treated with partial mastectomy and whole breast radiation, who were randomized to either SLND alone or completion ALND. There was no difference in overall survival or disease-free survival. One criticism is that the trial closed early before meeting accrual goals.

Giuliano AE, Hunt KK, Ballman KV, et al. Axillary dissection vs no axillary dissection in women with invasive breast cancer and sentinel node metastasis: a randomized clinical trial. *JAMA*. 2011;305:569–575.

Answer 87

The Hughes trial demonstrated that women with T1 N0 breast cancer treated with tamoxifen +/− radiation had 5-year IBTR rates of 1% and 4% with and without whole breast radiation, with no difference in overall survival between arms.

Hughes KS, Schnaper LA, Berry D, et al. Lumpectomy plus tamoxifen with or without irradiation in women 70 years of age or older with early breast cancer. *N Engl J Med*. 2004;351:971–977.

Question 88

What were the eligibility criteria and treatment arms for the ACOSOG Z0011 trial?

Question 89

What was the result of ACOSOG Z0011?

Question 90   **Locally Advanced Breast Cancer**

What type of breast cancer is associated with dermal lymphatic invasion?

Question 91

How is the diagnosis of inflammatory breast cancer made?

Answer 88

Clinical stage T1-T2 N0 breast cancer, with 1–2 sentinel lymph nodes positive following lumpectomy and SLNB, randomized to completion axillary lymph node dissection (ALND) or not. Patients who received neoadjuvant therapy or who underwent mastectomy were not included. All patients underwent lumpectomy and whole breast radiation, without regional nodal irradiation.

Giuliano AE, Hunt KK, Ballman KV, et al. Axillary dissection vs no axillary dissection in women with invasive breast cancer and sentinel node metastasis: a randomized clinical trial. *JAMA*. 2011;305:569–575.

Answer 89

The study closed early due to poor accrual, with a total of 891 patients enrolled. At median follow-up over 6 years, there was no difference in overall survival, disease-free survival, or locoregional recurrence, suggesting no benefit to completion ALND in patients meeting the eligibility criteria.

Giuliano AE, Hunt KK, Ballman KV, et al. Axillary dissection vs no axillary dissection in women with invasive breast cancer and sentinel node metastasis: a randomized clinical trial. *JAMA*. 2011;305:569–575.

Answer 90

Inflammatory breast cancer. However, dermal lymphatic invasion is neither sufficient nor required for the diagnosis of inflammatory breast cancer. Classical clinical findings of diffuse erythema and edema involving a third or more of the skin of the breast (peau d'orange) are needed to establish the diagnosis. The T staging for inflammatory breast cancer is T4d.

Merajver SD, Iniesta MD, Sabel MS. Inflammatory breast cancer. In: Harris J, Lippman ME, Morrow M, et al., eds. *Diseases of the Breast*. 4th ed. Philadelphia, PA: Lippincott Williams & Wilkins; 2010:762–773.

Answer 91

Inflammatory breast cancer is a clinical diagnosis, and patients typically present with rapid onset of peau d'orange, erythema and brawny induration over one-third of the breast. Although dermal lymphatic invasion is not necessary to make this diagnosis, histologic confirmation of invasive breast carcinoma is required.

Merajver SD, Iniesta MD, Sabel MS. Inflammatory breast cancer. In: Harris J, Lippman ME, Morrow M, et al., eds. *Diseases of the Breast*. 4th ed. Philadelphia, PA: Lippincott Williams & Wilkins; 2010:762–773.

Question 92

What is the most common site of locoregional recurrence after mastectomy?

Question 93

What are indications for post-mastectomy radiation therapy (PMRT)?

Question 94

What were the arms of the British Columbia post-mastectomy radiation phase III trial?

Question 95

What were the results of the British Columbia post-mastectomy radiation therapy (PMRT) phase III trial?

Answer 92

The chest wall (68%) is the most common site of failure following mastectomy with axillary dissection, followed by the supraclavicular lymph nodes (40%), and the axilla (14%).

Voogd AC, Nielsen M, Peterse JL, et al. Differences in risk factors for local and distant recurrence after breast-conserving therapy or mastectomy for stage I and II breast cancer: pooled results of two large European randomized trials. *J Clin Oncol.* 2001;19:1688–1697.

Answer 93

Patients with positive margins or pathologic stage III cancer (T3-T4N1, or any N2-N3) are candidates for PMRT. PMRT remains controversial for patients with T1-T2N1 breast cancer because of uncertain benefit in overall survival. However, locoregional control is improved by PMRT in N1 breast cancer.

Buchholz TA, Haffty BG. Breast cancer: locally advanced and recurrent disease, postmastectomy radiation, and systemic therapies. In: Halperin EC, Perez CA, Brady LW, eds. *Principles and Practice of Radiation Oncology.* 5th ed. New York, NY: Lippincott Williams and Wilkins; 2008:1292–1317.
Recht A, Edge SB, Solin LJ, et al. Postmastectomy radiotherapy: clinical practice guidelines of the American Society of Clinical Oncology. *J Clin Oncol.* 2001;19:1539–1569.
Taylor ME, Haffty BG, Rabinovitch R, et al. ACR appropriateness criteria on postmastectomy radiotherapy expert panel on radiation oncology-breast. *Int J Radiat Oncol Biol Phys.* 2009;73:997–1002.

Answer 94

Premenopausal patients with positive lymph nodes after mastectomy were randomized to receive CMF vs. CMF with post-mastectomy radiation therapy (PMRT) 37.5 Gy/16 fx.

Ragaz J, Jackson SM, Le N, et al. Adjuvant radiotherapy and chemotherapy in node-positive premenopausal women with breast cancer. *N Engl J Med.* 1997;337:956–962.

Answer 95

PMRT improved all endpoints including LRR (13% vs. 39%), disease-free survival (48% vs. 31%), and OS (47% vs. 37%).

Ragaz J, Olivotto IA, Spinelli JJ, et al. Locoregional radiation therapy in patients with high-risk breast cancer receiving adjuvant chemotherapy: 20-year results of the British Columbia randomized trial. *J Natl Cancer Inst.* 2005; 97:116–126.

Question 96

What were the arms of the Danish 82b post-mastectomy radiation therapy (PMRT) phase III trial?

Question 97

What were the findings of the Danish 82b post-mastectomy radiation trial?

Question 98

What were the arms of the Danish 82c post-mastectomy radiation phase III trial?

Question 99

What were the findings of the Danish 82c post-mastectomy radiation phase III trial?

Answer 96

Premenopausal patients with either positive lymph nodes, tumor > 5 cm, or skin/pectoralis fascia involvement after mastectomy were randomized to receive CMF vs. CMF with PMRT 48–50 Gy delivered by reverse hockey stick technique.

Overgaard M, Hansen PS, Overgaard J, et al. Postoperative radiotherapy in high-risk premenopausal women with breast cancer who receive adjuvant chemotherapy. Danish Breast Cancer Cooperative Group 82b Trial. *N Engl J Med.* 1997;337:949–955.

Answer 97

PMRT improved all endpoints including LRR (9% vs. 32%) and OS (54% vs. 45%). Multivariate analysis demonstrated that irradiation after mastectomy significantly improved disease-free survival and overall survival, irrespective of tumor size, the number of positive nodes, or the histopathological grade.

Overgaard M, Hansen PS, Overgaard J, et al. Postoperative radiotherapy in high-risk premenopausal women with breast cancer who receive adjuvant chemotherapy. Danish Breast Cancer Cooperative Group 82b Trial. *N Engl J Med.* 1997;337:949–955.

Answer 98

Post-menopausal patients with either positive lymph nodes, tumor > 5 cm, or skin/pectoralis fascia involvement after mastectomy were randomized to receive tamoxifen (1 year) vs. tamoxifen with PMRT 48–50 Gy delivered by reverse hockey stick technique.

Overgaard M, Jensen MB, Overgaard J, et al. Postoperative radiotherapy in high-risk postmenopausal breast-cancer patients given adjuvant tamoxifen: Danish Breast Cancer Cooperative Group DBCG 82c randomised trial. *Lancet.* 1999;353:1641–1648.

Answer 99

PMRT improved all endpoints including LRR (8% vs. 35%) and OS (45% vs. 36%).

Overgaard M, Jensen MB, Overgaard J, et al. Postoperative radiotherapy in high-risk postmenopausal breast-cancer patients given adjuvant tamoxifen: Danish Breast Cancer Cooperative Group DBCG 82c randomised trial. *Lancet.* 1999;353:1641–1648.

Question 100

What are some criticisms of the Danish PMRT trials?

Question 101

What were the treatment arms for the randomized phase III trial, NCIC-CTG MA.20—an intergroup trial of regional nodal irradiation for early stage breast cancer?

Question 102

At 5 years, what impact did the addition of regional nodal irradiation (RNI) have compared to whole breast irradiation (WBI) alone on isolated locoregional DFS, distant DFS, and OS, as demonstrated in NCIC-CTG MA.20?

Question 103

What were the rates of lymphedema and grade 2 or greater pneumonitis for WBI+RNI in comparison to WBI alone, as shown in NCIC-CTG MA.20?

Answer 100

Inadequate axillary dissection (median of only 7 LNs removed in each trial) and suboptimal systemic therapy by modern standards (CMF in 82b and tamoxifen for only 1 year in 82c) are some of the major criticisms of the Danish PMRT trial.

Overgaard M, Hansen PS, Overgaard J, et al. Postoperative radiotherapy in high-risk premenopausal women with breast cancer who receive adjuvant chemotherapy. Danish Breast Cancer Cooperative Group 82b Trial. *N Engl J Med*. 1997;337:949–955.

Overgaard M, Jensen MB, Overgaard J, et al. Postoperative radiotherapy in high-risk postmenopausal breast-cancer patients given adjuvant tamoxifen: Danish Breast Cancer Cooperative Group DBCG 82c randomised trial. *Lancet*. 1999;353:1641–1648.

Answer 101

Whole breast irradiation (50 Gy in 25 fx +/− boost) vs. whole breast + regional nodal irradiation (45 Gy in 25 fx to the internal mammary, supraclavicular, and high axillary lymph nodes).

Whelan TJ, Olivotto I, Ackerman I, et al. NCIC-CTG MA.20: an intergroup trial of regional nodal irradiation in early breast cancer. *J Clin Oncol*. 2011;29(18 suppl 1):LBA1003.

Answer 102

At 5 years, WBI+RNI demonstrated a statistically significant benefit in isolated locoregional DFS (96.8% vs. 94.5%, $p = .02$) and distant DFS (92.4% vs. 87.0%, $p = .002$). Overall DFS was also superior (89.7% vs. 84.0%, $p = .003$). A trend for improved OS was seen (92.3% vs. 90.7%, $p = .07$).

Whelan TJ, Olivotto I, Ackerman I, et al. NCIC-CTG MA.20: an intergroup trial of regional nodal irradiation in early breast cancer. *J Clin Oncol*. 2011;29(18 suppl 1):LBA1003.

Answer 103

WBI+RNI in comparison to WBI was associated with an increase in grade 2 or greater pneumonitis (1.3% vs. 0.2%, $p = .01$), and lymphedema (7.3% vs. 4.1%, $p = .004$).

Whelan TJ, Olivotto I, Ackerman I, et al. NCIC-CTG MA.20: an intergroup trial of regional nodal irradiation in early breast cancer. *J Clin Oncol*. 2011;29(18 suppl 1):LBA1003.

Question 104

What were the study characteristics of the patient population for NCIC-CTG MA.20, a phase III trial investigating WBI+RNI for high risk node-negative or node-positive breast cancer treated with BCS and adjuvant chemotherapy and/or endocrine therapy?

Question 105

What were the eligibility criteria for the "high-risk node-negative" group for NCIC-CTG MA.20, a phase III trial investigating WBI+RNI for high risk node-negative or node-positive breast cancer treated with BCS and adjuvant chemotherapy and/or endocrine therapy?

Question 106

NCIC-CTG MA.20, investigated WBI+RNI for high-risk node-negative or node-positive breast cancer treated with BCS and adjuvant chemotherapy and/or endocrine therapy?

At 5 years, where were the majority of the isolated locoregional recurrences located?

Answer 104

Of the 1,832 women enrolled, study characteristics were: Node negative patients, 10%; 1–3 positive nodes, 85%; > 4 positive nodes, 5%; adjuvant chemotherapy, 91%; and adjuvant endocrine therapy, 71%. Patient mean age was 53.3 years; median follow-up at the time of abstract publication was 62 months.

Whelan TJ, Olivotto I, Ackerman I, et al. NCIC-CTG MA.20: an intergroup trial of regional nodal irradiation in early breast cancer. *J Clin Oncol*. 2011;29(18 suppl 1):LBA1003.

Answer 105

The "high-risk node-negative" group consisted of women with tumors ≥ 5 cm, those with tumors ≥ 2 cm and fewer than 10 axillary nodes removed who were ER–negative, those who had histologic grade 3 tumors, or those with lymphovascular invasion.

Whelan TJ, Olivotto I, Ackerman I, et al. NCIC-CTG MA.20: an intergroup trial of regional nodal irradiation in early breast cancer. *J Clin Oncol*. 2011;29(18 suppl 1):LBA1003.

Answer 106

67% of the isolated regional recurrences were located in the axilla.
Only 1 isolated recurrence was in the internal mammary nodes.

Whelan TJ, Olivotto I, Ackerman I, et al. NCIC-CTG MA.20: an intergroup trial of regional nodal irradiation in early breast cancer. *J Clin Oncol*. 2011;29(18 suppl 1):LBA1003.

4

THORACIC CANCERS

JOHN GRESKOVICH AND SUSAN GUO

Question 1   NON-SMALL CELL LUNG CANCER—EARLY STAGE

What is the relative incidence of lung cancer worldwide and in developed countries?

Question 2

What percentage of patients with non-small cell lung cancer (NSCLC) present with localized, regional, and distant disease?

Question 3

What is the diagnostic sensitivity of three sputum cytology samples for central vs peripheral lung tumor?

Question 4

What were the changes or additions in the AJCC 7th edition (2010) TNM staging for lung cancer?

Answer 1

Lung cancer is the most common noncutaneous cancer worldwide, and leading cause of cancer death in males in 2008. In developed countries, second in cancer incidence in men after prostate, and third in women after breast and colorectal cancers.

Jemal A, Bray F, Center MM, et al. Global cancer statistics. *CA Cancer J Clin*. 2011;61:69–90.

Answer 2

Localized (confined to primary site) occurs in 15%. Regional (spread to regional lymph nodes) disease occurs in 22%. Distant (metastasized) disease occurs in 56%. Unknown (unstaged) disease occurs in 7%.

Howlader N, Noone AM, Krapcho M, et al. SEER Cancer Statistics Review, 1975–2008; National Cancer Institute. Bethesda, MD, http://seer.cancer.gov/csr/1975_2008/, based on November 2010 SEER data submission, posted to the SEER web site, 2011.

Answer 3

71% sensitivity for central tumors and 49% for peripheral tumors.

Sputum cytology is particularly useful for patients who present with centrally located tumors (i.e., small cell lung cancer or squamous cell carcinoma) and in those who present with hemoptysis. The sampling of sputum specimens should be the first step in a patient who presents with a central lesion with or without radiographic evidence of metastatic disease, in whom a semi-invasive procedure such as bronchoscopy may pose a higher risk.

Rivera MP, Detterbeck F, Mehta AC. Diagnosis of lung cancer: the guidelines. *Chest*. 2003;123:129S–136S.

Answer 4

T1 tumors separated into T1a (≤ 2 cm) and T1b (> 2 cm and ≤ 3 cm)

T2 tumors separated into T2a (> 3 cm and ≤ 5 cm) and T2b (> 5 cm and ≤ 7 cm)

T3 tumors included those > 7 cm (previously T2)

Separate tumor nodules in same lobe is a T3 (previously T4)

Separate tumor nodules in different ipsilateral lobes is a T4 (previously M1)

Separate tumor nodule in contralateral lobe is a M1a (previously M1)

Malignant pleural or pericardial effusion or malignant pleural nodules is a M1a (previously M1)

Distant metastatic disease is a M1b (previously M1)

Lung. Edge SB, Byrd DR, et al, eds. *AJCC Cancer Staging Handbook*. 7th ed. New York, NY: Springer; 2010:263.

Question 5

What features make a primary tumor a T1 and a T2 per the AJCC 7th edition TNM staging for lung cancer?

Question 6

What percent of detected lung cancers were stage I in the Early Lung Cancer Action Project (ELCAP) lung cancer screening trial?

Question 7

What is the role of low-dose, spiral CT screening according to the National Lung Screening Trial?

Answer 5

T1 tumors include any of the following:

- ≤ 3 cm (T1a: ≤ 2 cm; T1b: > 2 cm to ≤ 3 cm)
- must not invade visceral pleura or mainstem bronchus

T2 tumors include any of the following:

- > 3 cm to ≤ 7 cm (T2a: > 3 cm to ≤ 5 cm; T2b: > 5 cm to ≤ 7 cm)
- invades visceral pleura
- atelectasis or obstructing pneumonitis, extending to hila but not involving the entire lung
- involves mainstem bronchus, ≥ 2 cm distal to the carina

Lung. Edge SB, Byrd DR, et al, eds. *AJCC Cancer Staging Handbook*. 7th ed. New York, NY: Springer; 2010:263.

Answer 6

85% of lung cancer cases detected by low-dose, non-contrast, CT screening were stage I, 4% stage II, and 11% stage III.

Spiral CT detected abnormalities (non-calcified nodules) in 233 patients (23%) while CXR detected abnormalities in 68 patients (8%).

Biopsies were performed on 28 of 233 patients with non-calcified nodules; only 1 patient having a benign nodule.

Malignant tumors were discovered in 27 patients screened by low dose, spiral CT imaging followed by standard measures (high resolution, contrast CT, serial scans, biopsy, etc.) vs 7 malignant tumors if screened by CXR.

ELCAP was a prospective study of lung cancer screening begun in 1992 at New York University and Cornell Med Center using low-dose, non-contrast, spiral CT imaging (20 second acquisition time, single breath hold) in patients with the following entry criteria. ≥ 10 pack-yr cigarette use, ≥ 60 yrs old, no previous cancer, thoracic surgery candidate, symptom-free.

Henschke CI, McCauley DI, Yankelevitz DF, et al. Early lung cancer action project: overall design and findings from baseline screening. *Lancet*. 1999; 354:99–105.

Answer 7

- Low-dose CT screening reduces mortality from lung cancer.
- The National Lung Screening Trial randomized 54,454 patients at high risk for lung cancer to undergo 3 annual screenings with either low-dose CT or single-view CXR. There were 247 vs 309 deaths from lung cancer per 100,000 person-years in the low-dose CT group vs the CXR group, respectively, which represented a relative reduction in mortality from lung cancer of 20.0% (95% CI, 6.8 to 26.7; $p = .004$). The rate of death from any cause was also reduced in the low-dose CT group as compared with the CXR group by 6.7% (95% CI, 1.2 to 13.6; $p = .02$). However, the authors advise that more information with regard to cost effectiveness and rate of overdiagnosis are needed.

National Lung Screening Trial Research Team, Aberle DR, Adams AM, Berg CD, et al. Reduced lung-cancer mortality with low-dose computed tomographic screening. *N Engl J Med*. 2011;365:395–409.

Question 8

Which patients are considered appropriate candidates to undergo a sublobar resection (segmentectomy or wedge resection) by the 2010 NCCN guidelines for non-small cell lung cancer?

Question 9

Is minimally-invasive, video-assisted thoracic surgery (VATS) a reasonable and accepted alternative to open thoracotomy for early stage NSCLC pts?

Question 10

What were the outcomes for limited resection (segmentectomy or wedge resection) vs lobectomy in peripheral T1N0 non-small cell lung cancer in the Lung Cancer Study Group Trial 821?

Question 11

What are the common criteria to be considered a poor candidate for surgical resection of lung cancer?

Answer 8

Segmentectomy (preferred) or wedge resection is appropriate if:

- Poor pulmonary reserve or other major comorbidity that contraindicates lobectomy
- Peripheral nodule (outer third of lung) which is ≤ 2 cm in size with at least one of the following: (a) pure bronchoalveolar carcinoma, (b) nodule with ≥ 50% ground glass appearance, (c) long doubling time (≥ 400 days)

Sublobar resection should achieve parenchymal resection margins ≥ 2 cm (or ≥ the size of the nodule).

Sublobar resection should also sample appropriate N1 and N2 lymph node stations unless not technically feasible without substantially increasing the surgical risk.

NCCN Clinical Practice Guidelines in Oncology: Non-small cell lung cancer. Version 2.2010. National Comprehensive Cancer Network. March 5, 2010.

Answer 9

Yes. VATS is an accepted alternative. A meta-analysis of 21 comparative (2 which were randomized) studies showed no significant differences between VATS and open lobectomy with regards to prolonged air leak ($p = .71$), arrhythmia ($p = .86$), pneumonia ($p = .09$), and operative mortality ($p = .49$). VATS patients had reduced systemic recurrence rates ($p = .03$) and improved 5 year mortality ($p = .04$).

Yan TD, Black D, Bannon PG, et al. Systematic review and meta-analysis of randomized and non-randomized trials on the safety and efficacy of video-assisted thoracic surgery lobectomy for early-stage non-small cell lung cancer. *J Clin Oncol.* 2009; 27:2553–2562.

Answer 10

LCSG 821 was a prospective randomized trial of 247 patients with T1N0 NSCLC comparing limited resection vs lobectomy.

Patients undergoing lobectomy had statistically improved locoregional recurrence rate compared to limited resection (6% vs 17%; $p = .008$).

No statistically significant difference was noted in non-local recurrence, cancer specific mortality, or all cause mortality.

A minimum of 2 cm of clinically normal lung tissue was to be excised in limited resections.

Ginsberg RJ, Rubinstein LV. Randomized trial of lobectomy versus limited resection for T1N0 non-small cell lung cancer. Lung cancer study group. *Ann Thorac Surg.* 1995;60:615–622.

Answer 11

Baseline forced expiratory volume at one second (FEV_1) < 40% predicted

Predicted postoperative FEV_1 ≤ 30% predicted

Severely reduced diffusion capacity ≤ 40% predicted

Baseline hypoxemia and/or hypercapnia

Exercise oxygen consumption ≤ 50% predicted

Significant medical comorbidities: coronary artery disease, peripheral vascular disease, poorly controlled hypertension, and diabetes

Sinha B, McGarry RC. Stereotactic body radiotherapy for bilateral primary lung cancers: the Indiana University experience. *Int J Radiat Oncol Biol Phys.* 2006;66:1120–1124.

Question 12

What was the subject of the postoperative radiation therapy (PORT) meta-analysis?

Question 13

When all patients with stage I–IIIA were considered in the PORT meta-analysis, which group of patients showed a survival advantage?

Question 14

What was the cause of the excess mortality in the postoperative radiation patients evaluated in the PORT meta-analysis?

Question 15

Which stages of resected NSCLC showed a survival disadvantage for postoperative radiation in the PORT meta-analysis?

Answer 12

The PORT meta-analysis reviewed 2128 patients with stage I–IIIA NSCLC treated on 9 prospective trials and evaluated the outcomes of patients randomized between postoperative radiation vs no adjuvant radiation.

PORT Meta-analysis Trialists Group. Postoperative radiotherapy in non-small-cell lung cancer: systematic review and meta-analysis of individual patient data from nine randomized controlled trials. *Lancet* 1998;352:257–263.

Answer 13

Patients not receiving adjuvant radiation showed a survival advantage (55% vs 48%; $p = .001$).

PORT Meta-analysis Trialists Group. Postoperative radiotherapy in non-small-cell lung cancer: systematic review and meta-analysis of individual patient data from nine randomized controlled trials. *Lancet*. 1998;352:257–263.

Answer 14

Excess cardiac and respiratory deaths attributed to postoperative radiation therapy were the cause of excess mortality.

PORT Meta-analysis Trialists Group. Postoperative radiotherapy in non-small-cell lung cancer: systematic review and meta-analysis of individual patient data from nine randomized controlled trials. *Lancet*. 1998;352:257–263.

Answer 15

Stages I–II had a survival disadvantage when postoperative radiation therapy was used.

PORT Meta-analysis Trialists Group. Postoperative radiotherapy in non-small-cell lung cancer: systematic review and meta-analysis of individual patient data from nine randomized controlled trials. *Lancet*. 1998;352:257–263.

Question 16

What are the criticisms of the PORT meta-analysis?

Question 17

What is the range of overall survival rates for conventional, fractionated radiation therapy alone for early stage lung cancer?

Question 18

What randomized study showed improvement in disease-free and overall survival with adjuvant radiation in resected early stage lung cancer patients?

Question 19

What were the main inclusion criteria for tumors treated with SBRT on the phase II RTOG 0236 study?

Answer 16

Highly variable extent of surgical resection and nodal staging

27% of patients were stage I

Antiquated radiation techniques/large radiation fields with corresponding high V20/Cobalt-60 radiation allowed in 7 trials/variable radiation doses from 30–60 Gy/high dose fractions (2.5–3.0 Gy/fx) in some trials/2D planning in 8 trials/midline cord block allowed in 7 trials

PORT Meta-analysis Trialists Group. Postoperative radiotherapy in non-small-cell lung cancer: systematic review and meta-analysis of individual patient data from nine randomized controlled trials. *Lancet*. 1998;352:257–263.

Answer 17

Overall survival rates range from 17–55% at 3 years and 6–32% at 5 years.

Sandler HM, Curran WJ, Turrisi AT, et al. The influence of tumor size and pre-treatment staging on outcome following radiation therapy alone for stage I non-small cell lung cancer. *Int J Radiat Oncol Biol Phys*. 1990;19:9–13.
Sibley GS, Jamieson TA, Marks LB, et al. Radiotherapy alone for medically inoperable stage I non-small-cell lung cancer: the Duke experience. *Int J Radiat Oncol Biol Phys*. 1998;40:149–154.
Zhang HW, Yin WB, Zhang LJ, et al. Curative radiotherapy of early operable non-small cell lung cancer. *Radiother Oncol*. 1989;14:80–94.
Krol AD, Aussems P, Noordijk EM, et al. Local irradiation alone for peripheral stage I lung cancer: could we omit the elective nodal irradiation? *Int J Radiat Oncol Biol Phys*. 1996;34:297–302.

Answer 18

An Italian prospective, randomized trial published by Trodella et al. in 2002 evaluating adjuvant radiation vs observation in completed resected (R0), pathological stage I NSCLC patients showed a statistically significant disease-free survival (71% vs 60%, $p = .039$) and overall survival (67% vs 58%, $p = .048$) benefit for adjuvant radiation.

Adjuvant radiation dose was 50.4 Gy in 28 fractions, and the target volume was defined as the bronchial stump and ipsilateral hilum.

Trodella L, Granone P, Valente S, et al. Adjuvant radiotherapy in non-small cell lung cancer with pathological stage I: definitive results of a phase III randomized trial. *Radiother Oncol*. 2002;62:11–19.

Answer 19

Medically inoperable NSCLC, T1-2N0M0 (≤ 5 cm), ≥ 2 cm from the proximal bronchial tree, and mandatory staging PET and CT.

T3 (≤ 5 cm peripheral tumors only) tumors were allowed but ultimately none were enrolled.

Timmerman R, Paulus R, Galvin J, et al. Stereotactic body radiation therapy for inoperable early stage lung cancer. *JAMA*. 2010;303:1070–1076.

Question 20

What was the 3-year local control rate per RTOG 0236?

Question 21

What are commonly used dose and fractionation schemes for lung SBRT?

Question 22   NON-SMALL CELL LUNG CANCER—LOCALLY ADVANCED

What triad of symptoms makes up Horner's syndrome?

Question 23

What signs/symptoms can result from a Pancoast (superior sulcus) tumor and what structures are compressed or invaded that cause these signs/symptoms?

Answer 20

The estimated 3-year primary tumor control rate was 97.6% (95% CI, 84.3–99.7%).

Rates for disease-free survival and overall survival at 3 years were 48.3% (95% CI, 34.4%–60.8%) and 55.8% (95% CI, 41.6%–67.9%), respectively.

Timmerman R, Paulus R, Galvin J, et al. Stereotactic body radiation therapy for inoperable early stage lung cancer. *JAMA*. 2010;303:1070–1076.

Answer 21

60 Gy in 3 fractions, 50 Gy in 5 fractions, and 48 Gy in 4 fractions have all been reported to be safe and effective.

Timmerman R, Paulus R, Galvin J, et al. Stereotactic body radiation therapy for inoperable early stage lung cancer. *JAMA*. 2010;303:1070–1076.
Uematsu M, Shioda A, Suda A, et al. Computed tomography-guided frameless stereotactic radiotherapy for stage I non-small cell lung cancer: a 5-year experience. *Int J Radiat Oncol Biol Phys*. 2001;51:666–670.
Nagata Y, Matsuo Y, Takayama K, et al. Current status of stereotactic body radiotherapy for lung cancer. *Int J Clin Oncol*. 2007;12:3–7.

Answer 22

Ipsilateral ptosis (superior tarsal muscle), miosis (dilator pupillae muscle), anhidrosis.

Symptoms result from tumor compression of sympathetic trunk or inferior cervical (stellate) ganglion.

Chang JY, Bradley JD, Govindan R, et al. Lung. In: Halperin EC, Perez CA, Brady LW, eds. *Perez and Brady's Principles and Practice of Radiation Oncology*. 5th ed. Philadelphia, PA: Lippincott Williams & Wilkins; 2008:1076–1108.

Answer 23

Shoulder or back pain/invasion of parietal pleura, ribs, intercostals muscles, vertebral bodies

Weakness, paresthesias, or atrophy of intrinsic muscles of hand or numbness in ulnar nerve distribution/compression of brachial plexus

Horner's syndrome/compression of the sympathetic trunk or inferior cervical (stellate) ganglion

Hoarseness/compression of recurrent laryngeal nerve

SVC syndrome/compression of SVC

Chang JY, Bradley JD, Govindan R, et al. Lung. In: Halperin EC, Perez CA, Brady LW, eds. *Perez and Brady's Principles and Practice of Radiation Oncology*. 5th Ed. Philadelphia, PA: Lippincott Williams & Wilkins; 2008:1076–1108.

Question 24

What features make a primary tumor a T3 and a T4 per the AJCC 7th edition TNM staging for lung cancer?

Question 25

How are involved lymph nodes staged as per the AJCC 7th edition TNM staging for lung cancer?

Question 26

Does the addition of endosonography improve the detection of mediastinal nodal metastases in NSCLC?

Answer 24

T3 tumors include any of the following:

- > 7 cm
- invasion of the following (resectable) structures: chest wall, diaphragm, parietal or mediastinal pleura, pericardium
- involvement of mainstem bronchus within 2 cm of carina but not involving carina
- atelectasis or obstructive pneumonitis of entire lung
- separate tumor nodules within the same lobe

T4 tumors include any of the following:

- invasion of the following ("unresectable") structures: mediastinum, great vessels, heart, trachea, esophagus, recurrent laryngeal nerve, vertebral body
- invasion of carina
- separate tumor nodules within a different ipsilateral lobe

Lung. Edge SB, Byrd DR, et al, eds. *AJCC Cancer Staging Handbook*. 7th ed. New York, NY: Springer; 2010:263.

Answer 25

N1 nodes include any of the following:
- ipsilateral intrapulmonary, peribronchial, or hilar

N2 nodes include any of the following:
- ipsilateral mediastinal or subcarinal

N3 nodes include any of the following:
- contralateral hilar or mediastinal,
- ipsilateral or contralateral scalene or supraclavicular

There were no changes in nodal staging from the AJCC 6th edition

Lung. Edge SB, Byrd DR, et al, eds. *AJCC Cancer Staging Handbook*. 7th ed. New York, NY: Springer; 2010:263.

Answer 26

Yes. The prospective, phase III, randomized trial, Assessment of Surgical Staging vs Endoscopic Ultrasound (ASTER) trial, showed that EUS or EBUS followed by mediastinoscopy if EUS/EBUS was negative detected more nodal metastases than surgical staging with mediastinoscopy alone in 241 randomized patients.

62 pts (50%) had nodal metastasis detected by EUS/EBUS compared to 41 pts (35%) detected with surgical staging mediastinoscopy alone ($p = .019$).

Of the 62 positive nodal pts in the EBUS/EUS/mediastinoscopy arm, 56 of 62 (90%) pts had metastasis detected on EBUS or EUS. Therefore, 90% of pts were spared a mediastinoscopy.

The sensitivity for detecting nodal metastasis was 94% (95% CI 85–98) vs 80% (95% CI 68–89), significantly favoring EUS/EBUS ($p = .042$).

Complication rates were similar 6% vs 7% but 12 of 13 complications were related to surgical mediastinal staging.

Annema JT, va Meerbeeck JP, Rintoul RC, et al. Mediastinoscopy vs endosonography for mediastinal nodal staging of lung cancer. *JAMA*. 2010;204:2245–2252.

Question 27

What percent of patients with stage I–III NSCLC by CT-based staging are upstaged to stage IV (M1b) disease by FDG PET-CT?

Question 28

What are the most commonly detected distant metastatic disease sites by FDG PET-CT, which were undetectable by CT-based staging?

Question 29

What common mutations are seen in NSCLC patients?

Question 30

What is median survival and 2-year overall survival in stage III NSCLC patients treated with radiation alone?

Answer 27

Patients with stages IA, IB, IIA, IIB, IIIA, IIIB were found to have distant metastases in 0%, 17%, 17%, 18%, 26%, 21% of the cases, respectively.

Grouping of stages gives the following risk of upstaging on FDG PET: stage IA: 0%, stages Ib–II: 17%, stage III: 24%.

Mac Manus MP, Hicks RJ, Matthews JP, et al. High rate of detection of unsuspected distant metastases by PET in apparent stage III non-small-cell lung cancer: implications for radical radiation therapy. *Int J Radiat Oncol Biol Phys.* 2001;50:287–293.

Answer 28

The most commonly detected distant metastatic disease sites by FDG PET-CT previously undetected by CT-based staging are: lung (31%), adrenal (22%), bone (19%), and liver (13%). Other abdominal sites were seen in 18%.

No false positives reported in Mac Manus study.

Mac Manus MP, Hicks RJ, Matthews JP, et al. High rate of detection of unsuspected distant metastases by PET in apparent stage III non-small-cell lung cancer: implications for radical radiation therapy. *Int J Radiat Oncol Biol Phys.* 2001;50:287–293.

Answer 29

p53 mutations (50%), k-ras mutations common if adenocarcinoma

Ahrendt SA, Hu Y, Buta M, et al. p53 mutations and survival in stage I non-small-cell lung cancer: results of a prospective study. *J Natl Cancer Inst.* 2003;95:961–970.

Ahrendt SA, Decker PA, Alawi EA, et al. Cigarette smoking is strongly associated with mutation of the K-ras gene in patients with primary adenocarcinoma of the lung. *Cancer.* 2001;92:1525–1530.

Answer 30

Median survival is 9–13 month

2-year overall survival is 15–20%

Chang JY, Bradley JD, Govindan R, et al. Lung. In: Halperin EC, Perez CA, Brady LW. eds. *Perez and Brady's Principles and Practice of Radiation Oncology.* 5th ed. Philadelphia, PA: Lippincott Williams & Wilkins; 2008:1076–1108.

Curran Jr WJ, Stafford PM. Lack of apparent difference in outcome between clinically staged IIIA and IIIB non-small-cell lung cancer treated with radiation therapy. *J Clin Oncol.* 1990;8:409–415.

Question 31
What is the recommended limit for dose to the brachial plexus with conventional fractionation?

Question 32
What are the 5 RPA subgroups and corresponding median survivals reported by Werner-Wasik et al. developed from analysis of patients on nine RTOG unresectable NSCLC trials?

Question 33
What were the two arms of the Dillman randomized trial (CALGB 84-33) in unresectable stage III NSCLC?

Question 34
What were the results of the Dillman randomized trial (CALGB 84-33) in unresectable stage III NSCLC?

Answer 31

Per RTOG 0619, 95% of the brachial plexus volume should receive ≤ 60 Gy and the maximum dose should be no more than 66 Gy.

RTOG 0619. A randomized phase II trial of chemoradiotherapy versus chemoradiotherapy and vandetanib for high-risk postoperative advanced squamous cell carcinoma of the head and neck. www.rtog.org

Answer 32

RPA class 1	KPS ≥ 90, +chemo	MST: 16.2 mo
RPA class 2	KPS ≥ 90, −chemo, −effusion	MST: 11.9 mo
RPA class 3	KPS < 90, < 70 yr old, −large cell	MST: 9.7 mo
RPA class 4	All three subgroups below	MST: 6.1 mo
	(a) KPS ≥ 90, −chemo, +effusion	MST: 6.4 mo
	(b) KPS < 90, > 70 yr old, −effusion	MST: 6.3 mo
	or (c) KPS < 90, < 70 yr old, +large cell	MST: 5.6 mo
RPA class 5	> 70 yr old, +effusion	MST: 2.9 mo

Werner-Wasik M, Scott C, Cox JD, et al. Recursive partitioning analysis of 1999 Radiation Therapy Oncology Group (RTOG) patients with locally-advanced non-small-cell lung cancer (LA-NSCLC): identification of five groups with different survival. *Int J Radiat Oncol Biol Phys*. 2000;48:1475–1482.

Answer 33

Arm 1: Definitive radiation alone, 60 Gy in 30 fx, *versus*

Arm 2: Induction chemotherapy using CDDP, 100 mg/m^2 IV, days 1, 29 and Vinblastine, 5 mg/m^2 IV, weekly on days 1, 8, 15, 22, 29 followed by definitive radiation 60 Gy in 30 fx.

Dillman R, Seagren S, Herndon J, et al. A randomized trial of induction chemotherapy plus high-dose radiation versus radiation alone in stage III non-small cell lung cancer. *N Eng J Med*. 1990;323:940–945.

Answer 34

Induction chemotherapy (CDDP, 100 mg/m^2 IV, days 1, 29; Vinblastine, 5 mg/m^2 IV, weekly on days 1, 8, 15, 22, 29) followed by definitive radiation (60 Gy in 30 fx) starting day 50 showed an improvement in median and overall survival over definitive radiation alone (60 Gy in 30 fx).

Median survival was 13.7 vs 9.6 months for the CT > RT, and RT alone arms, respectively.

1-, 5-, 7-year overall survival was 54% vs 40%, 17% vs 6%, and 13% vs 6%, for the CT > RT and RT alone arms, respectively.

Dillman R, Seagren S, Herndon J, et al. A randomized trial of induction chemotherapy plus high-dose radiation versus radiation alone in stage III non-small cell lung cancer. *N Eng J Med*. 1990;323:940–945.

Question 35

What major randomized trials demonstrated the superiority of concurrent over sequential chemoradiation in medically or surgically inoperable stage II–III NSCLC?

Question 36

What were the arms of the RTOG 94-10 randomized trial in medically or surgically inoperable stage II–III NSCLC?

Question 37

What were the survival results of the RTOG 94-10 randomized trial in medically or surgically inoperable stage II–III NSCLC?

Answer 35

RTOG 94-10 and West Japan Lung Cancer Study Group trials both showed the superiority of concurrent chemoradiation over sequential treatment in terms of median survival and 5-year overall survival.

RTOG 94-10 showed an advantage to concurrent CDDP/Vinblastine/RT (63 Gy) over sequential CDDP/Vinblastine > RT (63 Gy) in terms of median survival (17 vs 14.6 months) and 5-year overall survival (16 vs 10%; $p = .046$).

West Japan Lung Cancer Study Group showed an advantage to concurrent CDDP/Vindesine/MMC/RT (28 Gy × 2, split course) over sequential CDDP/Vindesine/MMC>RT (28 Gy × 2, split course) in terms of median survival (16.5 vs 13.3 months) and 5-year overall survival (16 vs 9%; $p = .039$).

Curran W, Paulus R, Langer C, et al. Sequential vs concurrent chemoradiation for stage III non-small cell lung cancer: Randomized phase III trial RTOG 9410. *JNCI.* 2011;103:1–9.

Furuse K, Fukuoka M, Kawahar M, et al. Phase III study of concurrent versus sequential thoracic radiotherapy in combination with mitomycin, vindesine, and cisplatin in unresectable stage III non-small cell lung cancer. *J Clin Oncol.* 1999;17:2692–2699.

Answer 36

Arm 1 ("Dillman arm"): Induction chemotherapy using CDDP, 100 mg/m^2 IV, days 1, 29 and Vinblastine, 5 mg/m^2 IV, weekly on days 1, 8, 15, 22, 29 followed by definitive radiation 63 Gy in 34 fx (45 Gy in 25 fx of 1.8 Gy/fx, then 18 Gy in 9 fx of 2.0 Gy/fx).

Arm 2 ("Concurrent Dillman arm"): Concurrent chemoradiation using CDDP, 100 mg/m^2 IV, days 1, 29 and Vinblastine, 5 mg/m^2 IV, weekly on days 1, 8, 15, 22, 29 concurrent with definitive radiation 63 Gy in 34 fx (45 Gy in 25 fx of 1.8 Gy/fx, then 18 Gy in 9 fx of 2.0 Gy/fx).

Arm 3 ("Hyperfractionated arm"): Concurrent chemoradiation using CDDP, 50 mg/m^2 IV, days 1, 8, 29, 36 and Etoposide orally, 50 mg tablets, taken twice daily on days 1–5, 8–12, 15–19, 22–26, 29–33, 36–40 (days of radiation) concurrent with definitive, hyperfractionated radiation, 69.6 Gy in 58 fx of 1.2 Gy/fx twice daily with at least 6 hours between fractions.

Curran W, Paulus R, Langer C, et al. Sequential vs concurrent chemoradiation for stage III non-small cell lung cancer: randomized phase III trial RTOG 9410. *JNCI.* 2011;103:1–9.

Answer 37

The "Concurrent Dillman" arm had a statistically significant improved median and 5-year overall survival (med surv = 17.0 months, 5-yr OS: 16%) vs the "Dillman arm" (med surv = 14.6 months, 5-yr OS: 10%; $p = .046$) and "Hyperfractionated arm" (med surv = 15.6 months; 5-yr OS: 13%; $p = .046$)

Arm 1 ("Dillman"): Sequential CDDP/Vinblastine > RT (63 Gy)

Arm 2 ("Concurrent Dillman"): Concurrent CDDP/Vinblastine/RT (63 Gy)

Arm 3 ("Hyperfractionated"): Concurrent CDDP/Etoposide/HfxRT (69.6 Gy)

Curran W, Paulus R, Langer C, et al. Sequential vs concurrent chemoradiation for stage III non-small cell lung cancer: randomized phase III trial RTOG 9410. *JNCI.* 2011;103:1–9.

Question 38

What were the rates of acute and chronic grade ≥ 3esophagitis in the treatment arms of RTOG 94-10 randomized trial in medically or surgically inoperable stage II–III NSCLC?

Question 39

What were the rates of acute and chronic grade ≥ 3 pulmonary toxicities in the treatment arms of RTOG 94-10 randomized trial in medically or surgically inoperable stage II–III NSCLC?

Question 40

What was the rate and major etiology of acute and late fatal toxicity in the RTOG 94-10 randomized trial in medically or surgically inoperable stage II–III NSCLC?

Question 41

Was there any statistically significant differences in patterns of first failure between the treatment arms of RTOG 94-10 randomized trial in medically or surgically inoperable stage II–III NSCLC?

Answer 38

The two concurrent arms had statistically significant higher rates of acute grade ≥ 3 esophagitis. The "Hyperfractionated arm" had the highest rate of acute grade ≥ 3 esophagitis (45%) followed by the "Concurrent Dillman" arm (22%) with the sequential "Dillman" arm (4%) having the lowest ($p < .001$ for arm 1 vs 2 and arm 2 vs 3).

There was no difference in the rates of late esophagitis (4% for concurrent arms; 1% for sequential arm).

Arm 1 ("Dillman"): Sequential CDDP/Vinblastine > RT (63 Gy)

Arm 2 ("Concurrent Dillman"): Concurrent CDDP/Vinblastine/RT (63 Gy)

Arm 3 ("Hyperfractionated"): Concurrent CDDP/Etoposide/HfxRT (69.6 Gy)

Curran W, Paulus R, Langer C, et al. Sequential vs concurrent chemoradiation for stage III non-small cell lung cancer: randomized phase III trial RTOG 9410. *JNCI*. 2011;103:1–9.

Answer 39

The two concurrent arms (2.1–3.6%) had lower rates of acute grade ≥ 3 pulmonary toxicity compared to the sequential arm (8.7%); no *p*-value given in manuscript.

There was no difference in the rates of late grade ≥ 3 pulmonary toxicity (13–17%).

Arm 1 ("Dillman"): Sequential CDDP/Vinblastine > RT (63 Gy)

Arm 2 ("Concurrent Dillman"): Concurrent CDDP/Vinblastine/RT (63 Gy)

Arm 3 ("Hyperfractionated"): Concurrent CDDP/Etoposide/HfxRT (69.6 Gy)

Curran W, Paulus R, Langer C, et al. Sequential vs concurrent chemoradiation for stage III non-small cell lung cancer: randomized phase III trial RTOG 9410. *JNCI*. 2011;103:1–9.

Answer 40

The rate of acute fatal toxicity was 2% with 13 of 14 acute deaths from neutropenic sepsis. No difference seen between treatment arms; no *p*-value given in manuscript.

The rate of late fatal toxicity was 1% with 7 of 8 late deaths from pulmonary toxicity. No difference seen between treatment arms.

Arm 1 ("Dillman"): Sequential CDDP/Vinblastine > RT (63 Gy)

Arm 2 ("Concurrent Dillman"): Concurrent CDDP/Vinblastine/RT (63 Gy)

Arm 3 ("Hyperfractionated"): Concurrent CDDP/Etoposide/HfxRT (69.6 Gy)

Curran W, Paulus R, Langer C, et al. Sequential vs concurrent chemoradiation for stage III non-small cell lung cancer: randomized phase III trial RTOG 9410. *JNCI*. 2011;103:1–9.

Answer 41

Yes. Fewer patients had disease progression within the thoracic radiation therapy target volume who were treated on the "Hyperfractionated arm" compared to the "Dillman arm (20% vs 30%; $p = .03$)." The "Concurrent Dillman" arm had 25% in-field failure rate.

Arm 1 ("Dillman"): Sequential CDDP/Vinblastine > RT (63 Gy)

Arm 2 ("Concurrent Dillman"): Concurrent CDDP/Vinblastine/RT (63 Gy)

Arm 3 ("Hyperfractionated"): Concurrent CDDP/Etoposide/HfxRT (69.6 Gy)

Curran W, Paulus R, Langer C, et al. Sequential vs concurrent chemoradiation for stage III non-small cell lung cancer: randomized phase III trial RTOG 9410. *JNCI*. 2011;103:1–9.

Question 42

What study established 60 Gy as the minimum "standard" dose in stage III NSCLC?

Question 43

What was the randomization and the results of the Adjuvant Navelbine International Trialist Association (ANITA) trial?

Question 44

Was adjuvant radiation allowed in the Adjuvant Navelbine International Trialist Association (ANITA) trial?

Answer 42

RTOG 73-01 was a dose-escalation trial of radiation therapy alone in stage III NSCLC patients which escalated doses from 40 Gy to 50 Gy to 60 Gy, all at 2 Gy/fx, compared to 40 Gy in 20 fx split course.

Median and 3-year overall survival for 60 Gy/30 fx were ~10 months and 15%, respectively.

Perez CA, Stanley K, Rubin P, et al. A prospective randomized study of various irradiation doses and fractionation schedules in the treatment of inoperable non-oat-cell carcinoma of the lung. Preliminary report by the Radiation Therapy Oncology Group. *Cancer*. 1980;45:2744–2753.

Answer 43

840 patients were randomized between adjuvant vinorelbine (30 mg/m^2) and CDDP (100 mg/m^2) vs observation in resected stage IB–IIIA NSCLC

Adjuvant vinorelbine + CDDP improved median survival (65.7 vs 43.7 months; p = .017) and 5-year survival by 8.6% over observation in resected stage IB–IIIA NSCLC.

On subset analysis, only patients with stage II–III NSCLC (not stage IB) had a statistically significant improvement in survival.

Douillard JY, Rosell R, De Lena M, et al. Adjuvant vinorelbine plus cisplatin versus observation in patients with completely resected stage IB–IIIA non-small cell lung cancer (Adjuvant Navelbine International Trialist Association [ANITA]): a randomized controlled trial. *Lancet Oncol*. 2006;7:719–727.
Douillard JY, Rosell R, De Lena M, et al. Impact of postoperative radiation therapy on survival in patients with complete resection and stage I, II, or IIIA non-small-cell lung cancer treated with adjuvant chemotherapy: the adjuvant Navelbine International Trialist Association (ANITA) Randomised Trial. *Int J Radiat Oncol Biol Phys*. 2008;72:695–701.

Answer 44

Yes. Radiation was allowed but not randomized. Adjuvant radiation was at the discretion of the treating physicians. Radiation doses varied from 45–60 Gy.

Douillard JY, Rosell R, De Lena M, et al. Adjuvant vinorelbine plus cisplatin versus observation in patients with completely resected stage IB–IIIA non-small cell lung cancer (Adjuvant Navelbine International Trialist Association [ANITA]): a randomized controlled trial. *Lancet Oncol*. 2006;7:719–727.
Douillard JY, Rosell R, De Lena M, et al. Impact of postoperative radiation therapy on survival in patients with complete resection and stage I, II, or IIIA non-small-cell lung cancer treated with adjuvant chemotherapy: the adjuvant Navelbine International Trialist Association (ANITA) Randomised Trial. *Int J Radiat Oncol Biol Phys*. 2008;72:695–701.

Question 45
Which subset(s) of patients benefited from adjuvant radiation in the Adjuvant Navelbine International Trialist Association (ANITA) trial?

Question 46
What was the randomization and results of the International Adjuvant Lung Cancer Trial (IALT)?

Question 47
What is the role of chemotherapy in resected lung cancer according to the Lung Adjuvant Cisplatin Evaluation (LACE) meta-analysis?

Answer 45

pN1 patients in the observation arm who received adjuvant radiation had improved 5-year overall survival (42.6 vs 31.4%).

pN2 patients in the observation arm who received adjuvant radiation had improved 5-year overall survival (21.3 vs 16.6%).

pN2 patients in the adjuvant vinorelbine + CDDP arm who also received adjuvant radiation had improved 5-year overall survival (47.4 vs 34.0%).

Note: pN1 patients in the adjuvant vinorelbine + CDDP arm who also received adjuvant radiation had 5-year overall survival detriment (40.0 vs 56.3%).

Note: pN0 patients who received radiation had 5-year survival detriment in both the observation (43.8 vs 62.3%) and vinorelbine + CDDP (44.4 vs 59.7%) arms.

Douillard JY, Rosell R, De Lena M, et al. Adjuvant vinorelbine plus cisplatin versus observation in patients with completely resected stage IB–IIIA non-small cell lung cancer (Adjuvant Navelbine International Trialist Association [ANITA]): a randomized controlled trial. *Lancet Oncol.* 2006;7:719–727.

Douillard JY, Rosell R, De Lena M, et al. Impact of postoperative radiation therapy on survival in patients with complete resection and stage I, II, or IIIA non-small-cell lung cancer treated with adjuvant chemotherapy: the adjuvant Navelbine International Trialist Association (ANITA) Randomised Trial. *Int J Radiat Oncol Biol Phys.* 2008;72:695–701.

Answer 46

Prospective, randomized trial in 1,867 pts of 3–4 cycles of CDDP-based chemo vs observation in resected stage I–III NSCLC.

2- and 5-overall survival rates were statistically improved in the adjuvant chemotherapy arms: 70 vs 67% at 2 yrs; 45 vs 40% at 5 yrs; $p < .03$.

5-year disease-free survival better in adjuvant chemo arm: 39 vs 34%; $p < .003$

Subsequent analyses, however, showed that the benefits of adjuvant chemotherapy decreased as time progressed and were no longer statistically different after 7.5 years of follow-up.

Arriagada R, Bergman B, Dunant A, et al. Cisplatin-based adjuvant chemotherapy in patients with completely resected non-small cell lung cancer. *N Eng J Med.* 2004;350:351–360.

Arriagada R, Dunant A, Pignon J-P, et al. Long-term results of the International Adjuvant Lung Cancer Trial evaluating adjuvant cisplatin-based chemotherapy in resected lung cancer. *J Clin Oncol.* 2010;28:35–42.

Answer 47

Adjuvant cisplatin-based chemotherapy significantly improved survival in NSCLC patients with an overall HR of 0.89 ($p = .005$), which corresponded to a 5-year absolute survival benefit of 5.4%.

The survival benefit varied with stage: detrimental for stage IA (HR 1.4), nonsignificant for stage IB (HR 0.93), and significant for stage II (HR 0.83) and stage III (HR 0.8).

The LACE meta-analysis pooled individual data from 4,584 patients from five prospective randomized trials evaluating adjuvant cisplatin-based chemotherapy in resected NSCLC pts.

Pignon JP, Tribodet H, Scagliotti GV, et al. Lung adjuvant cisplatin evaluation: a pooled analysis by the LACE Collaborative Group. *J Clin Oncol.* 2008; 26:3552–3559.

Question 48

Have there been any prospective randomized trials showing a benefit for adjuvant non-cisplatin–based chemotherapy in resected NSCLC pts?

Question 49

Is there a defined role for adjuvant docetaxel after definitive chemoradiation for stage III NSCLC?

Question 50

Is there a significant benefit to the addition of surgical resection following induction chemoradiation over chemoradiation alone for technically resectable stage IIIA NSCLC?

Answer 48

Yes (and No). CALGB 9633 was a prospective randomized trial comparing 4 cycles of adjuvant carboplatin (AUC 6) and paclitaxel (200 mg/m^2) every 3 weeks vs observation in resected stage IB NSCLC.

Initially, the adjuvant arm showed a statistically significant 3-year overall survival benefit (79 vs 70%; $p = .045$) but at 5 years the overall survival was the same (60 vs 57%; $p = .32$).

Subgroup analysis showed that the early statistical survival benefit was limited to patients with tumors > 4 cm.

Strauss GM, Herndon J II, Maddaus MA, et al. Randomized clinical trial of adjuvant chemotherapy with paclitaxel and carboplatin following resection for stage IB non-small cell lung cancer (NSCLC): report of Cancer and Leukemia Group B (CALGB) protocol 9633. *J Clin Oncol.* 2004;22(July 15 supplement):7019 (ASCO Annual Meeting Proceedings (Post-Meeting Edition)).

Strauss GM, Herndon J II, Maddaus MA, et al. Adjuvant paclitaxel plus carboplatin compared with observation in stage IB non-small cell lung cancer: CALGB 9633 with the Cancer and Leukemia Group B, Radiation Therapy Oncology Group and North Central Cancer Treatment Study Groups. *J Clin Oncol.* 2008;26:5043–5051.

Answer 49

SWOG 9504, a phase II prospective trial showed encouraging results with a median survival time of 26 months and 5-year overall survival of 29% in stage IIIB patients using concurrent radiation (61 Gy), cisplatin, and etoposide followed by adjuvant taxotere for 2–3 cycles.

Unfortunately, a phase III prospective, Hoosier Oncology Group randomized trial evaluating RT/cisplatin/etoposide +/– adjuvant docetaxel did not show any benefit for adjuvant docetaxel in stage III NSCLC pts (median survival: 21.2 months vs 23.2 months in adjuvant vs no adjuvant arms, respectively; $p = .883$).

Gandara DR, Chansky K, Albain KS, et al. Consolidation docetaxel after concurrent chemoradiotherapy in stage IIIB non-small-cell lung cancer: phase II Southwest Oncology Group Study S9504. *J Clin Oncol.* 2003;21:2004–2010.

Gandara DR, Chansky K, Albain KS, et al. Long-term survival with concurrent chemoradiation therapy followed by consolidation docetaxel in stage IIIB non-small-cell lung cancer: a phase II Southwest Oncology Group Study S9504. *Clin Lung Cancer.* 2006; 8:116–121.

Hanna N, Neubauer M, Yiannoutsos C, et al. Phase III study of cisplatin, etoposide, and concurrent chest radiation with or without consolidation docetaxel in patients with inoperable stage III non-small-cell lung cancer: the hoosier oncology group and U.S. oncology. *J Clin Oncol.* 2008;26:5755–5760.

Answer 50

Controversial. INT-0139 reported no difference in median survival between induction chemoradiation followed by surgery vs chemoradiation alone (23.6 vs 22.2 months; p = ns).

The intergroup trial, INT-0139, was a phase III, randomized, prospective trial in 396 surgically staged N2+ pts., evaluating induction chemoradiation (cisplatin 50 mg/m^2 d1, 8, 29, 36; etoposide, 50 mg/m^2, d1-5, 29–33; RT, 45 Gy/25 fx) followed by surgery vs definitive chemoradiation (cisplatin 50 mg/m^2 d1, 8, 29, 36; etoposide, 50 mg/m^2, d1-5, 29–33; RT, 61 Gy/33 fx).

Both arms received two additional cycles of cisplatin and etoposide after concurrent chemoradiation.

The median progression-free survival was improved in the surgical patients (12.8 vs 10.5 months; $p = .017$).

A high rate of perioperative mortality was seen in the surgical arm with 16 deaths (8%). 14 of 16 deaths occurred in pneumonectomy patients. Most perioperative mortality was from ARDS.

Subset analysis of 90 patients undergoing chemoradiaton followed by lobectomy matched by patient characteristics to 90 patients undergoing chemoradiation showed a statistically significant survival benefit for lobectomy (33.6 vs 21.7 months).

Albain KS, Swann RS, Rusch VW, et al. Radiotherapy plus chemotherapy with or without surgical resection for stage III non-small cell lung cancer: a phase III randomized controlled trial. *Lancet.* 2009;374:379–386.

Question 51

What was included within the initial CTV per the SWOG 9416 protocol for Pancoast tumors?

Question 52

What stage patients with Pancoast tumors were eligible for the SWOG 9416 protocol?

Question 53

What preoperative regimen of radiation therapy and chemotherapy was given in the SWOG 9416 protocol for Pancoast tumors?

Question 54

What was the pathologic complete response (pCR) and minimal microscopic disease (MMD) rates reported in the SWOG 9416 protocol for Pancoast tumors?

Answer 51

Primary GTV

Ipsilateral level 2 (upper paratracheal) lymph nodes

Ipsilateral supraclavicular lymph nodes

Rusch VW, Giroux DJ, Kraut MJ, et al. Induction chemoradiation and surgical resection for non-small cell lung carcinomas of the superior sulcus: initial results of Southwest Oncology Group Trial 9416 (Intergroup Trial 0160). *J Thorac Cardiovasc Surg*. 2001;121:472–483.

Rusch VW, Giroux DJ, Kraut MJ, et al. Induction chemoradiation and surgical resection for superior sulcus non-small-cell lung carcinomas: long-term results of Southwest Oncology Group Trial 9416 (Intergroup Trial 0160). *J Clin Oncol*. 2007;25:313–318.

Answer 52

T3-4N0-1 patients were eligible for SWOG 9416 and had to undergo a negative staging mediastinoscopy.

Rusch VW, Giroux DJ, Kraut MJ, et al. Induction chemoradiation and surgical resection for non-small cell lung carcinomas of the superior sulcus: initial results of Southwest Oncology Group Trial 9416 (Intergroup Trial 0160). *J Thorac Cardiovasc Surg*. 2001;121:472–483.

Rusch VW, Giroux DJ, Kraut MJ, et al. Induction chemoradiation and surgical resection for superior sulcus non-small-cell lung carcinomas: long-term results of Southwest Oncology Group Trial 9416 (Intergroup Trial 0160). *J Clin Oncol*. 2007;25:313–318.

Answer 53

Preoperative radiation was 45 Gy in 25 fx.

Concurrent chemotherapy was CDDP (50 mg/m^2) days 1, 8, 29, 36, and Etoposide (50 mg/m^2) days 1–5, 29–33.

Rusch VW, Giroux DJ, Kraut MJ, et al. Induction chemoradiation and surgical resection for non-small cell lung carcinomas of the superior sulcus: initial results of Southwest Oncology Group Trial 9416 (Intergroup Trial 0160). *J Thorac Cardiovasc Surg*. 2001;121:472–483.

Rusch VW, Giroux DJ, Kraut MJ, et al. Induction chemoradiation and surgical resection for superior sulcus non-small-cell lung carcinomas: long-term results of Southwest Oncology group Trial 9416 (Intergroup Trial 0160). *J Clin Oncol*. 2007;25:313–318.

Answer 54

Pathologic complete response (pCR) was 36%.

Minimal microscopic disease (MMD) was 30%.

Rusch VW, Giroux DJ, Kraut MJ, et al. Induction chemoradiation and surgical resection for non-small cell lung carcinomas of the superior sulcus: initial results of Southwest Oncology Group Trial 9416 (Intergroup Trial 0160). *J Thorac Cardiovasc Surg*. 2001;121:472–483.

Rusch VW, Giroux DJ, Kraut MJ, et al. Induction chemoradiation and surgical resection for superior sulcus non-small-cell lung carcinomas: long-term results of Southwest Oncology group Trial 9416 (Intergroup Trial 0160). *J Clin Oncol*. 2007;25:313–318.

Question 55

Did patients with minimal microscopic disease (MMD) at surgery in the SWOG 9416 protocol for Pancoast tumors have median survival closer to patients with pathologic complete response (pCR) or patients with gross residual disease (GRD)?

Question 56

What was the reported local control rate in the SWOG 9416 protocol for Pancoast tumors?

Question 57

What percent of patients treated on SWOG 9416 protocol for Pancoast tumors underwent a R0 resection?

What was the 5-year overall survival?

Question 58

What was the reported rate of brain-only distant failure in the SWOG 9416 protocol for Pancoast tumors?

Answer 55

Patients with MMD had survivals similar to those with gross residual disease.

pCR: 94 month median survival ($p = .02$)

MMD: 30 month median survival

GRD: 29 month median survival

Rusch VW, Giroux DJ, Kraut MJ, et al. Induction chemoradiation and surgical resection for non-small cell lung carcinomas of the superior sulcus: initial results of Southwest Oncology Group Trial 9416 (Intergroup Trial 0160). *J Thorac Cardiovasc Surg*. 2001;121:472–483.

Rusch VW, Giroux DJ, Kraut MJ, et al. Induction chemoradiation and surgical resection for superior sulcus non-small-cell lung carcinomas: long-term results of Southwest Oncology group Trial 9416 (Intergroup Trial 0160). *J Clin Oncol*. 2007;25:313–318.

Answer 56

Local control was 90% in the SWOG 9416 trial.

Rusch VW, Giroux DJ, Kraut MJ, et al. Induction chemoradiation and surgical resection for non-small cell lung carcinomas of the superior sulcus: initial results of Southwest Oncology Group Trial 9416 (Intergroup Trial 0160). *J Thorac Cardiovasc Surg*. 2001;121:472–483.

Rusch VW, Giroux DJ, Kraut MJ, et al. Induction chemoradiation and surgical resection for superior sulcus non-small-cell lung carcinomas: long-term results of Southwest Oncology Group Trial 9416 (Intergroup Trial 0160). *J Clin Oncol*. 2007;25:313–318.

Answer 57

93% of patients underwent a R0 resection.

5-year overall survival for R0 patients was 54% vs 44% for all patients on study.

Rusch VW, Giroux DJ, Kraut MJ, et al. Induction chemoradiation and surgical resection for non-small cell lung carcinomas of the superior sulcus: initial results of Southwest Oncology Group Trial 9416 (Intergroup Trial 0160). *J Thorac Cardiovasc Surg*. 2001;121:472–483.

Rusch VW, Giroux DJ, Kraut MJ, et al. Induction chemoradiation and surgical resection for superior sulcus non-small-cell lung carcinomas: long-term results of Southwest Oncology group Trial 9416 (Intergroup Trial 0160). *J Clin Oncol*. 2007;25:313–318.

Answer 58

Brain-only distant failure rate was 41% in the SWOG 9416 study.

Rusch VW, Giroux DJ, Kraut MJ, et al. Induction chemoradiation and surgical resection for non-small cell lung carcinomas of the superior sulcus: initial results of Southwest Oncology Group Trial 9416 (Intergroup Trial 0160). *J Thorac Cardiovasc Surg*. 2001;121:472–483.

Rusch VW, Giroux DJ, Kraut MJ, et al. Induction chemoradiation and surgical resection for superior sulcus non-small-cell lung carcinomas: long-term results of Southwest Oncology group Trial 9416 (Intergroup Trial 0160). *J Clin Oncol*. 2007;25:313–318.

Question 59

What treatment paradigm is used for treating stage I–IIIA, typical and atypical carcinoid tumors of the lung?

Question 60

What is the role of bevacizumab in advanced stage, recurrent, or metastatic non-small cell lung cancer?

Answer 59

Surgical resection is the mainstay of therapy for resectable, stage I–IIIA, typical and atypical carcinoid tumors.

No adjuvant radiation is recommended for completed resected, stage I–IIIA typical and stage I atypical, carcinoid tumors.

Adjuvant radiation is recommended for completely resected, stage II–IIIA, atypical carcinoid tumors.

NCCN Clinical Practice Guidelines in Oncology: Non-small cell lung cancer. Version 2.2010. National Comprehensive Cancer Network. March 5, 2010.

Answer 60

Bevacizumab in combination with paclitaxel and carboplatin is listed as 1st line therapy for PS 0–1, advanced stage, recurrent, or metastatic NSCLC per the 2010 NCCN guidelines for NSCLC.

Patients must meet the following criteria:

* nonsquamous NSCLC
* no history of hemoptysis ($\geq$ ½ teaspoon per event)

Other relative exclusion criteria are:

* brain metastasis
* uncontrolled hypertension
* therapeutic anticoagulation
* aspirin use > 325 mg/d
* use of NSAIDs known to inhibit platelet function

In 2006, the FDA approved bevacizumab for patients with unresectable, locally advanced, recurrent, or metastatic nonsquamous NSCLC.

ECOG recommends bevacizumab in combination with paclitaxel and carboplatin for select patients with advanced nonsquamous NSCLC based on the results of a phase III clinical trials (ECOG 4599).

Bevacizumab blocks the vascular endothelial growth factor and inhibits angiogenesis.

In squamous histology patients, a phase II trial showed a prohibitive rate of pulmonary hemorrhage (Johnson DH et al.).

Sandler A, Gray P, Perry MC, et al. Paclitaxel-carboplatin alone or with bevacizumab for non-small cell lung cancer. *N Engl J Med*. 2006;355:2542–2550.

NCCN Clinical Practice Guidelines in Oncology: Non-small cell lung cancer. Version 2.2010. National Comprehensive Cancer Network. March 5, 2010.

Johnson DH, Fehrenbacher L, Novotny W, et al. Randomized phase II trial comparing bevacizumab plus carbopatin and paclitaxel with carboplatin and paclitaxel alone in previously untreated locally advanced or metastatic non-small cell lung cancer. *J Clin Oncol*. 2004;21:1804–1809.

Question 61

Is there a role for continuation maintenance therapy in NSCLC patients with response or stable disease after 4–6 cycles of chemotherapy?

Question 62

What is the difference between continuation maintenance chemotherapy vs switch maintenance chemotherapy?

Answer 61

For continuation maintenance therapy, biologic agents should be continued until evidence of disease progression or unacceptable toxicity.

Bevacizumab (category 1) may be continued beyond 4 to 6 cycles of initial therapy (e.g., platinum-doublet chemotherapy given with bevacizumab).

Cetuximab (category 1) may be continued beyond 4 to 6 cycles of initial therapy (e.g., cisplatin, vinorelbine, and cetuximab therapy).

Pemetrexed (category 2B) may also be given as continuation maintenance therapy in <u>nonsquamous</u> histology.

No randomized trials support the continuation maintenance of conventional cytotoxic agents beyond 4 to 6 cycles of therapy.

Sandler A, Gray P, Perry MC, et al. Paclitaxel-carboplatin alone or with bevacizumab for non-small cell lung cancer. *N Engl J Med*. 2006;355:2542–2550.

Patel JD, Hensing TA, Rademaker A, et al. Phase II study of pemetrexed and carboplatin plus bevacizumab with maintenance pemetrexed and bevacizumab as first-line therapy for nonsquamous non-small-cell lung cancer. *J Clin Oncol*. 2009;27:3284–3289.

Pirker R, Pereira JR, Szczesna A, et al. Cetuximab plus chemotherapy in patients with advanced non-small-cell lung cancer (FLEX): an open-label randomised phase III trial. *Lancet*. 2009;373:1525–1531.

NCCN Clinical Practice Guidelines in Oncology: Non-small cell lung cancer. Version 2.2010. National Comprehensive Cancer Network. March 5, 2010.

Answer 62

Continuation maintenance refers to the use of at least one of the agents given in first-line chemotherapy.

Switch maintenance refers to the initiation of a different agent, not included as part of the first-line regimen.

Gerber DE, Schiller JH. Carcinoma of the lung. In: Skeel RT, Khleif SN, eds. *Handbook of Cancer Chemotherapy*. 8th ed. Philadelphia, PA: Lippincott Williams & Wilkins; 2011:109–110.

Question 63

Is there a role for switch maintenance therapy in NSCLC patients with response or stable disease after 4–6 cycles of chemotherapy?

Question 64   SMALL CELL LUNG CANCER

What is the role of surgical resection in small cell lung cancer patients?

Question 65

If a patient undergoes surgical resection (lobectomy and mediastinal node dissection) of a clinical T1N0 small cell lung cancer, what is the appropriate adjuvant therapy for a pathologic stage T1N0 patient?

How about for a pathologic T1N2 patient?

Question 66

What is the recommended chemotherapy regimen/doses to be given concurrent with radiation in limited stage small cell lung cancer patients?

Answer 63

Switch maintenance therapy has shown a benefit in progression-free and overall survival with the initiation of pemetrexed or erlotinib in patients who did not progress after 4–6 cycles of first-line chemotherapy.

Pemetrexed (category 2B) may be initiated after 4 to 6 cycles of first-line platinum-doublet chemotherapy in nonsquamous histologies.

Erlotinib (category 2B) may be initiated after 4 to 6 cycles of first-line platinum-doublet chemotherapy.

Ciuleanu T, Brodowicz T, Zielinski C, et al. Maintenance pemetrexed plus best supportive care versus placebo plus best supportive care: a randomized, double-blind, phase 3 study. *Lancet*. 2009;374:1432–1440.

Cappuzzo F, Ciuleanu T, Stelmakh L, et al. SATURN: a double-blind, randomized, phase III study of maintenance erlotinib versus placebo following nonprogression with first-line platinum-based chemotherapy in patients with advanced NSCLC [abstract]. *J Clin Oncol*. 2009;27(Suppl 1):Abstract 8001.

Answer 64

Surgical resection is appropriate for properly staged, T1-2N0M0 patients.

Patients should have CT chest and upper abdomen, FDG PET-CT, brain imaging, and surgical mediastinal staging to document clinical N0M0 disease.

Resection should be a lobectomy with mediastinal dissection or sampling.

Patients with stage > T1-2N0M0 do not benefit from surgery.

Kalemkerian GP, Akerley W, Bogner P, et al. Small cell lung cancer. *J Natl Compr Canc Netw*. 2011;9:1086–1113.

Lad T, Piantadosi S, Thomas P, et al. A prospective randomized trial to determine the benefit of surgical resection of residual disease following response of small cell lung cancer to combination chemotherapy. *Chest*. 1994;106:320S–323S.

Answer 65

Appropriate adjuvant therapy for a pathologic T1N0 small cell carcinoma patient after lobectomy and mediastinal nodal dissection would be adjuvant chemotherapy alone.

Appropriate adjuvant therapy for a pathologic T1N2 small cell carcinoma patient after lobectomy and mediastinal nodal dissection would be adjuvant, concurrent chemotherapy and mediastinal radiotherapy.

Kalemkerian GP, Akerley W, Bogner P, et al. Small cell lung cancer. *J Natl Compr Canc Netw*. 2011;9:1086–1113.

Answer 66

Cisplatin, 60 mg/m^2 day 1, and Etoposide, 120 mg/m^2 day 1–3, on weeks 1, 4 of radiation.

A maximum of 4–6 cycles of chemotherapy are given for limited stage patients.

Turrisi AT III, Kim K, Blum R, et al. Twice-daily compared with once-daily thoracic radiotherapy in limited small-cell lung cancer treated concurrently with cisplatin and etoposide. *N Engl J Med*. 1999;340:265–271.

Question 67

What radiation dose-fractionation regimens are recommended by the 2011 Small Cell Lung Cancer NCCN Guidelines for limited stage patients?

Question 68

What radiation dose-fractionation schedules were tested in the landmark, phase III randomized trial, INT 0096 (RTOG 8815), in limited stage small cell lung cancer?

What were the results of this trial?

Question 69

What is the main criticism of the phase III randomized trial, INT 0096 (RTOG 8815), in limited stage small cell lung cancer?

Answer 67

Limited stage patients should receive either 45 Gy in 30 fractions of 1.5 Gy per fraction delivered twice daily with at least a 6 hour interfraction interval, or 60–70 Gy in 30–35 fractions of 2 Gy per fraction delivered once daily.

Kalemkerian GP, Akerley W, Bogner P, et al. Small cell lung cancer. *J Natl Compr Canc Netw.* 2011;9:1086–1113.
Turrisi AT III, Kim K, Blum R, et al. Twice-daily compared with once-daily thoracic radiotherapy in limited stage small-cell lung cancer. *Int J Radiot Oncol Biol Phys.* 2004;59:943–951.

Answer 68

412 limited stage, small cell lung patients were randomized between 45 Gy in 30 fractions of 1.5 Gy per fraction delivered twice daily with at least a 6 hour interfraction interval, vs 45 Gy in 25 fractions of 1.8 Gy per fraction delivered once daily.

The twice daily arm had improved median survival (23 mo. vs 19 mo.; $p = .04$) and 5-year overall survival (26% vs 16%; $p = .04$).

There was a significantly higher rate of acute grade 3 esophagitis in the twice daily arm (27% vs 11%; $p < .001$).

There were fewer local failures within the twice daily arm (36% vs 52%; $p = .06$)

Both arms received the same concurrent chemotherapy, CDDP (60 mg/m^2) on day 1 and Etoposide (120 mg/m^2) on days 1–3, repeated every 3 weeks for four cycles

All patients achieving a complete response to chemoradiation received prophylactic cranial radiation, 25 Gy in 10 fractions.

Turrisi AT III, Kim K, Blum R, et al. Twice-daily compared with once-daily thoracic radiotherapy in limited stage small-cell lung cancer. *Int J Radiat Oncol Biol Phys.* 2004;59:943–951.

Answer 69

The once daily arm of 45 Gy in 25 fractions of 1.8 Gy per fraction is less biologically effective (lower BED) than the twice daily arm of 45 Gy in 30 fractions of 1.5 Gy per fraction.

The twice daily arm had improved median survival (23 mo. vs 19 mo.) and 5-year overall survival (26% vs 16%).

There were fewer local failures within the twice daily arm (36% vs 52%; $p = .06$)

There was a significantly higher rate of acute grade 3 esophagitis in the twice daily arm (27% vs 11%; $p < .001$).

Both arms received the same concurrent chemotherapy, CDDP (60 mg/m^2) on day 1 and Etoposide (120 mg/m^2) on days 1–3, repeated every 3 weeks for four cycles.

All patients achieving a complete response to chemoradiation received prophylactic cranial irradiation, 25 Gy in 10 fractions.

Turrisi AT III, Kim K, Blum R, et al. Twice-daily compared with once-daily thoracic radiotherapy in limited stage small-cell lung cancer. *Int J Radiot Oncol Biol Phys.* 2004;59:943–951.

Question 70

What is the improvement in overall survival and local control when thoracic radiation therapy is added to chemotherapy in limited stage small cell lung cancer patients?

Question 71

When combining chemotherapy and radiation for limited stage small cell lung cancer, what is the optimal timing of the two therapies?

Question 72

Is there a role for thoracic radiation in extensive stage small cell lung cancer patients?

Answer 70

Two meta-analyses have been done evaluating the benefit of adding thoracic radiation therapy to chemotherapy for limited stage small cell lung cancer patients, both showing an overall survival benefit of 5.4%, and a local control benefit of 25–30%.

Warde et al. evaluated 11 randomized trials showing a 2-year overall survival benefit (20% vs 15%) and a local control benefit (47% vs 24%).

Pignon et al. evaluated 13 randomized trials containing 2140 patients showing a 3-year overall survival benefit (8.9% vs 14.3%).

Warde P, Payne D. Does thoracic irradiation improve survival and local control in limited-stage small-cell carcinoma of the lung? A meta-analysis. *J Clin Oncol.* 1992;10:890–895.

Pignon JP, Arriagade R, Ihde DC, et al. A meta-analysis of thoracic radiotherapy for small-cell lung cancer. *N Engl J Med.* 1992;327:1618–1624.

Answer 71

Concurrent chemoradiation is better than sequential therapy and early institution of radiation with cycle 1 or 2 of chemotherapy is recommended.

Takada et al. reported a phase III randomized trial of concurrent vs sequential chemoradiation using 4 cycles of CDDP/Etoposide with radiation starting cycle 1 vs after completing all chemotherapy. The 2-, 3-, and 5-year survival rates favored the concurrent, early radiation (54%, 30%, 24% vs 35%, 20%, 18%; p = ns). This 231 patient trial was underpowered to detect a statistically significant survival difference (median survival favored concurrent radiation: 27 month vs 20 month; p = .07).

Meta-analysis of trials using platinum-containing chemotherapy showed significant benefit to early radiation.

Takada M, Rukuoka M, Kawahara M, et al. Phase III study of concurrent versus sequential thoracic radiotherapy in combination with cisplatin and etoposide for limited-stage small-cell lung cancer: results of the Japan Clinical Oncology Group Study 9104. *J Clin Oncol.* 2002;20:3054–3060.

Pijils-Johannesma M, De Ruysscher D, Vansteenkiste J, et al. Timing of chest radiotherapy in patients with limited stage small cell lung cancer: a systematic review and meta-analysis of randomized controlled trials. *Cancer Treat Rev.* 2007;33:461–473.

Answer 72

Yes. A phase III, prospective randomized trial by Jeremic et al. showed a benefit to adding accelerated, twice-daily radiation, 54 Gy in 36 fx at 1.5 Gy/fx, to chemotherapy in extensive stage patients who achieved a complete response at distant sites after 3 cycles of cisplatin and etoposide chemotherapy.

Median survival (17 vs 11 months) and 5-year overall survival (9.1% vs 3.7%; p = .04) favored the addition of thoracic radiation.

All randomized patients had a CR to EPx3 at distant sites and were randomized between:

· Arm 1: 54 Gy/36fx/1.5 Gy BID + ECx2 > EPx2
· Arm 2: EPx4

Concurrent chemotherapy during radiation was etoposide and carboplatin.

All randomized patients also received prophylactic cranial irradiation, 25 Gy in 10 fx.

Jeremic B, Shibamoto Y, Nikolic N, et al. Role of radiation therapy in the combined-modality treatment of patients with extensive disease small cell lung cancer: a randomized study. *J Clin Oncol.* 1999;17:2092–2099.

Question 73

What benefits does tobacco cessation hold for small cell lung cancer patients?

Question 74

What are the 2011 Small Cell Lung Cancer NCCN guidelines for radiation therapy constraints for mean lung dose (MLD) and V20 (volume of normal lung receiving greater than or equal to 20 Gy)?

Question 75

What is the 2011 Small Cell Lung Cancer NCCN guidelines for radiation therapy constraints for mean esophagus dose?

Question 76

What is the 2011 Small Cell Lung Cancer NCCN guidelines for radiation therapy constraints for the heart?

Answer 73

First, it has been shown in a retrospective review (Videtic GMM et al.) that small cell lung cancer patients who quit smoking tobacco prior to treatment have improved survival and less toxicity than those who continue to smoke.

Second, patients who continue to smoke have a higher rate of secondary malignancies (Richardson GE et al.).

Videtic GMM, Stitt LW, Dar AR, et al. Continued cigarette smoking by patients receiving concurrent chemoradiotherapy for limited-stage small-cell lung cancer is associated with decreased survival. *J Clin Oncol*. 2003;21:1544–1549.
Richardson GE, Tucker MA, Venzon DJ, et al. Smoking cessation after successful treatment of small-cell lung cancer is associated with fewer smoking-related second primary cancers. *Ann Intern Med*. 1993;119:383–390.

Answer 74

Mean Lung Dose (MLD) should be less than or equal to 20 Gy; V20 should be less than 40%.

Kalemkerian GP, Akerley W, Bogner P, et al. Small cell lung cancer. *J Natl Compr Canc Netw*. 2011;9:1086–1113.
Kim TH, Cho KH, Pyo HR, et al. Dose-volumetric parameters for predicting severe radiation pneumonitis after three-dimensional conformal radiation therapy for lung cancer. *Radiology*. 2005;235:208–215.

Answer 75

Mean esophagus dose should be less than 34 Gy.

Kalemkerian GP, Akerley W, Bogner P, et al. Small cell lung cancer. *J Natl Compr Canc Netw*. 2011;9:1086–1113.
Rose J, Rodrigues G, Yaremko B, et al. Systematic review of dose-volume parameters in the prediction of esophagitis in thoracic radiotherapy. *Radiother Oncol*. 2009;91:282–287.

Answer 76

Up to one-third of the heart can receive 60 Gy, two-thirds 45 Gy, and whole heart 40 Gy.

Kalemkerian GP, Akerley W, Bogner P, et al. Small cell lung cancer. *J Natl Compr Canc Netw*. 2011;9:1086–1113.

Question 77

What are the limits for the maximum spinal cord dose when using an accelerated hyperfractionated regimen (45 Gy/30 fx at 1.5 Gy BID) and when using a standard, once-daily fractionation scheme for limited stage small cell lung cancer patients?

Question 78

What are the median survival rates for limited and extensive stage small cell lung cancer (SCLC) patients?

Question 79

What percentage of patients with small cell lung cancer have brain metastases at the time of diagnosis?

What is the cumulative incidence of brain metastases at two years in these patients?

Question 80

What was the difference in outcomes seen in the Auperin meta-analysis of prophylactic cranial irradiation (PCI) for small cell lung cancer (SCLC) patients in complete remission?

Answer 77

The maximum spinal cord dose limit for the accelerated, hyperfractionated regimen is 41 Gy, and for the standard fractionated, once-daily regimen is 50 Gy.

Answer 78

Limited stage patients have median survival rate of 23 months while extensive stage patients have median survival rate of 7 months.

Slotman B, Faivre-Finn C, Kramer G, et al. Prophylactic cranial irradiation in extensive small-cell lung cancer. *N Engl J Med*. 2007;357:664–672.

Turrisi AT III, Kim K, Blum R, et al. Twice-daily compared with once-daily thoracic radiotherapy in limited stage small-cell lung cancer. *Int J Radiot Oncol Biol Phys*. 2004;59:943–951.

Answer 79

Ten percent of small cell lung cancer patients have brain metastasis at the time of diagnosis, with a cumulative incidence of more than 50% at 2 years.

Arriagada R, Le Chevalier T, Borie F, et al. Prophylactic cranial irradiation for patients with small-cell lung cancer in complete remission. *J Natl Cancer Inst*. 1995;87:183–190.

Komaki R. Prophylactic cranial irradiation for small cell carcinoma of the lung. *Cancer Treat Symp*. 1985;2:35–39.

Answer 80

The Auperin meta-analysis reviewed seven randomized trials that included 987 SCLC patients in complete remission who received PCI between 1977 and 1995. PCI decreased the incidence of brain metastases by half (58.6% vs 33.3%) and improved 3-year overall survival from 15.3% to 20.7%.

Auperin A, Arriagada R, Pignon JP, et al. Prophylactic cranial irradiation for patients with small-cell lung cancer in complete remission. Prophylactic Cranial Irradiation Overview Collaborative Group. *N Engl J Med*. 1999;341:476–484.

Question 81

What is the effect of the timing of prophylactic cranial irradiation (PCI) after initiating chemotherapy for small cell lung cancer (SCLC)?

Question 82

What is the rationale for prophylactic cranial irradiation (PCI) for extensive stage small cell lung cancer (SCLC)?

Question 83

What were some critiques of the Slotman EORTC 08993 study investigating the role of prophylactic cranial irradiation (PCI) in extensive stage small cell lung cancer (SCLC)?

Question 84

What were the most common acute effects after prophylactic cranial irradiation (PCI) in the Slotman EORTC 08993 trial in extensive stage small cell lung cancer (SCLC)?

Answer 81

According to the Auperin meta-analysis, there was a decrease in risk of brain metastases with earlier PCI (< 4–6 months vs > 6 months) without an effect on risk of death.

The Auperin meta-analysis reviewed seven randomized trials that included 987 SCLC patients in complete remission who received PCI between 1977 and 1995. PCI decreased the incidence of brain metastases by half (58.6% vs 33.3%) and improved 3-year overall survival from 15.3% to 20.7%.

Auperin A, Arriagada R, Pignon JP, et al. Prophylactic cranial irradiation for patients with small-cell lung cancer in complete remission. Prophylactic Cranial Irradiation Overview Collaborative Group. *N Engl J Med.* 1999;341:476–484.

Answer 82

Slotman et al. investigated the role of PCI in patients with extensive SCLC who had a response to chemotherapy in EORTC 08993. Median survival was 5.4 months without PCI and 6.7 months with PCI. Incidence of symptomatic brain metastases was decreased with PCI (15% vs 40%). Disease-free survival was also improved.

Slotman B, Faivre-Finn C, Kramer G, et al. Prophylactic cranial irradiation in extensive stage small cell lung cancer. *N Engl J Med.* 2007;357:664–672.

Answer 83

No pre-treatment MRI was done.

The RT group was more likely to receive chemotherapy at the time of extracranial progression (68% vs 45%).

Only 59% of patients in the control group received whole brain radiation therapy for intracranial progression of disease.

Slotman B, Faivre-Finn C, Kramer G, et al. Prophylactic cranial irradiation in extensive stage small cell lung cancer. *N Engl J Med.* 2007;357:664–672.

Answer 84

At 3 months, the largest negative impact of PCI was fatigue and hair loss.

Worsening role, emotional, and cognitive function based on health-related quality of life assessments were also seen after PCI.

Slotman B, Mauer ME, Bottomley A, et al. Prophylactic cranial irradiation in extensive disease small-cell lung cancer: short-term health-related quality of life and patient reported symptoms: results of an international Phase III randomized controlled trial by the EORTC Radiation Oncology and Lung Cancer Groups. *J Clin Oncol.* 2009;27:78–84.

Question 85

What is (are) the appropriate dose and fractionation scheme(s) for whole brain radiation used for prophylactic cranial irradiation in small cell lung cancer patients?

Question 86

Has dose escalation proven to improve outcomes of prophylactic cranial irradiation (PCI) for small cell lung cancer (SCLC) patients?

Question 87

Were there any differences in quality of life or chronic neurotoxicity in different doses of prophylactic cranial irradiation (PCI) for small cell lung cancer (SCLC) patients according to RTOG 0212?

Question 88

What is the rate of cognitive dysfunction in small cell lung cancer (SCLC) patients before and after prophylactic cranial irradiation (PCI)?

Answer 85

Two regimens are recommended by the NCCN guidelines for limited stage patients: 30 Gy in 15 fx or 25 Gy in 10 fx.

Kalemkerian GP, Akerley W, Bogner P, et al. Small cell lung cancer. *J Natl Compr Canc Netw.* 2011;9:1086–1113.
Le Pechoux C, Dunant A, Senan S, et al. Standard dose versus higher dose prophylactic cranial irradiation (PCI) in patient with limited stage small cell lung cancer in complete remission after chemotherapy and thoracic radiotherapy. *Lancet Oncol.* 2009; 10:467–474.

Answer 86

RTOG (Radiation Therapy Oncology Group) 0212 was a prospective randomized trial, which assessed the effect of dose and fractionation schedule of PCI on the incidence of chronic neurotoxicity (CNt) and changes in quality of life for patients with limited-stage SCLC. Patients were randomized to PCI with 25 Gy in 10 fx, and 36 Gy delivered either in 18 fx (one fraction per day) or 24 fx (two fractions per day).

No differences in the 2-year incidence of brain metastases were seen.

There was an overall survival and chest relapse advantage for the 25 Gy in 10 fx arm (42% vs 37%) due to increased cancer-related mortality in the high-dose group.

Le Pechoux C, Dunant A, Senan S, et al. Standard-dose versus higher-dose prophylactic cranial irradiation (PCI) in patients with limited-stage small-cell lung cancer in complete remission after chemotherapy and thoracic radiotherapy (PCI99-01, EORTC 22003-08004, RTOG 0212, and IFCT 99-01): a randomized clinical trial. *Lancet Oncol.* 2009;467–474.

Answer 87

No significant differences were seen in quality of life. However, the 36 Gy cohort exhibited increased chronic neurotoxicity at 12 months. Because of this increased risk, 25 Gy remains the standard of care for patients with limited stage SCLC who have a complete response to initial chemoradiation.

RTOG (Radiation Therapy Oncology Group) 0212 randomized patients to PCI with 25 Gy in 10 fx, and 36 Gy delivered either in 18 fx (one fraction per day) or 24 fx (two fractions per day).

Wolfson AH, Bae K, Komaki R, et al. Primary analysis of a phase II randomized trial RTOG 0212: impact of different total doses and schedules of prophylactic cranial irradiation on chronic neurotoxicity and quality of life or patients with limited-disease small-cell lung cancer. *Int J Radiat Oncol Biol Phys.* 2011;81:77–84.

Answer 88

High rates of cognitive dysfunction are seen in this patient population prior to PCI. In a prospective series of 30 patients with limited SCLC who had complete response to definitive treatment to the primary tumor, 29 of 30 patients (97%) had cognitive deficits on neuropsychological testing prior to PCI. No significant difference was seen in evaluation after PCI.

Komaki R, Meyers CA, Shin DM, et al. Evaluation of cognitive function in patients with limited small cell lung cancer prior to and shortly following prophylactic cranial irradiation. *Int J Radiat Oncol Biol Phys.* 1995;33:179–182.

Question 89

Is there any role for prophylactic cranial irradiation (PCI) for non-small cell lung cancer (NSCLC)?

Question 90   **THYMOMA**

How is the mediastinum subdivided into compartments, and what structures are in each?

In which compartment are thymomas most commonly found?

Question 91

What is the mechanism of myasthenia gravis, and what percentage of patients with thymoma also have myasthenia gravis?

Question 92

What paraneoplastic syndromes are commonly seen in patients with thymoma?

Answer 89

No. There has been no difference in 1-year overall survival or disease-free survival in 4 randomized trials.

PCI did improve CNS relapse rate at 1 year (7.7% vs 18%; $p = .004$) in RTOG 0214.

RTOG 0214 investigated the role of PCI vs observation in patients with stage IIIA–B, non-small cell lung cancer without disease progression after definitive treatment.

Gore EM, Bae K, Wong SJ, et al. Phase III comparison of prophylactic cranial irradiation versus observation in patients with locally advanced non-small-cell lung cancer: primary analysis of radiation therapy oncology group study RTOG 0214. *J Clin Oncol.* 2011;29:272–278.

Kalemkerian GP, Akerley W, Bogner P, et al. Small Cell Lung Cancer. *J Natl Compr Canc Netw.* 2011;9:1086–1113.

Answer 90

Anterior mediastinum (anterior to pericarcium and great vessels): thymus, lymph nodes, small vessels

Middle mediastinum: heart, proximal great vessels, central airway structures, lymph nodes

Posterior mediastinum (posterior to heart and great vessels): sympathetic chain ganglia, vagus nerve, thoracic duct, esophagus

Thymomas are most commonly found in the anterior mediastinum.

Hung AY, Eng TY, Scarbrough TJ, et al. Mediastinum and Trachea. In: Halperin EC, Perez CA, Brady LW, eds. *Perez and Brady's Principles and Practice of Radiation Oncology.* 5th ed. Philadelphia, PA: Lippincott Williams & Wilkins; 2008:1109–1130.

Answer 91

Myasthenia gravis is an autoimmune disease characterized by the presence of antibodies that react with postsynaptic nicotinic acetylcholine receptors at the neuromuscular junction. Thirty to forty percent of thymoma patients have myasthenia gravis. Conversely, only 10–15% of patients with myasthenia gravis have a thymoma.

Hung AY, Eng TY, Scarbrough TJ, et al. Mediastinum and trachea. In: Halperin EC, Perez CA, Brady LW, eds. *Perez and Brady's Principles and Practice of Radiation Oncology.* 5th ed. Philadelphia, PA: Lippincott Williams & Wilkins; 2008:1109–1130.

Lara Jr PN. Malignant thymoma: current status and future directions. *Cancer Terat Rev.* 2000;26:127–131.

Drachman DB. Myasthenia gravis. *N Engl J Med.* 1994;330:1797–1810.

Answer 92

Myasthenia gravis is the most common, and other syndromes include benign cytopenia, hypogamma-globulinemia, and polymyositis.

Lewis JE, Wick MR, Scheithauer BW, et al. Thymoma. A clinicopathologic review. *Cancer.* 1987;60:2727–2743.

Souadjian JV, Enriquez P, Silverstein MN, et al. The spectrum of diseases associated with thymoma. Coincidence or syndrome. *Arch Intern Med.* 174;134:374–379.

Question 93

What is the Masaoka staging system for thymomas?

Question 94

What is the treatment paradigm for thymoma?

Question 95

How does the clinical behavior of thymic carcinomas differ from thymomas?

How are thymic carcinomas treated?

Answer 93

The Masaoka staging system is the most widely used staging system for thymomas.

I. Macroscopically completely encapsulated, with no microscopic capsular invasion

II.
   a. Macroscopic invasion into surrounding mediastinal fatty tissue or mediastinal pleura
   b. Microscopic invasion into the capsule

III. Macroscopic invasion into surrounding organs
   a. Pleural or pericardial implants/dissemination
   b. Lymphogenous or hematogenous metastases

Hung AY, Eng TY, Scarbrough TJ, et al. Mediastinum and trachea. In: Halperin EC, Perez CA, Brady LW, eds. *Perez and Brady's Principles and Practice of Radiation Oncology.* 5th ed. Philadelphia, PA: Lippincott Williams & Wilkins; 2008:1109–1130.

Answer 94

Surgical resection is the mainstay of treatment for thymomas, and a complete en bloc surgical resection remains the treatment of choice for all thymomas regardless of extent of invasion, except in rare advanced cases with extensive intra- or extrathoracic metastasis. Adjuvant radiation should be considered for any residual disease or incomplete resection regardless of stage. For stage I patients and possibly stage II (controversial), the recurrence rates are low enough that the benefit from radiation is marginal. For patients with stage III disease, recurrence rates are high enough that adjuvant radiation should be strongly considered although the literature is not conclusive.

Hung AY, Eng TY, Scarbrough TJ, et al. Mediastinum and trachea. In: Halperin EC, Perez CA, Brady LW, eds. *Perez and Brady's Principles and Practice of Radiation Oncology.* 5th ed. Philadelphia, PA: Lippincott Williams & Wilkins; 2008:1109–1130.

Kondo K, Monden Y. Therapy for thymic epithelial tumors: a clinical study of 1320 patients from Japan. *Ann Thorac Surg.* 2003;76(3):878–884; discussion 884–885.

Curran Jr WJ, Kornstein MJ, Brooks JJ, et al. Invasive thymoma: the role of mediastinal irradiation following complete or incomplete surgical resection. *J Clin Oncol.* 1988;6:1722–1727.

Maggi G, Casadio C, Cavallo A, et al. Thymoma: results of 241 operated cases. *Ann Thorac Surg.* 1991;51:152–156.

Answer 95

Thymic carcinomas are more aggressive than thymomas and have a higher propensity for capsular invasion. Patients frequently present with advanced disease and have a poorer 5-year survival than with thymomas.

Complete surgical resection is the preferred method of treatment, although recurrence is common. Incomplete resections followed by adjuvant radiation and/or chemotherapy have shown some benefits without increased morbidity and mortality. Despite aggressive treatments, most patients do poorly; overall 5-year survival according to one report was 1%, with all 14 patients dead after 9 years.

Hung AY, Eng TY, Scarbrough TJ, et al. Mediastinum and Trachea. In: Halperin EC, Perez CA, Brady LW, eds. *Perez and Brady's Principles and Practice of Radiation Oncology.* 5th ed. Philadelphia, PA: Lippincott Williams & Wilkins; 2008:1109–1130.

Kondo K, Monden Y. Therapy for thymic epithelial tumors: a clinical study of 1320 patients from Japan. *Ann Thorac Surg* 2003;76:878–884; discussion 884–885.

Wick MR, Scheithauer BW, Weiland LH, et al. Primary thymic carcinomas. *Am J Pathol.* 1982;6:613–630.

De Montpreville V, Macchiarini P, Dulmet E. Thymic neuroendocrine carcinoma (carcinoid): a clinicopathologic study of fourteen cases. *J Thorac Cardiovasc Surg.* 1996;111:134–141.

Question 96

What are common tumors that arise from the heart and pericardium?

What percentage are benign vs malignant?

Question 97

What is the most common primary pericardial tumor, and how is it generally treated?

Question 98

What is the median survival of patients with malignant primary tumors of the heart?

Answer 96

Primary cardiac tumors are exceedingly rare, with an overall incidence of 0.021% (range 0%–0.19%). Approximately 75% are benign, consisting mostly of atrial myxomas, lipomas, papillary fibroelastomas, and rhabdomyomas, and 25% are malignant, consisting mostly of malignant mesothelioma, fibrosarcoma, angiosarcoma, and teratoma. Metastases to the heart and pericardium are over 20 times more common than primary cardiac tumors.

Reynen K. Frequency of primary tumors of the heart. *Am J Cardiol*. 1996;77:107.

Tendulkar RD, Chidel MA, Macklis RM. Tumors of the Heart and Great Vessels. In: Halperin EC, Perez CA, Brady LW, eds. *Perez and Brady's Principles and Practice of Radiation Oncology*. 5th ed. Philadelphia, PA: Lippincott Williams & Wilkins; 2008:1154–1161.

Lam KY, Dickens P, Lam Chan AC. Tumors of the heart: a 20-year experience with a review of 12,485 consecutive autopsies. *Arch Pathol Lab Med* 1993;117:1027–1031.

Answer 97

Mesothelioma is the most common pericardial neoplasm and may either be confined to the pericardial sac at diagnosis, or extend beyond it, involving the myocardium or mediastinal structures. Locally advanced or metastatic disease is common because these tumors are usually asymptomatic until they are more advanced. As with pleural mesothelioma, surgical resection of all gross disease is the treatment of choice in the definitive setting, and a high rate of local recurrence is expected without adjuvant therapy. Postoperative radiation therapy and chemotherapy should be considered. The radiation treatment volume should include the entire pericardial surface and middle mediastinal lymph nodes.

Aggarwal P, Wali JP, Aggarwal J. Pericardial mesothelioma presenting as a mediastinal mass. *Singapore Med J*. 1991;32:185–186.

Tendulkar RD, Chidel MA, Macklis RM. Tumors of the Heart and Great Vessels. In: Halperin EC, Perez CA, Brady LW, eds. *Perez and Brady's Principles and Practice of Radiation Oncology*. 5th ed. Philadelphia, PA: Lippincott Williams & Wilkins; 2008:1154–1161.

Answer 98

The median survival of patients with malignant primary tumors is approximately 1 year, and both local and distant relapse is common. Worse outcomes are seen for tumors with high mitotic activity, and the ability to resect all gross tumor and a left atrial site of origin predict for longer survival. The use of adjuvant radiation therapy has been associated with longer survival, whereas adjuvant chemotherapy has provided mixed results. However, all studies are retrospective and may be biased by patient selection.

Tendulkar RD, Chidel MA, Macklis RM. Tumors of the Heart and Great Vessels. In: Halperin EC, Perez CA, Brady LW, eds. *Perez and Brady's Principles and Practice of Radiation Oncology*. 5th ed. Philadelphia, PA: Lippincott Williams & Wilkins; 2008:1154–1161.

Burke AP, Cowan D, Virmani R. Primary sarcomas of the heart. *Cancer*. 1992;69:387–395.

Poole GV, Breyer RH, Holiday RH, et al. Tumors of the heart: surgical considerations. *J Cardiovasc Surg*. 1984;25:5.

Putnam JB, Sweeney MS, Colon R, et al. Primary cardiac sarcomas. *Ann Thorac Surg*. 1991;51:906–910.

Tazelaar HD, Locke TJ, McGregor CG. Pathology of surgically excised primary cardiac neoplasms. *Mayo Clin Proc*. 1992;57:957–965.

Question 99

How are malignant primary cardiac neoplasms managed?

Question 100

What are the doses, targets, and fractionation of adjuvant radiation therapy to the heart?

Question 101

What late toxicities may be seen with irradiation to the heart?

Answer 99

Surgical resection is the primary treatment of choice for patients with primary malignant cardiac tumors. However, local resection is often incomplete due to the extent and invasion of tumors. Sarcomas account for almost all primary malignant cardiac neoplasms, and treatment principles should be similar to those for soft tissue sarcoma arising from other areas of the body. After complete or incomplete resection of tumor, adjuvant radiation and chemotherapy may be used in an attempt to improve local and distant control. Anecdotal cases of orthotopic heart transplantation (OHT) for patients with malignant cardiac neoplasms have described in the literature; however, results have been mixed with some reports of long-term survivors, while many other patients have developed distant metastases and death within months of transplant.

Tendulkar RD, Chidel MA, Macklis RM. Tumors of the heart and great vessels. In: Halperin EC, Perez CA, Brady LW, eds. *Perez and Brady's Principles and Practice of Radiation Oncology.* 5th ed. Philadelphia, PA: Lippincott Williams & Wilkins; 2008:1154–1161.

Answer 100

For completely resected tumors with negative margins, doses of 45–50 Gy at 1.8–2 Gy per fraction should be considered. An additional 10–20 Gy boost should be considered to a smaller volume for microscopic or gross residual disease. The initial target should include all areas known to harbor tumor before surgery plus a margin of at least 2 cm. Among patients with pericardial mesothelioma, the entire pericardium should be included in the initial target volume.

Coverage of the middle and inferior mediastinal lymph nodes should be considered for tumors with high propensity for nodal involvement, such as mesothelioma, angiosarcoma, rhabdomyosarcoma, carcinoma, or lymphoma.

Tendulkar RD, Chidel MA, Macklis RM. Tumors of the heart and great vessels. In: Halperin EC, Perez CA, Brady LW, eds. *Perez and Brady's Principles and Practice of Radiation Oncology.* 5th ed. Philadelphia, PA: Lippincott Williams & Wilkins; 2008:1154–1161.

Answer 101

Radiation induced heart disease (RIHD) may manifest as pericarditis, myocarditis, conduction defects, or coronary heart disease. Risk factors for developing RIHD include total dose, dose per fraction, irradiated volume, radiation technique, age at exposure, and use of concurrent or anthracycline-based chemotherapy. Emami et al estimated the TD 5/5 for developing pericarditis to be 40 Gy for the whole heart, and 60 Gy for 1/3 of the heart. Other late toxicities include radiation pneumonitis and fibrosis. However, these effects have not been well-documented, likely as a result of poor overall survival in these patients.

Tendulkar RD, Chidel MA, Macklis RM. Tumors of the heart and great vessels. In: Halperin EC, Perez CA, Brady LW, eds. *Perez and Brady's Principles and Practice of Radiation Oncology.* 5th ed. Philadelphia, PA: Lippincott Williams & Wilkins; 2008:1154–1161.

Emami B, Lyman J, Brown A, et al. Tolerance of normal tissue to therapeutic irradiation. *Int J Radiat Oncol Biol Phys.* 1991;31:109–122.

Question 102

What is the most common cause of mesothelioma?

Question 103

What are the histologic subtypes of mesothelioma?

Which is the most common?

Which has the worst prognosis?

Question 104

What are the four EORTC poor prognostic factors for mesothelioma?

Question 105

What is the first-line chemotherapy in unresectable mesothelioma?

Answer 102

Asbestos exposure is the primary cause of pleural and peritoneal mesothelioma. The risk relates to duration and intensity of exposure. Asbestos exposure and smoking are synergistic for developing lung cancer; however, smoking alone is not associated with mesothelioma.

Antman KH. Natural history and epidemiology of malignant mesothelioma. *Chest*. 1993;103(4 Suppl):373S–376S.

Answer 103

Malignant mesothelioma is typically classified into three broad histologic subtypes: epithelioid, sarcomatoid, and biphasic (mixed).
The epithelioid variant is the most common, comprising about 60% of all mesotheliomas.
The sarcomatoid subtype has the worst prognosis.

Churg A, Inai K, Samet JM, et al. Tumours of the pleura. In: Travis WD, Brambilla E, Muller-Hermelink HK, et al., eds. *Pathology and Genetics of Tumours of the Lung, Pleura, Thymus, and Heart*. Lyon, France: IARC Press; 2004:125–144.

Answer 104

EORTC poor prognostic factors for mesothelioma are:

1. WBC $> 8.3 \times 10^9$/dL
2. Poor performance status
3. Sarcomatous histology
4. Male gender

Curran D, Sahmoud T, Therasse P, et al. Prognostic factors in patients with pleural mesothelioma: the European Organization for Research and Treatment of Cancer experience. *J Clin Oncol*. 1998;16:145–152.

Answer 105

Cisplatin and pemetrexed doublet. Combination therapy prolongs survival compared to cisplatin alone in patients with advanced mesothelioma.

Vogelzang NJ, Rusthoven JJ, Symanowski J, et al. Phase III study of pemetrexed in combination with cisplatin versus cisplatin alone in patients with malignant pleural mesothelioma. *J Clin Oncol*. 2003;21:2636–2644.

Question 106
What is the treatment paradigm for resectable mesothelioma?

Question 107
How is IMRT delivered for adjuvant therapy in the treatment of mesotheliomas?

What are the expected toxicities and outcomes?

Question 108
What should the contralateral lung V20 be restricted to when planning adjuvant radiation for mesotheliomas?

Answer 106

Failure of single-modality treatments to increase survival in mesothelioma patients has led to a variety of multimodality approaches. For carefully selected patients with localized disease who are seeking aggressive therapy, combined modality approach including surgical debulking with pleurectomy or radical extrapleural pneumonectomy, adjuvant radiation therapy, and pemetrexed-based chemotherapy is used. These approaches are associated with substantial treatment-related morbidity and mortality, and such treatment algorithms should be restricted to selected patients who are treated at centers with expertise in mesothelioma treatment.

Ceresoli GL, Gridelli C, Santoro A. Multidisciplinary treatment of malignant pleural mesothelioma. *Oncologist.* 2007;12:850–863.

Answer 107

MD Anderson Cancer Center reported their early experience using IMRT in delivering adjuvant radiation. The CTV included the surgically violated inner chest wall, insertion of diaphragm, pleural reflections, and deep margin of the incision. CTV delineation was facilitated by intraoperative radio-opaque marking. CTV doses were 45–50 Gy with boosts taken to 60 Gy for close or positive margins.

The most common toxicities were nausea/vomiting (89%) and dyspnea (90%). Esophagitis was absent (59%) or mild (34% grade 1–2). Results showed that in 63 adjuvant IMRT patients, the median survival was 14.2 months and 3-year overall survival was 20%. Distant recurrence was seen in 54% and local or regional relapse in 13%. Only 3 patients (5%) recurred within the irradiated volume resulting in excellent local control.

Ahamad A, Stevens CW, Smythe WR, et al. Promising early local control of malignant pleural mesothelioma following postoperative intensity modulated radiotherapy (IMRT) to the chest. *Cancer J.* 2003;9:476–484.

Rice DC, Stevens CW, Correa AM, et al. Outcomes after extrapleural pneumonectomy and intensity-modulated radiation therapy for malignant pleural mesothelioma. *Ann Thorac Surg.* 2007;84:1685–1692; discussion 1692–1693.

Answer 108

The V20 should be restricted to below 7%. Retrospective review from MD Anderson Cancer Center showed that patients with V20 > 7% had a 42-fold risk of pulmonary-related death ($p = .001$). The authors conclude that the mean V20 should be restricted to below 7% and the mean lung dose below 8.5 Gy, although both should be kept as low as possible.

Rice DC, Smythe WR, Liao Z. Dose-dependent pulmonary toxicity after postoperative intensity-modulated radiotherapy for malignant pleural mesothelioma. *Int J Radiat Oncol Biol Phys.* 2007;69:350–357.

5

GASTROINTESTINAL CANCERS

ANDREW VASSIL

Question 1   ESOPHAGEAL CANCER

What is the incidence of esophageal cancer in the United States and worldwide?

Question 2

What are risk factors for esophageal squamous cell carcinoma?

Question 3

What are risk factors for esophageal adenocarcinoma?

Question 4

In the RTOG 85-01 study, published by Herskovic et al., of radiation therapy alone (64 Gy) compared to radiation (50 Gy) combined with cisplatin and 5-fluorouracil for esophageal cancer, what was the difference in median and 5-year overall survival?

Turn page to see the answers.

Answer 1

In the United States, approximately 16,640 cases of esophageal cancer were diagnosed and 14,500 deaths occurred in 2010. Worldwide, there were approximately 482,300 cases of esophageal cancer diagnosed, and 406,800 deaths in 2008.

Jemal A, Siegel R, Xu J, et al. Cancer statistics, 2010. *CA Cancer J Clin*. 2010;60:277–300.
Jemal A, Bray F, Center MM, et al. Global cancer statistics. *CA Cancer J Clin*. 2011;61:69–90.

Answer 2

Tobacco and alcohol use are the most commonly associated risk factors.

Poverty

Achalasia

Caustic esophageal injury

Nonepidermolytic palmoplanta keratoderma (tylosis)

Plummer-Vinson syndrome

History of head and neck cancer

History of breast cancer treated with radiotherapy

Frequent consumption of extremely hot beverages.

Enzinger PC, Mayer RJ. Esophageal cancer. *N Engl J Med*. 2003;349:2241–2252.

Answer 3

Tobacco use and Barrett's esophagus are the most commonly associated risk factors.

Weekly reflux symptoms

Obesity

History of breast cancer treated with radiotherapy

Prior use of beta-blockers, anticholinergic agents, or aminophyllines

Enzinger PC, Mayer RJ. Esophageal cancer. *N Engl J Med*. 2003;349:2241–2252.

Answer 4

Outcomes favored the combination of radiation and chemotherapy.

- Median survival 14.1 months vs 9.3 months ($p < .0001$)
- 5-year overall survival 27% vs 0% ($p < .0001$)

Cooper JS, Guo MD, Herskovic A, et al. Chemoradiotherapy of locally advanced esophageal cancer: long-term follow-up of a prospective randomized trial (RTOG 85-01). Radiation Therapy Oncology Group. *JAMA*. 1999;281:1623–1627.
Herskovic A, Martz K, al-Sarraf M, et al. Combined chemotherapy and radiotherapy compared with radiotherapy alone in patients with cancer of the esophagus. *N Engl J Med*. 1992;326:1593–1598.

Question 5

In the RTOG 85-01 study, published by Herskovic et al., of radiation therapy alone (64 Gy) compared to radiation (50 Gy) combined with cisplatin and 5-fluorouracil for esophageal cancer, what were the doses and schedules of cisplatin and 5-fluorouracil?

Question 6

In the RTOG 85-01 study, published by Herskovic et al., of radiation therapy alone (64 Gy) compared to radiation (50 Gy) combined with cisplatin and 5-fluorouracil for esophageal cancer, what was the most common location of disease failure?

Question 7

Were there differences in outcomes based on histology for the RTOG 85-01 study, published by Herskovic et al., of radiation therapy alone (64 Gy) compared to radiation (50 Gy) combined with cisplatin and 5-fluorouracil for esophageal cancer?

Question 8

In the RTOG 94-05 (INT 0123) study, published by Minsky et al., of standard-dose (50.4 Gy) vs high-dose (64.8 Gy) radiation with concurrent cisplatin and 5-fluorouracil for esophageal cancer, what was the difference in median and 2-year overall survival?

Answer 5

- Cisplatin, 75 mg/m^2 intravenously, on the first day of weeks 1, 5, 8, and 11.
- 5-fluorouracil, two cycles, 1000 mg/m^2 per day, days 1 to 4 by continuous infusion, weeks 1 and 5.

Toxicity reported was severe in 44% and life-threatening in 20% of patients receiving combined therapy vs 25% and 3% for those treated with radiation alone.

Herskovic A, Martz K, al-Sarraf M, et al. Combined chemotherapy and radiotherapy compared with radiotherapy alone in patients with cancer of the esophagus. *N Engl J Med*. 1992;326:1593–1598.

Answer 6

Persistence of disease was the most common cause of treatment failure in all patients (37% for radiation alone; 25% and 28% after combined modality therapy in the randomized and nonrandomized cohorts, respectively).

Combined chemotherapy and radiation appeared to prevent, not just delay, the local growth of tumor.

Cooper JS, Guo MD, Herskovic A, et al. Chemoradiotherapy of locally advanced esophageal cancer: long-term follow- up of a prospective randomized trial (RTOG 85-01). Radiation Therapy Oncology Group. *JAMA*. 1999;281:1623–1627.

Answer 7

No. Twelve percent of patients included had adenocarcinoma, the remaining 88% had squamous cell carcinoma. There was no difference in outcomes based on histology.

Cooper JS, Guo MD, Herskovic A, et al. Chemoradiotherapy of locally advanced esophageal cancer: long-term follow-up of a prospective randomized trial (RTOG 85-01). Radiation Therapy Oncology Group. *JAMA*. 1999;281:1623–1627.

Answer 8

Higher radiation dose did not result in higher median (13 months for standard-dose vs 18 months for high-dose) or two-year survival (31% for standard-dose vs 40% for high-dose).

Note: results of this study have been criticized due to the presence of 7 out of 11 deaths in the high-dose cohort occurring at radiation doses below 50.4 Gy.

Minsky BD, Pajak TF, Ginsberg RJ, et al. INT 0123 (Radiation Therapy Oncology Group 94-05) phase III trial of combined-modality therapy for esophageal cancer: high-dose versus standard-dose radiation therapy. *J Clin Oncol*. 2002;20:1167–1174.

Question 9

In the RTOG 94-05 (INT 0123) study, published by Minsky et al., of standard-dose (50.4 Gy) vs high-dose (64.8 Gy) radiation with concurrent cisplatin and 5-fluorouracil for esophageal cancer, what was the difference in persistence of locoregional disease?

Question 10

What is the significance of pathologic response to induction therapy for esophageal cancer?

Question 11

What is the role of surgery after induction chemoradiotherapy (tri-modality therapy) compared to chemo-radiotherapy alone for squamous cell carcinoma of the esophagus?

Question 12

What is the utility of a post-induction therapy FDG-PET scan for esophageal cancer?

Answer 9

There was no statistically significant difference in local control between the two cohorts; 56% vs 52% for the high dose and control groups, respectively.

Minsky BD, Pajak TF, Ginsberg RJ, et al. INT 0123 (Radiation Therapy Oncology Group 94-05) phase III trial of combined-modality therapy for esophageal cancer: high-dose versus standard-dose radiation therapy. *J Clin Oncol*. 2002;20:1167–1174.

Answer 10

Data shows improved survival for patients achieving a pathologic complete response with induction therapy.

A study of neoadjuvant radiation and concurrent chemotherapy showed those achieving a pathologic complete response had a significant improvement in three-year survival rates compared to those with residual disease (64% vs 19%).

In the CALGB 9781/RTOG 97-16 study of induction radiation and concurrent chemotherapy, a 40% rate pathologic complete response occurred.

Tepper J, Krasna MJ, Niedzwiecki D, et al. Phase III trial of trimodality therapy with cisplatin, fluorouracil, radiotherapy, and surgery compared with surgery alone for esophageal cancer: CALGB 9781. *J Clin Oncol*. 2008;26:1086–1092.
Urba SG, Orringer MB, Turrisi A, et al. Randomized trial of preoperative chemoradiation versus surgery alone in patients with locoregional esophageal carcinoma. *J Clin Oncol*. 2001;19:305–313.

Answer 11

In a phase III study, surgery was shown to improve locoregional control: (2-year progression free survival 64.3% vs 40.7%).

No significant difference in survival was seen (note, these studies were restricted to patients with squamous cell carcinoma).

Median survival: 16.4 months (tri-modality therapy) vs 14.9 months (chemoradiotherapy).

Clinical tumor response to induction therapy was shown to be the single independent prognostic factor for overall survival ($p < .0001$).

Stahl M, Stuschke M, Lehmann N, et al. Chemoradiation with and without surgery in patients with locally advanced squamous cell carcinoma of the esophagus. *J Clin Oncol*. 2005;23:2310–2317.

Answer 12

Retrospective data suggest that post-induction chemoradiotherapy FDG-PET scans may select for patients in whom surgery could be avoided, however, this has not been studied prospectively.

In a retrospective study, patients with post-induction therapy FDG-PET SUV ≤ 3 in the tumor (38% of patients) had a 2-year overall survival of 71% vs 11% for those with post-induction therapy FDG-PET SUV ≥ 3.1. Two-year local failure was also improved for those with FDG-PET SUV ≤ 3 (75%) vs SUV > 3 (28%). For patients undergoing trimodality therapy, there was no difference in outcome.

Monjazeb AM, Riedlinger G, Aklilu M, et al. Outcomes of patients with esophageal cancer staged with [(1)F]fluorodeoxyglucose positron emission tomography (FDG-PET): can postchemoradiotherapy FDG-PET predict the utility of resection? *J Clin Oncol*. 2010;28:4714–4721.

Question 13

What is the role of brachytherapy in the management of esophageal cancer?

Question 14

What is the accuracy of esophageal cancer tumor staging with endoscopic ultrasound (EUS) compared to CT staging?

Question 15

What is the accuracy of esophageal cancer regional staging with endoscopic ultrasound (EUS) compared to CT staging?

Question 16

What is the sensitivity and specificity of a EUS-guided fine needle aspiration (FNA) for lymph node staging in esophageal cancer?

Answer 13

Palliation and dose intensification after external beam radiation

In a randomized study, brachytherapy has been shown to provide a more durable palliative response, but stent placement provides a more rapid relief of symptoms.

Brachytherapy after external beam radiation should only be used in select circumstances given the risk of toxicity, such as fistula formation. Contraindications include tracheal or bronchial involvement, cervical esophagus location, or stenosis that cannot be bypassed.

Gaspar LE, Nag S, Herskovic A, et al. American Brachytherapy Society (ABS) consensus guidelines for brachytherapy of esophageal cancer. Clinical Research Committee, American Brachytherapy Society, Philadelphia, PA. *Int J Radiat Oncol Biol Phys*. 1997;38:127–132.

Homs MY, Steyerberg EW, Eijkenboom WM, et al. Single-dose brachytherapy versus metal stent placement for the palliation of dysphagia from oesophageal cancer: multicentre randomised trial. *Lancet*. 2004;364:1497–1504.

Answer 14

Overall tumor depth staging accuracy of EUS is 85–90%, compared with 50–80% for CT.

EUS provides better regional staging the CT, MRI or PET scanning, particularly for lymph node evaluation.

Additionally, EUS allows for fine needle aspiration to improve the accuracy of lymph node assessment.

A learning curve has been reported for EUS staging.

Tio TL, Coene PP, den Hartog Jager FC, et al. Preoperative TNM classification of esophageal carcinoma by endosonography. *Hepatogastroenterology*. 1990;37:376–381.

van Vliet EP, Eijkemans MJ, Poley JW, et al. Staging of esophageal carcinoma in a low-volume EUS center compared with reported results from high-volume centers. *Gastrointest Endosc*. 2006;63:938–947.

Ziegler K, Sanft C, Zeitz M, et al. Evaluation of endosonography in TN staging of oesophageal cancer. *Gut*. 1991;32:16–20.

Answer 15

The accuracy of regional nodal staging is 70–80% for EUS and 50–70% for CT.

Fine-needle aspiration improves EUS accuracy.

Tio TL, Coene PP, den Hartog Jager FC, et al. Preoperative TNM classification of esophageal carcinoma by endosonography. *Hepatogastroenterology*. 1990;37:376–381.

Ziegler K, Sanft C, Zeitz M, et al. Evaluation of endosonography in TN staging of oesophageal cancer. *Gut*. 1991;32:16–20.

Answer 16

Based on retrospective series, there is a reported 93% sensitivity and 100% specificity of regional nodal staging with EUS-FNA.

EUS-guided fine-needle aspiration (FNA) for lymph node staging is under prospective evaluation.

Vazquez-Sequeiros E, Norton ID, Clain JE, et al. Impact of EUS-guided fine-needle aspiration on lymph node staging in patients with esophageal carcinoma. *Gastrointest Endosc*. 2001;53:751–757.

Question 17

What is the role of Barrett's esophagus management in prevention of esophageal cancer?

Question 18

What proportion of patients with advanced distal esophageal and gastroesophageal junction adenocarcinoma harbor HER2 overexpression?

Question 19

What is the benefit to the addition of trastuzumab to fluoropyrimidine–based chemotherapy in patients with advanced gastroesophageal and gastric cancer?

Question 20

What brachytherapy dose is used for esophageal cancer after 5-fluorouracil–based chemotherapy and 45–50 Gy external beam radiation are used?

Answer 17

A prospective, randomized study of radiofrequency ablation for patients with dysplastic Barrett's esophagus reduced risk of disease progression, with fewer cancers (1.2% vs 9.3%, p = .045).

A small randomized study showed regression in Barrett's esophagus with aggressive acid reflux management. It is unclear if this translates into a reduction in cancer risk.

Peters FT, Ganesh S, Kuipers EJ, et al. Endoscopic regression of Barrett's oesophagus during omeprazole treatment; a randomised double blind study. *Gut.* 1999;45:489–494.

Shaheen NJ, Sharma P, Overholt BF, et al. Radiofrequency ablation in Barrett's esophagus with dysplasia. *N Engl J Med.* 2009;360:2277–2288.

Answer 18

In a phase III study for patients with adenocarcinoma of the gastroesophageal junction and distal esophagus, the HER2 positivity rate was 32.2%.

HER2 is human epidermal growth factor receptor 2 and is under investigation as a for treatment with targeted therapy. RTOG 1010 is testing the addition of trastuzumab to trimodality therapy for of HER2 overexpressing esophageal adenocarcinoma in the upfront setting.

Bang Y, Chung H, Sawaki A, et al. HER2-positivity rates in advanced gastric cancer (GC): results from a large international phase III trial. *J Clin Oncol.* 2008;26 (May 20 suppl). Abstract 4526.

www.rtog.org

Answer 19

Improved overall survival. The Trastuzumab for Gastric Cancer (ToGA) trial evaluated the addition of trastuzumab to cisplatin and 5-fluorouracil or capecitabine for patients with advanced gastroesophageal and gastric cancer. Median overall survival was improved with trastuzumab and chemotherapy as compared to chemotherapy alone, 13.8 vs 11.1 months, respectively [p = .0046].

The addition of trastuzumab to trimodality therapy for esophageal adenocarcinoma is being tested by the RTOG.

Bang YJ, Van Cutsem E, Feyereislova A, et al. Trastuzumab in combination with chemotherapy versus chemotherapy alone for treatment of HER2-positive advanced gastric or gastro-oesophageal junction cancer (ToGA): a phase 3, open-label, randomised controlled trial. *Lancet.* 2010;376:687–697.

Answer 20

HDR 10 Gy in 2 weekly fractions of 5 Gy

LDR 20 Gy in a single course at 0.4–1 Gy/hr

All doses are specified to 1 cm from the midsource or mid-dwell position.

Concurrent chemotherapy should not be given.

The most significant toxicity is esophageal fistula.

Gaspar LE, Nag S, Herskovic A, et al. American Brachytherapy Society (ABS) consensus guidelines for brachytherapy of esophageal cancer. Clinical Research Committee, American Brachytherapy Society, Philadelphia, PA. *Int J Radiat Oncol Biol Phys.* 1997;38:127–132.

Question 21

What are felt to be risk factors for gastric cancer?

Question 22

What benefits were found in the United States phase III intergroup trial (INT-0116) testing adjuvant chemotherapy and concurrent radiation therapy for resected gastric cancer?

Answer 21

Smoking is recognized as the most important behavioral risk factor for gastric cancer.

- *Helicobacter pylori* gastric infection
- Advanced age
- Male gender
- Diet low in fruits and vegetables
- Diet high in salted, smoked, or preserved foods
- Chronic atrophic gastritis
- Intestinal metaplasia
- Pernicious anemia
- Gastric adenomatous polyps
- Family history of gastric cancer
- Menetrier disease (giant hypertrophic gastritis)
- Familial adenomatous polyposis

American Cancer Society. *Cancer Facts and Figures*. Atlanta, GA: American Cancer Society; 2010.

Ladeiras-Lopes R, Pereira AK, Nogueira A, et al. Smoking and gastric cancer: systematic review and meta-analysis of cohort studies. *Cancer Causes Control*. 2008;19:689–701.

Answer 22

Although localized gastric cancer is treated with radical surgery, local (tumor bed), regional (nodal) and distant failure remain high. Thus, adjuvant therapies have been tested. INT-0116 assessed adjuvant 5-fluorouracil and leucovorin, followed by concurrent radiation (4500 cGy) with 5-fluorouracil, followed by additional 5-fluorouracil and leucovorin versus observation. This study showed that adjuvant therapy resulted in:

- improved median survival (36 months vs 27 months, $p = .005$)
- improved 3-year overall survival (50% vs 41%, $p = .005$)
- improved relapse free survival (48% vs 31%, $p < .001$)

Macdonald JS, Smalley SR, Benedetti J, et al. Chemoradiotherapy after surgery compared with surgery alone for adenocarcinoma of the stomach or gastroesophageal junction. *N Engl J Med*. 2001;345:725–730.

Question 23

What benefits were found in the European phase III trial (MRC-ST02) testing neoadjuvant and adjuvant chemotherapy for stage II or higher adenocarcinoma of the stomach or lower third of the esophagus?

Question 24

What lymph node groups are removed in "D1" and "D2" lymph node dissection for gastric cancer?

Question 25

In the Dutch phase III study randomizing patients with adenocarcinoma of the stomach without evidence of distant metastasis to D1 or D2 lymph node dissection, what was the difference in 5-year overall and relapse free survival?

Answer 23

European investigators tested three cycles of epirubicin, cisplatin and continuous infusion 5-fluorouracil before and after radical surgery. The addition of neoadjuvant and adjuvant chemotherapy resulted in:

- improved progression-free survival (HR for progression 0.66, 95% confidence interval 0.53–0.81, $p < .001$)
- improved overall survival (HR for death 0.75, 95% confidence interval 0.60–0.93, $p = .009$)
- improved 5-year overall survival (36.3% vs 23%)
- tumor downstaging, with greater proportion of stage T1 and T2 tumors (51.7% vs 36.8%, $p = .002$), N0 or N1 disease (84.4% vs 70.5%, $p = .01$)
- smaller median maximum diameter of the resected tumor (3 cm vs 5 cm, $p < .001$)

Cunningham D, Allum WH, Stenning SP, et al. Perioperative chemotherapy versus surgery alone for resectable gastroesophageal cancer. *N Engl J Med*. 2006;355:11–20.

Answer 24

- D1 dissection includes removal of N1 lymph nodes groups, including the perigastric lymph nodes along the lesser curvature and greater curvature of the stomach.
- D2 dissections remove N1 lymph node groups, and N2 lymph node groups along regional vasculature; including those along the left gastric artery, common hepatic artery, celiac artery, and splenic artery.

The Japanese Research Society for the Study of Gastric Cancer have described these nodal groups. These groupings can be modified slightly, depending on the location of the primary tumor. It is recommended that at least 16 regional lymph nodes be assessed pathologically for a pN0 determination to be made.

Stomach. In: Edge SB, Byrd DR, Compton CC, et al., eds. *AJCC Cancer Staging Handbook*: from the AJCC Cancer Staging Manual. 7th ed. New York, NY: Springer; 2010:119.

Kajitani T. The general rules for the gastric cancer study in surgery and pathology. Part I. Clinical classification. *Jpn J Surg*. 1981;11:127–139.

Answer 25

There were no significant differences in overall survival or relapse rates at 5 years.

D2 dissection resulted in:

- higher rates of complications (43 vs 25%, $p < .001$)
- more postoperative deaths (10% vs 4%, $p = .004$)
- longer hospital stays (median 16 vs 14 days, $p < .001$)

After long term follow-up (11 years), there was still no statistically significant difference in overall survival rates. Despite this trial and similar outcomes from the MRC study, the extent of lymph node dissection remains controversial. Patients with N2 disease may derive a benefit from D2 dissection after long-term follow-up in the Dutch study.

Bonenkamp JJ, Hermans J, Sasako M, et al. Extended lymph-node dissection for gastric cancer. *N Engl J Med*. 1999;340:908–914.

Hartgrink HH, van de Velde CJ, Putter H, et al. Extended lymph node dissection for gastric cancer: who may benefit? Final results of the randomized Dutch gastric cancer group trial. *J Clin Oncol*. 2004;22:2069–2077.

Question 26

When considering worldwide cancer death, where does gastric cancer rank?

Question 27

What is the most common location for gastric cancer?

Question 28

Which organism has been strongly associated with gastric adenocarcinoma?

Question 29

What were the outcomes in a French multicenter trial of preoperative and postoperative chemotherapy (5-fluorouracil and cisplatin) vs surgery alone for resectable stage II or greater adenocarcinoma of the stomach or distal esophagus?

Answer 26

Gastric cancer is the second most common cause of cancer death worldwide, representing approximately 9.7% of cancer deaths. Lung cancer is the most common (18.2% of cancer deaths), and liver cancer is the third most common cause (9.2% of cancer deaths).

Ferlay J, Shin HR, Bray F, et al. Estimates of worldwide burden of cancer in 2008: GLOBOCAN 2008. *Int J Cancer*. 2010;127:2893–2917.

Answer 27

The proximal stomach and gastroesophageal junction are the most common locations for gastric cancer. This is due to a combination of an increase in incidence in the location, and decrease in incidence of distal tumors. Approximately 34% occur in the cardia, 22% in the pyloric antrum, 17% at the body, 27% at other sites.

Blot WJ, Devesa SS, Kneller RW, et al. Rising incidence of adenocarcinoma of the esophagus and gastric cardia. *JAMA*. 1991;265:1287–1289.

Powell J, McConkey CC. Increasing incidence of adenocarcinoma of the gastric cardia and adjacent sites. *Br J Cancer*. 1990;62:440–443.

Answer 28

Helicobacter pylori (H. pylori) was discovered in the 1980's, can cause chronic active gastritis and atrophic gastritis (carcinogenic steps), and has been clearly associated with gastric adenocarcinoma (both intestinal and diffuse types).

Meta-analysis of seven controlled trials (all in areas with a high incidence of gastric cancer) found significantly lower rates of gastric cancer (1.1% vs 1.7%) in patients randomized to eradication (RR 0.65, 95% CI 0.43–0.98).

Two to four drug combinations are used to eradicate H. pylori. Drugs typically include omeprazole, amoxicillin and clavulanate potassium, and metronidazole.

Huang JQ, Sridhar S, Chen Y, et al. Meta-analysis of the relationship between *Helicobacter pylori* seropositivity and gastric cancer. *Gastroenterology*. 1998;114:1169–1179.

Answer 29

Treatment with chemotherapy resulted in:

- Improved R0 (microscopically complete) resection: 84% vs 73%
- Trend towards fewer node-positive tumors (67% vs 80%)
- Improved 5-year disease free survival (34% vs 19%)
- Improved 5-year overall survival (38% vs 24%)

This study supports the findings in the MAGIC study.

Huang JQ, Sridhar S, Chen Y, et al. Meta-analysis of the relationship between *Helicobacter pylori* seropositivity and gastric cancer. *Gastroenterology*. 1998;114:1169–1179.

Cunningham D, Allum WH, Stenning SP, et al. Perioperative chemotherapy versus surgery alone for resectable gastroesophageal cancer. *N Engl J Med*. 2006;355:11–20.

Question 30

Based on patterns of failure after surgery for gastric cancer, what regions are at risk for disease recurrence?

Question 31

What is the overall accuracy of tumor depth of invasion assessment with endoscopic ultrasound for gastric cancer?

Question 32

What are the most common symptoms of gastric cancer?

Answer 30

The anastomoses, gastric remnant and/or duodenal stump and regional lymph node beds are regions at highest risk for disease recurrence.

Initial lymph node drainage is to nodes along the lesser and greater curvatures (gastric and gastroepiploic nodes)

- Celiac axis
- Porta hepatic
- Splenic spurapancreatic
- Pancreaticodudenal
- Adjacent para-aortic
- Distal paraesphageal

Gunderson LL, Sosin H. Adenocarcinoma of the stomach: areas of failure in a re-operation series (second or symptomatic look) clinicopathologic correlation and implications for adjuvant therapy. *Int J Radiat Oncol Biol Phys*. 1982;8:1–11.

Answer 31

Approximately 80%

Accompanying fibrosis and metastatic perigastric nodes are the main reasons for overestimating the extent of disease.

Saito N, Takeshita K, Habu H, et al. The use of endoscopic ultrasound in determining the depth of cancer invasion in patients with gastric cancer. *Surg Endosc*. 1991;5:14–19.

Answer 32

Weight loss and persistent abdominal pain are the most common symptoms at initial diagnosis.

At presentation:

- Weight loss: 62%
- Abdominal pain: 52%
- Nausea: 34%
- Dysphagia: 26%
- Melena: 20%
- Early satiety: 18%
- Ulcer-type pain: 17%

Wanebo HJ, Kennedy BJ, Chmiel J, et al. Cancer of the stomach. A patient care study by the American College of Surgeons. *Ann Surg*. 1993;218:583–592.

Question 33

What are common indications, radiation dose and outcomes for palliative radiation therapy for gastric cancer?

Question 34

What did the CALGB 80101 (RTOG 0571) study test for patients with either resected gastric or gastroesophageal junction cancers?

Question 35

What were the dose planning goals for the liver, kidneys, heart and spinal cord in the CALGB 80101 (RTOG 0571) study [postoperative epirubicin, cisplatin, 5-fluorouracil vs 5-fluorouracil and leucovorin, before and after adjuvant radiation therapy with concurrent 5-fluorouracil and leucovorin in resected gastric cancer]?

Answer 33

Palliative radiation therapy for gastric cancer is generally well tolerated.

- Indications: bleeding, obstruction, pain
- Dose: 30 Gy in 10 fractions (other dosing may include 8 Gy in a single fraction to 40 Gy in 16 fractions)
- Survival at one year is approximately 8%
- Approximately 50–70% of patients with bleeding respond to radiation therapy
- Approximately 25–81% of patients have improvement in obstructive symptoms
- Approximately 25–86% of patients achieve improvement in pain

Kim MM, Rana V, Janjan NA, et al. Clinical benefit of palliative radiation therapy in advanced gastric cancer. *Acta Oncol.* 2008;47:421–427.

Tey J, Back MF, Shakespeare TP, et al. The role of palliative radiation therapy in symptomatic locally advanced gastric cancer. *Int J Radiat Oncol Biol Phys.* 2007;67:385–388.

Answer 34

Given the high rate of local failure in the chemotherapy arm of the MAGIC trial, adding radiation therapy to ECF (epirubicin, cisplatin, 5-fluorouracil) was tested in the CALGB 80101 study.

Patients with either resected gastric or gastroesophageal junction cancers were eligible for the CALGB study comparing:

- Postoperative epirubicin, cisplatin, 5-fluorouracil before and after 5-fluorouracil plus concurrent radiation
- Postoperative 5-fluorouracil and leucovorin before and after 5-fluoruracil plus concurrent radiation (per INT 0116 protocol)

Accrual to this trial is complete and the data are maturing. Preliminary report of toxicity favors epirubicin, cisplatin, 5-fluorouracil.

www.rtog.org

Fuchs C, Tepper JE, Niedwiecki D, et al. Postoperative adjuvant chemoradiation for gastric or gastroesophageal adeno-carcinoma using epirubicin, cisplatin, and infusional (CI) 5-FU (ECF) before and after CI 5-FU and radiotherapy (RT): interim toxicity results from Intergroup trial CALGB 80101. [Abstract] American Society of Clinical Oncology Gastrointestinal Cancers Symposium; January 26–28, 2006; San Francisco, CA.; 2006: A-61.

Answer 35

Liver: < 30 Gy to 30%

Kidneys: < 20 Gy to 50% of combined volume

Heart: < 25 Gy to 50%

Spinal cord: < 45 Gy

www.rtog.org

http://www.cancer.gov/clinicaltrials/search/view?cdrid=258787&version=HealthProfessional

Question 36

BILIARY TRACT MALIGNANCY

What are considered risk factors for the development of cholangiocarcinoma?

Question 37

What is the incidence of cholangiocarcinoma in patients with primary sclerosing cholangitis?

Question 38

Which histologic variant of cholangiocarcinoma has the best prognosis?

Question 39

What are common signs and symptoms of cholangiocarcinoma?

Answer 36

Hepatolithiasis, pyogenic cholangitis, liver fluke infestation, choledochal cysts, past exposure to thorium dioxide, typhoid carrier state, ulcerative colitis, and primary sclerosing cholangitis.

In the United States and Europe, primary sclerosing cholangitis and choledochal cyst represent the most commonly identified risk factors. However for many patients, a risk factor is not identified.

Chapman RW. Risk factors for biliary tract carcinogenesis. *Ann Oncol*. 1999;10(Suppl 4):308–311.

Jesudian AB, Jacobson IM. Screening and diagnosis of cholangiocarcinoma in patients with primary sclerosing cholangitis. *Rev Gastroenterol Disord*. 2009;9:E41–E47.

Nagorney DM, Gigot JF. Primary epithelial hepatic malignancies: etiology, epidemiology, and outcome after subtotal and total hepatic resection. *Surg Oncol Clin N Am*. 1996;5:283–300.

Van Leeuwen DJ, Huibregtse K, Tytgat GN. Carcinoma of the hepatic confluence 25 years after Klatskin's description: diagnosis and endoscopic management. *Semin Liver Dis*. 1990;10:102–113.

Answer 37

For patients with primary sclerosing cholangitis, approximately 20–30% have a synchronous diagnosis of cholangiocarcinoma, and 50% develop cholangiocarcinoma in 1 year.

Close surveillence with CA 19-9, ultrasound, and endoscopic retrograde cholangiopancreatography (ERCP) may be considered for patients with primary sclerosing cholangitis given their high risk of developing cholangiocarcinoma.

de Groen PC, Gores GJ, LaRusso NF, et al. Biliary tract cancers. *N Engl J Med*. 1999;341:1368–1378.

Fevery J, Verslype C, Lai G, et al. Incidence, diagnosis, and therapy of cholangiocarcinoma in patients with primary sclerosing cholangitis. *Dig Dis Sci*. 2007;52:3123–3135.

Answer 38

Papillary adenocarcinoma is associated with the best prognosis, but is the rarest form.

More than 90% of cholangiocarcinomas are adenocarcinoma; variants include nodular, sclerosing and papillary.

The remaining cases are usually squamous cell carcinoma.

Fevery J, Verslype C, Lai G, et al. Incidence, diagnosis, and therapy of cholangiocarcinoma in patients with primary sclerosing cholangitis. *Dig Dis Sci*. 2007;52:3123–3135.

Nakeeb A, Pitt HA, Sohn TA, et al. Cholangiocarcinoma. A spectrum of intrahepatic, perihilar, and distal tumors. *Ann Surg*. 1996;224:463–473; discussion 73–75.

Answer 39

Jaundice, hepatomegaly, right upper quadrant mass.

Clay-colored stools, dark urine, pruritus, right upper quadrant abdominal pain, weight loss, fever.

Nakeeb A, Pitt HA, Sohn TA, et al. Cholangiocarcinoma. A spectrum of intrahepatic, perihilar, and distal tumors. *Ann Surg*. 1996;224:463–473; discussion 73–75.

Nagorney DM, Donohue JH, Farnell MB, et al. Outcomes after curative resections of cholangiocarcinoma. *Arch Surg*. 1993;128:871–877; discussion 7–9.

Question 40

What technique is most useful to aid in determining resectability of cholangiocarcinoma?

Question 41

How are biliary tumors classified anatomically?

Question 42

When is radiation therapy typically used for cholangiocarcinoma?

Answer 40

Staging laparoscopy. After tissue diagnosis is made, and staging imaging studies such as magnetic resonance cholangiopancreatography and multi-phase computed tomography are used to assess portal vein or hepatic arterial involvement, staging laparoscopy can select the majority of patients with unresectable cholangiocarcinoma, thus reducing unnecessary laparotomies.

Callery MP, Strasberg SM, Doherty GM, et al. Staging laparoscopy with laparoscopic ultrasonography: optimizing resectability in hepatobiliary and pancreatic malignancy. *J Am Coll Surg*. 1997;185:33–39.

Weber SM, DeMatteo RP, Fong Y, et al. Staging laparoscopy in patients with extrahepatic biliary carcinoma. Analysis of 100 patients. *Ann Surg*. 2002;235:392–399.

Answer 41

Cholangiocarcinoma is the term used for primary tumors of the bile ducts. Tumors are defined as intrahepatic, perihilar, and distal extrahepatic. A "Klatskin" tumor involves the bifurcation of the hepatic duct.

de Groen PC, Gores GJ, LaRusso NF, et al. Biliary tract cancers. *N Engl J Med*. 1999;341:1368–1378.

Klatskin G. Adenocarcinoma of the hepatic duct at its bifurcation within the porta hepatis. An unusual tumor with distinctive clinical and pathological features. *Am J Med*. 1965;38:241–256.

Answer 42

Palliation and adjuvant settings. Radiation therapy may be used for palliation, and its use in the adjuvant setting is controversial as prospective, randomized studies are lacking.

Most retrospective studies indicate a local control benefit to radiation therapy, given the high propensity for local failure with surgery alone. Patients with positive margins and/or lymph node involvement may be considered for adjuvant radiation therapy. Typically the radiation dose used is approximately 45–50.4 Gy, and combined with 5-fluorouracil based chemotherapy. A retrospective review of patients treated at the MD Anderson Cancer Center showed similar survival and local control for patients with positive margins or lymph nodes, treated with adjuvant radiation therapy, compared to patients treated with surgery alone who had negative margins and no lymph node involvement.

Borghero Y, Crane CH, Szklaruk J, et al. Extrahepatic bile duct adenocarcinoma: patients at high-risk for local recurrence treated with surgery and adjuvant chemoradiation have an equivalent overall survival to patients with standard-risk treated with surgery alone. *Ann Surg Oncol*. 2008;15:3147–3156.

Question 43

What radiation therapy techniques are used for patients with locally advanced cholangiocarcinoma?

Question 44   **PANCREATIC CANCER**

What are risk factors for pancreatic cancer?

Question 45

Approximately how many new cases and deaths from pancreatic cancer were estimated for 2010?

Answer 43

External beam radiation therapy, brachytherapy and stereotactic body radiotherapy techniques have all been applied to patients with locally advanced cholangiocarcinoma. 80–90% of patients present with unresectable disease.

Commonly used doses include:

- 50.4 Gy for adjuvant therapy (with or without concurrent chemotherapy, typically 5-fluorouracil)
- 30 Gy to 50.4 Gy for palliation
- 5 Gy HDR fractions (six fractions over 3 days for brachytherapy alone, 4 fractions over 2 days when combined with external beam radiation)
- Stereotactic delivery of 24–54 Gy in six fractions, e.g., 36 Gy in 6 fractions per Princess Margaret Hospital phase I/II protocol

Brunner TB, Eccles CL. Radiotherapy and chemotherapy as therapeutic strategies in extrahepatic biliary duct carcinoma. *Strahlenther Onkol*. 2010;186:672–680.

Dawson LA, Eccles C, Craig T. Individualized image guided iso-NTCP based liver cancer SBRT. *Acta Oncol*. 2006;45:856–864.

Answer 44

Smoking – This is considered the most important risk factor for pancreatic cancer.

Family history of chronic pancreatitis

Advancing age

Male sex

Diabetes mellitus

Obesity

Non-O blood group

Occupational exposures (chlorinated hydrocarbon solvents and nickel)

African-American ethnicity

High-fat diet; diets high in meat and low in vegetables and folate

Possibly Helicobacter pylori infection and periodontal disease

Vincent A, Herman J, Schulick R, et al. Pancreatic cancer. *Lancet*. 2011;378:607–620.

Answer 45

New cases: 43,140

Deaths: 36,800

Only approximately 10–15% of patients have disease amenable to attempts at a curative resection.

Jemal A, Siegel R, Xu J, et al. Cancer statistics *CA Cancer J Clin*. 2010;60:277–300.

Question 46

What local tumor factors establish resectability for pancreatic cancer?

Question 47

What is involved in a Whipple procedure for pancreatic cancer?

Question 48

The RTOG 97-04 phase III study compared gemcitabine to 5-fluorouracil, before and after concurrent chemoradiation for patients with resected pancreatic adenocarcinoma. Which group of patients had the highest survival?

Answer 46

Localized disease, small cancers (< 2 cm) with no lymph node metastases, and no extension beyond the capsule of the pancreas are most suitable for surgical resection.

Complete surgical resection can yield actuarial 5-year survival rates of 18% to 24%.

Yeo CJ, Abrams RA, Grochow LB, et al. Pancreaticoduodenectomy for pancreatic adenocarcinoma: postoperative adjuvant chemoradiation improves survival. A prospective, single-institution experience. *Ann Surg*. 1997;225:621–633; discussion 33–36.

Answer 47

Removal of:

- Distal half of the stomach
- Gall bladder and its cystic duct
- Common bile duct
- Head of the pancreas
- Duodenum
- Proximal jejunum
- Regional lymph nodes.

As the head of the pancreas and the duodenum share the same arterial blood supply (the gastroduodenal artery), if only the head of the pancreas were removed it would compromise blood flow to the duodenum. This procedure results in a 5-year survival of approximately 20% for selected patients.

Yeo CJ, Cameron JL, Lillemoe KD, et al. Pancreaticoduodenectomy for cancer of the head of the pancreas. 201 patients. *Ann Surg*. 1995;221:721–731; discussion 31–33.

Answer 48

Patients with pancreatic head cancers treated with gemcitabine and chemoradiation had a median survival of 20.5 months and a 3-year survival rate of 31% compared with those treated with fluorouracil and chemoradiation who had a median survival of 16.9 months and a 3-year survival rate of 22% ($p = .09$).

Regine WF, Winter KA, Abrams RA, et al. Fluorouracil versus gemcitabine chemotherapy before and after fluorouracil-based chemoradiation following resection of pancreatic adenocarcinoma: a randomized controlled trial. *JAMA*. 2008;299:1019–1026.

Question 49

The RTOG 97-04 phase III study compared gemcitabine to 5-fluoruracil, before and after concurrent chemoradiation for patients with resected pancreatic adenocarcinoma. What was the significance of postoperative CA 19-9 levels?

Question 50

What is CA 19-9?

Question 51

What imaging studies are typically undertaken prior to conducting a Whipple procedure for pancreatic cancer?

Answer 49

A prospectively determined protocol specific secondary endpoint of the RTOG 97-04 study evaluated the ability of postresection CA 19-9 to predict survival.

No patient with a CA 19-9 > 180 U/mL survived more than 3 years.

Median survival was 9 months for patients with CA 19-9 ≥ 180 compared with 21 months for those with CA 19-9 lower than 180 ($p < .0001$).

Berger AC, Garcia M Jr, Hoffman JP, et al. Postresection CA 19-9 predicts overall survival in patients with pancreatic cancer treated with adjuvant chemoradiation: a prospective validation by RTOG 9704. *J Clin Oncol.* 2008;26:5918–5922.

Answer 50

CA 19-9 is monosialo-ganglioside/glycolipid and sialyl derivative of lacto-N-fucopentaose II (sialyl-Lewis(a), hapten of human Lewis(a) blood group determinant).

It is detected in serum of healthy individuals at low concentration < 40 U/ml.

CA 19-9 requires the presence of the Lewis blood group antigen (a glycosyl transferase) to be expressed. For individuals with a Lewis-negative phenotype (an estimated 5–10% of the population), CA 19-9 levels are not a useful tumor marker.

Lamerz R. Role of tumour markers, cytogenetics. *Ann Oncol.* 1999;10(Suppl 4):145–149.
Tempero MA, Uchida E, Takasaki H, et al. Relationship of carbohydrate antigen 19-9 and Lewis antigens in pancreatic cancer. *Cancer Res.* 1987;47:5501–5503.

Answer 51

Tri-phase computed tomographic scans

Magnetic resonance imaging

Positron emission tomographic scan

Endoscopic ultrasound examination

Laparoscopic staging

All of these can aid in the diagnosis and staging and help identify patients with disease that is not amenable to resection.

Riker A, Libutti SK, Bartlett DL. Advances in the early detection, diagnosis, and staging of pancreatic cancer. *Surg Oncol.* 1997;6:157–169.

Question 52

What were the outcomes for patients with unresectable pancreatic cancer treated in the Gastrointestinal Tumor Study Group (GITSG) 9273 study of 60 Gy vs 40 Gy + 5-fluorouracil vs 60 Gy + 5-fluorouracil?

Question 53

What outcomes were seen in the Eastern Cooperative Oncology Group phase III study of gemcitabine alone vs gemcitabine plus 50.4 Gy for patients with unresectable pancreatic cancer?

Question 54

In the European 2000–01 FFCD/SFRO study of gemcitabine alone vs 60 Gy with cisplatin and 5-fluorouracil followed by gemcitabine for patients with unresectable pancreatic cancer, what were the differences in outcomes?

Answer 52

Chemotherapy improved:

- Time to progression: 12.6 weeks (radiation alone) vs 30.4–33 weeks (combination arms).
- Median survival: 22.9 weeks (radiation alone) vs 40.3–42.2 weeks (combination arms).

A split-course radiation technique was used by the GITSG (2–3 courses of 20 Gy separated by 2 week breaks).

Note, the Eastern Cooperative Oncology Group phase III study (E8282) tested the addition of 5-fluorouracil and mitomycin C to 59.4 Gy radiation for patients with unresectable pancreatic cancer showed no improvement in outcomes with the addition of chemotherapy.

Cohen SJ, Dobelbower Jr R, Lipsitz S, et al. A randomized phase III study of radiotherapy alone or with 5-fluorouracil and mitomycin-C in patients with locally advanced adenocarcinoma of the pancreas: Eastern Cooperative Oncology Group study E8282. *Int J Radiat Oncol Biol Phys.* 2005;62:1345–1350.

Moertel CG, Frytak S, Hahn RG, et al. Therapy of locally unresectable pancreatic carcinoma: a randomized comparison of high dose (6000 rads) radiation alone, moderate dose radiation (4000 rads + 5-fluorouracil), and high dose radiation + 5-fluorouracil: The Gastrointestinal Tumor Study Group. *Cancer.* 1981;48:1705–1710.

Answer 53

No significant difference in progression free survival: 6.7 months (gemcitabine alone) vs 6 months (gemcitabine plus radiation)

Significantly improved median survival: 9.2 months (gemcitabine alone) vs 11.1 months (gemcitabine plus radiation therapy)

Grade 4/5 toxicities were significantly worse with radiation therapy: 9% (gemcitabine alone) vs 41% (gemcitabine plus radiation).

No statistical differences were seen in quality of life measurements at 6, 15 to 16, and 36 weeks.

Note, this study was terminated early due to poor accrual; prevention of distant recurrences remains a problem.

Loehrer Sr PJ, Feng Y, Cardenes H, et al. Gemcitabine alone versus gemcitabine plus radiotherapy in patients with locally advanced pancreatic cancer: an eastern cooperative oncology group trial. *J Clin Oncol.* 2011;29:4105–4112.

Answer 54

- Median survival was shorter in the radiation arm: 8.6 vs 13 months.
- 1-year survival was worse in the radiation arm: 32% vs 53%.
- More patients experienced grade 3–4 toxicities in the radiation arm.

Of note, this study used higher doses of radiation (60 Gy) than are used in most trials. The addition of cisplatin may have increased toxicity profiles. Median survival was in the radiation arm was worse than that seen with other modern studies including radiation therapy.

Chauffert B, Mornex F, Bonnetain F, et al. Phase III trial comparing intensive induction chemoradiotherapy (60 Gy, infusional 5-FU and intermittent cisplatin) followed by maintenance gemcitabine with gemcitabine alone for locally advanced unresectable pancreatic cancer. Definitive results of the 2000–01 FFCD/SFRO study. *Ann Oncol.* 2008;19:1592–1599.

Question 55

What are the arms in the phase III RTOG 0848 study for patients with resected head of pancreas adenocarcinoma?

Question 56

In the RTOG 0848 study of adjuvant therapy for patients with resected head of pancreas adenocarcinoma, what lymph node groups are treated in patients receiving radiation therapy?

Answer 55

Patients are first randomized to:

- 5 cycles of Gemcitabine alone

vs

- Gemcitabine + Erlotinib

  - Each Gemcitabine cycle consists of: 1000 mg/m² Gemcitabine, IV over thirty minutes, once a week for three weeks, then off one week = one cycle).
  - Erlotinib is a tyrosine kinase inhibitor of the epidermal growth factor receptor; given at a dose of 100 mg by mouth daily without breaks.

If no progression is found after 5 cycles of therapy, patients undergo a second randomization to:

- 1 additional cycle of chemotherapy (assigned in the first randomization) alone

vs

- 1 additional cycle of chemotherapy (assigned in the first randomization) followed by 50.4 Gy with either capecitabine or 5-fluorouracil

  - 5-fluorouracil is given at a dose of 250 mg/m²/day, 7 days per week by continuous IV infusion via an outpatient infusion pump.
  - Capecitabine is given as 825 mg/m² orally, twice daily Monday through Friday.
  - Concurrent chemotherapy is started on day one of radiation for 5.5 weeks or until radiation is completed.

This study will avoid using radiation for patients who develop metastatic disease during gemcitabine.

www.rtog.org

Answer 56

Lymph nodes in the region of portions of the following vessels are included (see protocol for specific details):

- Celiac
- Superior mesenteric artery
- Portal vein
- Para-aortic

Pancreaticojejunostomy and pre-operative tumor bed regions are also treated.

www.rtog.org

Question 57

What was the outcome of the European Study Group for Pancreatic Cancer 1 Trial (ESPAC-1) of observation, chemoradiation, chemotherapy alone, chemoradiation followed by chemotherapy for patients with resected pancreatic cancer?

Question 58

Has stereotactic body radiotherapy been shown to improve outcomes for patients with unresectable pancreatic cancer?

Question 59

What benefit does chemoradiation provide over best supportive care for patients with locally advanced pancreatic cancer?

Answer 57

This study showed improved survival with chemotherapy alone and a detrimental effect with the addition of radiation therapy.

This study is highly criticized for multiple reasons:

- Poor quality assurance.
- Selection bias (physicians allowed to select one of 3 parallel trials).
- Background treatment was allowed (nearly 1/3 of patients in observation and chemotherapy arms received chemotherapy and radiation).
- Radiation dose was inconsistent (designed for 40 Gy, but choice of 60 Gy offered).
- Only 70% of patients in the radiation arm received radiation.
- No treatment information was obtained for 10% of patients.

Neoptolemos JP, Stocken DD, Friess H, et al. A randomized trial of chemoradiotherapy and chemotherapy after resection of pancreatic cancer. *N Engl J Med*. 2004;350:1200–1210.

Answer 58

Three small reports have shown:

- Relatively high toxicity rates: 25% gastrointestinal ulceration rate in one study.
- No survival benefit compared to modern series with conventionally fractionated radiation therapy and chemotherapy.
- Example of doses that have been tested include 45 Gy in 3 fractions over 5–10 days and 25 Gy in a single fraction.

Hoyer M, Roed H, Sengelov L, et al. Phase-II study on stereotactic radiotherapy of locally advanced pancreatic carcinoma. *Radiother Oncol*. 2005;76:48–53.

Chang DT, Schellenberg D, Shen J, et al. Stereotactic radiotherapy for unresectable adenocarcinoma of the pancreas. *Cancer*. 2009;115:665–672.

Schellenberg D, Goodman KA, Lee F, et al. Gemcitabine chemotherapy and single-fraction stereotactic body radiotherapy for locally advanced pancreatic cancer. *Int J Radiat Oncol Biol Phys*. 2008;72:678–686.

Answer 59

A Japanese study of 31 patients with locally unresectable pancreatic cancer randomized between 50.4 Gy in 28 fractions with concurrent 5-fluorouracil or no chemoradiation.

Treatment resulted in:

- Improved median survival: 6.4 months vs 13.2 months ($p = .0009$).
- One-year survival: 0% vs 53% ($p = .0009$).

Shinchi H, Takao S, Noma H, et al. Length and quality of survival after external-beam radiotherapy with concurrent continuous 5-fluorouracil infusion for locally unresectable pancreatic cancer. *Int J Radiat Oncol Biol Phys*. 2002;53:146–150.

Question 60

What percent of colorectal cancers felt to be caused by microsatellite instability?

Question 61

What genetic pathway is defective in patients with hereditary nonpolyposis colorectal cancer (HNPCC)?

Question 62

What are the most common presenting symptoms of rectal cancer?

Answer 60

Approximately 15% of colorectal cancers are due to replication errors known as microsatellite instability.

The remaining 85% of colorectal cancers thought to arise from chromosomal instability.

The genetic defect is only found in 5–6% of cases of colorectal in families where an inherited risk has been identified.

Kinzler KW, Vogelstein B. Landscaping the cancer terrain. *Science*. 1998;280:1036–1037.
Lengauer C, Kinzler KW, Vogelstein B. Genetic instabilities in human cancers. *Nature*. 1998;396:643–649.
Lindblom A. Different mechanisms in the tumorigenesis of proximal and distal colon cancers. *Curr Opin Oncol*. 2001;13:63–69.

Answer 61

Patients with HNPCC or Lynch syndrome have a genetic defect in mismatch repair (MMR) genes.

The most common mutations involve hMSH2, hMLH1, hPMS1, hPMS2, or hMSH6 and account for approximately 3% to 5% of all colorectal malignancies. Of these, most involve hMSH2 and hMLH1, with 15% to 60% of affected family members having one of these two mutations.

Strate LL, Syngal S. Hereditary colorectal cancer syndromes. *Cancer Causes Control*. 2005;16:201–213.
Syngal S, Fox EA, Li C, et al. Interpretation of genetic test results for hereditary nonpolyposis colorectal cancer: implications for clinical predisposition testing. *JAMA*. 1999;282:247–253.

Answer 62

Gastrointestinal bleeding

Change in bowel habits

Abdominal pain

Intestinal obstruction

Weight loss

Change in appetite

Weakness

Stein W, Farina A, Gaffney K, et al. Characteristics of colon cancer at time of presentation. *Fam Pract Res J*. 1993;13:355–363.

Question 63

Which staging modalities are used in the evaluation of rectal cancer?

Question 64

What is the number of lymph nodes that should be examined for patients entered on node negative rectal cancer trials?

Question 65

Surgical technique for rectal cancer varies depending on tumor location, stage, and presence or absence of high-risk features. What are the surgical techniques used for rectal cancer?

Answer 63

Digital-rectal examination (and rectovaginal exam) in conjunction with rigid proctoscopy is used to determine if sphincter-sparing surgery is feasible.

Complete colonoscopy is used to rule out synchronous lesions.

Computed tomography of the chest, abdomen and pelvis is used to rule out metastatic disease.

Magnetic resonance imaging of the abdomen and pelvis aids in determining depth of invasion, nodal and distant metastases, and feasibility of achieving negative circumferential margins.

Endorectal ultrasound aids in determining depth of invasion and identification of nodal metastases.

Positron emission tomography may improve the sensitivity and specificity for identifying distant metastatic spread.

Schmidt CR, Gollub MJ, Weiser MR. Contemporary imaging for colorectal cancer. *Surg Oncol Clin N Am.* 2007;16:369–388.

Answer 64

In *Guidelines 2000 for Colon and Rectal Cancer Surgery*, for entry to node negative surgical and adjuvant trials, the recommendation was that a minimum of 12 nodes was to be examined.

Lymph node resection is both prognostic and therapeutic.

Accurate staging is essential for patient management and clinic research.

Nelson H, Petrelli N, Carlin A, et al. Guidelines 2000 for colon and rectal cancer surgery. *J Natl Cancer Inst.* 2001;93:583–596.

Answer 65

Polypectomy is used for select T1 cancers without high-risk features.

Transanal local excision and transanal endoscopic microsurgery for select clinically staged T1/T2 N0 rectal cancers without high-risk features.

Total mesorectal excision (TME) with autonomic nerve preservation via low anterior resection.

TME via abdominoperineal resection (APR) with a permanent end-colostomy is used if sphincter-preservation is not feasible.

Balch GC, De Meo A, Guillem JG. Modern management of rectal cancer: a 2006 update. *World J Gastroenterol.* 2006;12:3186–3195.

Baxter NN, Garcia-Aguilar J. Organ preservation for rectal cancer. *J Clin Oncol.* 2007;25:1014–1020.

Question 66

When is neoadjuvant therapy recommended for rectal cancer and what are the potential benefits?

Question 67

For rectal cancer, does T stage still influence outcomes for patients with N2 disease?

Question 68

In the Mayo Clinic/NCCTG 86-47-51 study, patients with stage II or III rectal cancer were treated with adjuvant 5-fluorouracil based chemotherapy and radiation therapy (50.4 Gy) randomized to receive either protracted venous infusion [PVI] (225 mg/m^2 continuously throughout radiation) or bolus 5-fluorouracil (500 mg/m^2 on the first three, and last three days of radiation). What difference in disease outcomes was seen?

Answer 66

Patients with clinical T3, T4 or node positive rectal cancer were included in the German phase III study of neoadjuvant vs adjuvant radiation therapy (5040 cGy) with concurrent chemotherapy (5-fluorouracil, weeks 1 and 5, 5 days per week, 1000 mg/m²).

Compared to adjuvant chemoradiation, neoadjuvant chemoradiation resulted in:

- improved tumor regression
- improved downstaging (8% complete pathological response; 25% compared to 40% lymph node positive rate, $p < .001$)
- improved resectability and higher rate of sphincter preservation (39% sphincter preserving surgery vs 19%, $p = .004$)
- reduced rate of local recurrence (6% vs 13%, $p = .006$)
- no difference in 5 year overall survival

Sauer R, Becker H, Hohenberger W, et al. Preoperative versus postoperative chemoradiotherapy for rectal cancer. *N Engl J Med*. 2004;351:1731–1740.

Answer 67

Yes. On pooled analysis of 2551 patients on three prospective trials (NCCTG 79-47-51, NCCTG 86-47-51, and INT 114) survival was influence by T stage. All patients received postoperative radiation, and 96% received concurrent and maintenance chemotherapy.

Among N2 patients, T stage influenced 5-yr OS as follows:

- T1–2, 69%
- T3, 48%
- T4, 38%

Gunderson LL, Sargent DJ, Tepper JE, et al. Impact of T and N substage on survival and disease relapse in adjuvant rectal cancer: a pooled analysis. *Int J Radiat Oncol Biol Phys*. 2002;54:386–396.

Answer 68

Tumor recurrence 47% for bolus vs 37% for PVI ($p = .01$)

Distant metastases 40% for bolus vs 31% for PVI ($p = .03$)

4-year overall survival 60% for bolus vs 60% for PVI ($p = .005$)

No difference in local recurrence was found ($p = .11$)

O'Connell MJ, Martenson JA, Wieand HS, et al. Improving adjuvant therapy for rectal cancer by combining protracted-infusion fluorouracil with radiation therapy after curative surgery. *N Engl J Med*. 1994;331:502–507.

Question 69

What is the prognostic significance of tumor response, as seen in the German Rectal Cancer Group trial comparing neoadjuvant to adjuvant chemoradiation?

Question 70

What is the prognostic significance of nodal response, as seen in the German Rectal Cancer Group trial?

Question 71

What is involved with a total mesorectal excision (TME)?

Answer 69

Prognosis can be related to the extent of post treatment tumor regression and the final tumor stage in the surgical specimen. The 5-year disease free survival are:

- ypT0: 86%
- ypT1: 95%
- ypT2: 81%
- ypT3: 65%
- ypT4: 42%

Rodel C, Martus P, Papadoupolos T, et al. Prognostic significance of tumor regression after preoperative chemoradiotherapy for rectal cancer. *J Clin Oncol*. 2005;23:8688–8696.

Answer 70

The presence of involved lymph nodes in the surgical specimen affected 5-year disease free survival rates:

ypN0: 85%

ypN1: 65%

ypN2: 18%

Rodel C, Martus P, Papadoupolos T, et al. Prognostic significance of tumor regression after preoperative chemoradiotherapy for rectal cancer. *J Clin Oncol*. 2005;23:8688–8696.

Answer 71

Sharp dissection within the areolar plane of loose connective tissue outside (lateral to) the visceral mesorectal fascia.

With this approach, all mesorectal soft tissues encasing the rectum, including mesentery and all regional nodes are removed intact.

Colon and Rectum. In: Edge SB, Byrd DR, Compton CC, et al., eds. *AJCC Cancer Staging Handbook: from the AJCC Cancer Staging Manual*. 7th ed. New York, NY: Springer; 2010:152–153.

Question 72

What is the benefit of the addition of chemotherapy to pre-operative radiation therapy for rectal cancer?

Question 73

What is the difference in gastrointestinal toxicity and anastomotic stricture rates with preoperative vs postoperative radiation therapy for rectal cancer?

Question 74

What is the risk of sacral fracture risk after preoperative radiation therapy for rectal cancer?

Answer 72

Multiple randomized trials have assessed if concurrent administration of chemotherapy with conventional fractionation RT improves outcomes. Meta-analysis showed concomitant chemotherapy with neoadjuvant radiotherapy, compared to radiation alone, increases:

- Complete pathologic response rates: 11.8% vs 3.5%
- Local control: 16.5% vs 9.4%
- At the expense of higher rates of grade 3 or 4 treatment related toxicity with chemoradiotherapy: 15% vs 5%
- No significant impact on rates of sphincter preservation, disease-free survival, or overall survival is seen.

Ceelen WP, Van Nieuwenhove Y, Fierens K. Preoperative chemoradiation versus radiation alone for stage II and III resectable rectal cancer. *Cochrane Database Syst Rev.* 2009:CD006041.

Answer 73

Preoperative chemoradiotherapy does not appear to increase the complication rate from surgical resection.

In the German Rectal Cancer Group trial (preoperative vs postoperative chemoradiation), incidence of acute grade 3 or 4 gastrointestinal toxicity was: 28.8% vs 31.7%, respectively ($p = .001$). Long-term grade 3 or 4 toxicity was also favored pre-operative therapy (14% vs 24%, $p = .01$).

Postoperative morbidity rates were not higher with neoadjuvant therapy in the German Rectal Cancer Group trial.

Significantly fewer patients undergoing neoadjuvant therapy had chronic anastomotic strictures: 4% vs 12% ($p = .003$).

Sauer R, Becker H, Hohenberger W, et al. Preoperative versus postoperative chemoradiotherapy for rectal cancer. *N Engl J Med.* 2004;351:1731–1740.

Answer 74

Sacral insufficiency fractures are an uncommon late complication of pelvic radiation therapy.

In one report, the incidence of sacral insufficiency fractures at three years after preoperative chemoradiotherapy was 3% overall.

Women appeared to be at a higher risk (5.8% vs 1.6%).

Herman MP, Kopetz S, Bhosale PR, et al. Sacral insufficiency fractures after preoperative chemoradiation for rectal cancer: incidence, risk factors, and clinical course. *Int J Radiat Oncol Biol Phys.* 2009;74:818–823.

Question 75

For which patients with rectal cancer may local excision alone be considered?

Question 76

How many rectal cancers are estimated to have occurred in 2010?

Question 77

What serum tumor marker is useful to assess for patients with colorectal cancer?

When and how often should it be checked?

Answer 75

Generally accepted criteria include:

- Tumor size less than 4 cm
- Location 8 cm or less from the anal verge
- Well or moderately well differentiated histology
- Mobile, not ulcerated tumor
- No suspicion of perirectal or presacral nodes
- Tumor involves less than one-third of the circumference of the rectal wall
- Tumor stage ≤ T2

Blackstock W, Russo SM, Suh WW, et al. ACR Appropriateness Criteria: local excision in early-stage rectal cancer. *Curr Probl Cancer*. 2010;34:193–200.

Answer 76

39,670 cases of rectal cancer were estimated for 2010.

102,900 cases of colon cancer were estimated for 2010.

Cancers of the digestive system represented the organ system with the highest incidence of cancer in 2010 (274,330 cases).

Jemal A, Siegel R, Xu J, et al. Cancer statistics, 2010. *CA Cancer J Clin*. 2010;60:277–300.

Answer 77

Carcinoembryonic antigen (CEA).

Per ASCO 2006 update of recommendations for the use of tumor markers in gastrointestinal cancer, it is recommended that CEA be ordered preoperatively.

Postoperative CEA levels should be performed every 3 months for stage II and III disease for at least 3 years if the patient is a potential candidate for surgery or chemotherapy of metastatic disease.

CEA is the marker of choice for monitoring the response of metastatic disease to systemic therapy.

Locker GY, Hamilton S, Harris J, et al. ASCO 2006 update of recommendations for the use of tumor markers in gastrointestinal cancer. *J Clin Oncol*. 2006;24:5313–5327.

Question 78

Has a survival difference been seen with the addition of preoperative radiation therapy for rectal cancer?

Question 79

What are the outcome differences between pre-operative short-course radiation (5 Gy × 5 fractions) vs preoperative radiation (50.4 Gy in 28 fractions) with concurrent chemotherapy for rectal cancer?

Question 80

What constitutes a "T3" vs "T4" lesion for colorectal cancer according to the *American Joint Commission on Cancer 7th edition* staging manual?

Answer 78

Short-course radiation (5 Gy × 5 fractions) was found to improve local control and overall survival compared to surgery alone in a Swedish randomized study.

- 5-year local control: 89% vs 73%.
- 5-year overall survival: 58% vs 48%.

The Swedish study did not require total mesorectal excision. In a subsequent Dutch study requiring total mesorectal excision, preoperative short-course improved in 5-year local recurrence rates (5.6% vs 10.9%), but no difference in survival was found.

Swedish Rectal Cancer Trial. Improved survival with preoperative radiotherapy in resectable rectal cancer. *N Engl J Med*. 1997;336:980–987.

Kapiteijn E, Marijnen CA, Nagtegaal ID, et al. Preoperative radiotherapy combined with total mesorectal excision for resectable rectal cancer. *N Engl J Med*. 2001;345:638–646.

Peeters KC, Marijnen CA, Nagtegaal ID, et al. The TME trial after a median follow-up of 6 years: increased local control but no survival benefit in irradiated patients with resectable rectal carcinoma. *Ann Surg*. 2007;246:693–701.

Answer 79

A randomized study Poland directly comparing the two pre-operative treatment strategies in 316 patients with T3–4 rectal cancer showed no differences in outcomes at 4 years.

- Early radiation toxicity was higher in the chemoradiation group: 18.2% vs 3.2% ($p < .001$).
- 4-year overall survival: 67.2 % (short-course) vs 66.2% chemoradiation ($p = .960$)
- Disease-free survival: 58.4% vs 55.6% ($p = .820$)
- Crude incidence of local recurrence: 9.0% vs 14.2% ($p = .170$)
- Severe late toxicity: 10.1 vs 7.1% ($p = .360$)

(Note, this is a small study with limited power to detect small differences)

Bujko K, Nowacki MP, Nasierowska-Guttmejer A, et al. Long-term results of a randomized trial comparing preoperative short-course radiotherapy with preoperative conventionally fractionated chemoradiation for rectal cancer. *Br J Surg*. 2006;93:1215–1223.

Answer 80

T3 is defined as "tumor invades through the muscularis propria into pericolorectal tissues."

T4 is defined as "tumor penetrates to the surface of the visceral peritoneum (T4a)" or "directly invades or is adherent to other organs or structures (T4b)."

Colon and Rectum. In: Edge SB, Byrd DR, Compton CC, et al., eds. *AJCC Cancer Staging Handbook: from the AJCC Cancer Staging Manual*. 7th ed. New York, NY: Springer; 2010:155.

Question 81

According the *American Joint Commission on Cancer 7th edition* staging manual, for colorectal cancer, patients with 1–3 regional lymph nodes may be subcategorized into N1a, N1b, and N1c. What differentiates these subsets?

Question 82

According the *American Joint Commission on Cancer 7th edition* staging manual, what factors separate patients from group stage I-II vs stage III colorectal cancer?

Question 83   ANAL CANCER

What virus is known to be a causative agent for anal cancer?

Answer 81

N1a is "metastasis in one regional lymph node."

N1b is "metastases in 2–3 regional lymph nodes."

N1c is "tumor deposit(s) in the subserosa, mesentery, or nonperitonealized pericolic or perirectal tissues without regional nodal metastasis."

Colon and Rectum. In: Edge SB, Byrd DR, Compton CC, et al., eds. *AJCC Cancer Staging Handbook: from the AJCC Cancer Staging Manual.* 7th ed. New York, NY: Springer; 2010:155.

Answer 82

Patients with node positive disease are classified as stage group III if no distant metastatic disease is present.

Patients with the highest "T" stage (T4b), and no evidence of nodal or distant metastatic disease are classified as having stage IIC disease.

Colon and Rectum. In: Edge SB, Byrd DR, Compton CC, et al., eds. *AJCC Cancer Staging Handbook: from the AJCC Cancer Staging Manual.* 7th ed. New York, NY: Springer; 2010:155.

Answer 83

Human papillomavirus (HPV) type 16 is the subtype most frequently associated with anal cancer. Anal cancer incidence is rising; there were an estimated 5,260 new cases and 720 deaths from anal cancer in the United States in 2010.

Other risk factors include:

- Receptive anal intercourse
- High lifetime number of sexual partners
- Smoking
- Anogenital condylomata
- HIV (via increased HPV infection)

American Cancer Society. *Cancer Facts and Figures.* Atlanta, GA: American Cancer Society; 2010.

Ryan DP, Compton CC, Mayer RJ. Carcinoma of the anal canal. *N Engl J Med.* 2000;342:792–800.

Question 84

Based on primary tumor location, what nodal areas are at risk for regional spread of anal cancer?

Question 85

Where does nonkeratinizing squamous cell carcinoma of the anal canal occur?

Question 86

The EORTC 22861 study randomized patients with anal cancer to radiation therapy alone vs radiation therapy with concurrent 5-fluorouracil and mitomycin-C. What benefit(s) were seen with the addition of chemotherapy?

Question 87

The UKCCCR Anal Cancer Trial Working Party trial randomized patients to radiation alone vs radiation therapy with concurrent 5-fluorouracil and mitomycin-C. What benefit(s) were seen with the addition of chemotherapy?

Answer 84

Nodal regions spanning the superficial inguinal to internal iliac lymph nodes may be involved:

- Tumors of the perianal skin, distal anal canal to dentate line – superficial inguinal, femoral and external iliac nodes.
- Tumors above the dentate line – perirectal and internal iliac nodes (internal pudendal, hypogastric, and obturator).
- Proximal anal canal – perirectal and superior hemorrhoidal nodes.

Frost DB, Richards PC, Montague ED, et al. Epidermoid cancer of the anorectum. *Cancer*. 1984;53:1285–1293.
Greenall MJ, Quan SH, Stearns MW, et al. Epidermoid cancer of the anal margin. Pathologic features, treatment, and clinical results. *Am J Surg*. 1985;149:95–101.

Answer 85

Nonkeratinizing squamous cell carcinoma typically arises from the anal canal proximal to the dentate line.

The anal canal is 3–4 cm in length, extending proximally from the anal verge to the rectal mucosa. From the anal verge to the dentate line, the anal canal is lined by squamous mucosa, from which keratinizing squamous cell carcinoma typically arises. The dentate line marks a transition between the distal squamous mucosa and a transitional area of squamous and nonsquamous mucosa.

Ryan DP, Compton CC, Mayer RJ. Carcinoma of the anal canal. *N Engl J Med*. 2000;342:792–800.

Answer 86

In the EORTC study, combined modality therapy resulted in:

- improved locoregional control at 2 years (31% vs 22%, $p = .02$)
- improved colostomy-free interval ($p = .002$)
- no statistically significant difference in overall survival.

Bartelink H, Roelofsen F, Eschwege F, et al. Concomitant radiotherapy and chemotherapy is superior to radiotherapy alone in the treatment of locally advanced anal cancer: results of a phase III randomized trial of the European Organization for Research and Treatment of Cancer Radiotherapy and Gastrointestinal Cooperative Groups. *J Clin Oncol*. 1997;15:2040–2049.

Answer 87

In the UKCCCR study, combined modality therapy resulted in:

- reduced 3-year local failure rates (39% vs 61%, $p < .0001$)
- reduced death from anal cancer (relative risk 0.71, 0.53–0.95, $p = .02$)
- more frequent early ($p = .03$), but not late morbidity.
- no statistically significant difference in 3-year overall survival (65% for combined modality therapy, 58% for radiation alone)

UKCCCR Anal Cancer Trial Working Party. UK Co-ordinating Committee on Cancer Research. Epidermoid anal cancer: results from the UKCCCR randomised trial of radiotherapy alone versus radiotherapy, 5-fluorouracil, and mitomycin. *Lancet*. 1996;348:1049–1054.

Question 88

The intergroup study (ECOG 1289/RTOG 87-04) used radiation therapy (40–50.4 Gy) with concurrent 5-fluorouracil, randomizing patients to the addition of mitomycin-C. What benefit(s) were seen with the addition of mitomycin-C?

Question 89

The RTOG 98-11 trial randomized patients with anal cancer to standard concurrent 5-fluorouracil and mitomycin C vs induction cisplatin and 5-fluorouracil followed radiation (55–59 Gy) with concurrent cisplatin and 5-fluorouracil. What were the difference(s) in results between the two arms?

Question 90

When compared to continuous radiation therapy for anal cancer (RTOG 87-04), what effect does a planned 2-week treatment (RTOG 92-08) break with dose escalated radiation have on treatment outcomes?

Answer 88

The addition of mitomycin-C to radiation therapy with concurrent 5-fluorouracil resulted in:

- improved complete response rate (posttreatment biopsies were positive in 15% of patients in the 5-fluorouracil arm vs 7.7% in the mitomycin-C arm, $p = .135$)
- reduced need for colostomy (4-years colostomy rate 9% vs 22%, $p = .002$)
- improved colostomy-free survival (71% vs 59%; $p = .014$)
- improved disease-free survival (73% vs 51%, $p = .0003$)
- no significant difference in overall survival.
- higher grade 4 and 5 toxicity (23% vs 7%, $p \leq .001$)

Flam M, John M, Pajak TF, et al. Role of mitomycin in combination with fluorouracil and radiotherapy, and of salvage chemoradiation in the definitive nonsurgical treatment of epidermoid carcinoma of the anal canal: results of a phase III randomized intergroup study. *J Clin Oncol.* 1996;14:2527–2539.

Answer 89

Results overall favored standard therapy with concurrent 5-fluorouracil, mitomycin-C, and radiation. Standard therapy compared to induction followed by concurrent cisplatin and 5-fluorouracil resulted in:

- improved colostomy-free survival rates (10% vs 19%, $p = .02$)
- higher rate of Grade 3 or 4 hematologic toxicity (61% vs 42%, $p < .001$)
- similar rate of severe long-term toxic effects (11% vs 10%)
- no difference in 5-year disease-free survival rates (60% vs 54%, $p = .17$)
- no difference in 5-year overall survival rates (75% vs 70%, $p = .10$)
- no difference in 5-year local-regional recurrence rates (25% vs 33%, $p = .07$)
- no difference in 5-year distant metastasis rates (15% vs 19%, $p = .14$)

Ajani JA, Winter KA, Gunderson LL, et al. Fluorouracil, mitomycin, and radiotherapy versus fluorouracil, cisplatin, and radiotherapy for carcinoma of the anal canal: a randomized controlled trial. *JAMA.* 2008;299:1914–1921.

Answer 90

- Despite an effort to escalate radiation dose to 59.4 Gy with concurrent 5-fluorouracil and mitomycin C with a two week planned break in RTOG 92-08, compared to continuous radiation to 50.4 Gy, outcomes appeared to be worse. The two week break occurred after 36 Gy in 20 fractions.
- Disease-free and colostomy-free survivals were higher by approximately 30% in patients treated without a mandatory break, however the difference was not statistically significant.
- Of note, RTOG 92-08 was closed, then re-opened with treatment break removed, resulting in colostomy-free survival rates similar to subsequent protocols using continuous radiation.

Konski A, Garcia Jr M, John M, et al. Evaluation of planned treatment breaks during radiation therapy for anal cancer: update of RTOG 92-08. *Int J Radiat Oncol Biol Phys.* 2008;72:114–118.

Question 91

What nodal groups are included (elective or involved) in the clinical target volume for IMRT planning in the treatment of anal cancer?

Question 92

What is the estimated incidence of anal cancer in the United States for 2011?

Question 93

What is the estimated number of deaths from anal cancer in the United States for 2011?

Question 94

What is the most common, and second most common histologic type of anal canal tumors?

Answer 91

- Peri-rectal
- Inguinal
- External iliac
- Internal Iliac
- Pre-sacral

Myerson RJ, Garofalo MC, El Naqa I, et al. Elective clinical target volumes for conformal therapy in anorectal cancer: a radiation therapy oncology group consensus panel contouring atlas. *Int J Radiat Oncol Biol Phys.* 2009;74:824–830.

Answer 92

5820 new cases of anal cancer were estimated for 2011.

Anal cancer represents only 2.1% of digestive system cancers.

The incidence of anal cancer has increased in the past 30 years worldwide.

Siegel R, Ward E, Brawley O, et al. Cancer statistics, 2011: the impact of eliminating socioeconomic and racial disparities on premature cancer deaths. *CA Cancer J Clin.* 2011;61:212–236.

Answer 93

770 deaths from anal cancer are estimated for 2011.

Tumor diameter and nodal status influence survival.

Ajani JA, Winter KA, Gunderson LL, et al. Prognostic factors derived from a prospective database dictate clinical biology of anal cancer: the intergroup trial (RTOG 98-11). *Cancer.* 2010;116:4007–4013.
Siegel R, Ward E, Brawley O, et al. Cancer statistics: the impact of eliminating socioeconomic and racial disparities on premature cancer deaths. *CA Cancer J Clin.* 2011;61:212–236.

Answer 94

Squamous cell carcinoma represents approximately 75% and adenocarcinoma 20% of cases.

Other histologies include melanoma, neuroendocrine tumors, carcinoid tumor, Kaposi sarcoma, leiomyosarcoma, and lymphoma.

Klas JV, Rothenberger DA, Wong WD, et al. Malignant tumors of the anal canal: the spectrum of disease, treatment, and outcomes. *Cancer.* 1999;85:1686–1693.

Question 95

What represents the superior aspect of the anal canal?

Question 96

Based on the series published by Nigro et al., what percentage of patients were found to have no evidence of disease by biopsy after treatment with 3000 cGy in 15 fractions, combined with 5-fluorouracil and mitomycin-C?

Question 97

Are there differences in disease outcomes between IMRT and traditional 3D-CRT treatment combined with 5-fluoruracil and mitomycin-C for anal cancer?

Question 98

What treatment-related toxicities appear to be improved with the use of IMRT compared to traditional 3D-CRT techniques?

Answer 95

The anal canal begins where the rectum enters the puborectalis sling, at the apex of the anal sphincter musculature. This is approximately 1–2 cm above the dentate line.

Anus. Edge SB, Byrd DR, Compton CC, et al., eds. *AJCC Cancer Staging Handbook: from the AJCC Cancer Staging Manual*. 7th ed. New York, NY: Springer; 2010:165.

Answer 96

84% of patients had no biopsy proven evidence of disease after combined chemotherapy and radiation therapy.

This report from Wayne State University concluded that chemotherapy combined with radiation therapy without abdominoperineal may be offered for patients with anal canal cancer.

Leichman L, Nigro N, Vaitkevicius VK, et al. Cancer of the anal canal. Model for preoperative adjuvant combined modality therapy. *Am J Med*. 1985;78:211–215.

Nigro ND, Seydel HG, Considine B, et al. Combined preoperative radiation and chemotherapy for squamous cell carcinoma of the anal canal. *Cancer*. 1983;51:1826–1829.

Answer 97

No differences in 2 year local-regional failure, colostomy failure, disease-free survival, overall survival or colostomy-free survival was seen in review of data from RTOG 0529 (dose-painted IMRT, 50.4–54 Gy) compared to data from RTOG 9811 (standard concurrent 5-fluorouracil and mitomycin C vs induction cisplatin and 5-fluorouracil followed radiation with concurrent cisplatin and 5-fluorouracil).

Kachnic LA, Winter KA, Myerson RJ, et al. RTOG 0529: A phase II study of dose-painted IMRT (DP-IMRT), 5-fluorouracil, and mitomycin-C for the reduction of acute morbidity in anal cancer. In: American Society of Clinical Oncology 2010 Gastrointestinal Cancers Symposium, 22–24 January 2010, Orlando, FL.; 2010: A-405.

Answer 98

Based on a retrospective comparison of data from RTOG 0529 (dose-painted IMRT) compared to data from RTOG 9811 (3D-CRT), acute grade 3 or higher toxicities favored IMRT:

- Dermatologic toxicity: 20% with IMRT vs 50% with 3D-CRT
- Gastrointestinal toxicity: 20% with IMRT vs 35% with 3D-CRT

Kachnic LA, Winter KA, Myerson RJ, et al. RTOG 0529: A phase II study of dose-painted IMRT (DP-IMRT), 5-fluorouracil, and mitomycin-C for the reduction of acute morbidity in anal cancer. In: American Society of Clinical Oncology 2010 Gastrointestinal Cancers Symposium, 22–24 January 2010, Orlando, FL.; 2010: A-405.

Question 99

Can chemotherapy be avoided for patients with early stage anal cancer (T1/2N0M0)?

Question 100

What dose and schedule of 5-fluorouracil is given concurrently with radiation therapy per RTOG 0529 and RTOG 9811 (dose-painted IMRT for anal cancer)?

Question 101

What dose and schedule of mitomycin-C is given concurrently with radiation therapy per RTOG 0529 and RTOG 9811 (dose-painted IMRT for anal cancer)?

Question 102

What are the mechanisms of action and common toxicities of 5-fluorouracil?

Answer 99

One randomized trial (UKCCCR) included patients with T1 and 2 tumors, however results were not analyzed according to primary tumor stage, thus it is unclear if treatment with chemotherapy can be eliminated.

Retrospective data shows mixed results for the elimination of concurrent chemotherapy.

Randomized data showed combined chemotherapy and radiation therapy improves disease-free survival, local control and colostomy-free survival.

Concurrent chemotherapy is currently recommended for this patient population by the National Comprehensive Cancer Network.

UKCCCR Anal Cancer Trial Working Party. UK Co-ordinating Committee on Cancer Research. Epidermoid anal cancer: results from the UKCCCR randomised trial of radiotherapy alone versus radiotherapy, 5-fluorouracil, and mitomycin. *Lancet*. 1996;348:1049–1054.

Answer 100

Intravenous 1000 mg/m^2/day, for 96 hours (Monday–Friday), starting day 1 of radiation.

A second, and final, cycle is repeated on day 29.
www.rtog.org

Answer 101

Intravenous 10 mg/m^2/day on day 1 and day 29.

Myelosuppresion is a common dose-limiting toxicity of mitomycin-C.

www.rtog.org

Answer 102

Antimetabolite fluoropyrimidine analog of the nucleoside pyrimidine

The active metabolites of 5-fluorouracil inhibit RNA processing, deplete thymidine triphosophate (thus inhibit DNA synthesis) and incorporate into both RNA and DNA.

Lansiaux A. Antimetabolites. *Bull Cancer*. 2011;98:1263–1274.

Question 103

What are the 5-year overall survival for patients with stage I, II, III, and IV squamous cell carcinoma of the anal canal?

Answer 103

Based on data from the National Cancer Database (1985–2000), 5-year overall survival is:

- Stage I – 70%
- Stage II – 59%
- Stage III – 41%
- Stage IV – 19%

Other than T, N, M factors, other predictors of a higher risk of death were male sex, ≥ 65 years old, African-American race, living in lower median income areas, and poorly differentiated cancer.

Bilimoria KY, Bentrem DJ, Rock CE, et al. Outcomes and prognostic factors for squamous-cell carcinoma of the anal canal: analysis of patients from the National Cancer Data Base. *Dis Colon Rectum*. 2009;52:624–631.

6

GENITOURINARY CANCERS

KEVIN L. STEPHANS AND ARYAVARTA M.S. KUMAR

Question 1 PROSTATE CANCER—GENERAL

What is the circulating half-life of prostate-specific antigen (PSA) in a normal male?

Question 2

What has been the effect of PSA screening upon the incidence and stage distribution of patients with prostate cancer?

Question 3

What has been the effect of PSA screening upon the incidence of prostate cancer–specific mortality?

Question 4

Along with stage migration, have there been other changes in the way we assess important prognostic disease parameters (i.e., Gleason score) over time?

Answer 1

PSA is generally accepted as having a half life of 2–3 days.

Lotan Y, Roehrborn CG. Clearance rates of total prostate specific antigen (PSA) after radical prostatectomy in African-Americans and Caucasians. *Prostate Cancer Prostatic Dis*. 2002;5:111–114.

Answer 2

The incidence of prostate cancer increased dramatically more than doubling in the years after screening (from 100/100,000 people to over 240/100,000 people), and now has again decreased to 160/100,000 people with just over 217,000 new diagnosis in 2010.

The stage distribution has likewise changed with a far greater percentage of patients presenting with early stage disease, with only 4% of patients presenting with metastatic disease at presentation.

Cooperberg MR, Moul JW, Carroll PR. The changing face of prostate cancer. *J Clin Oncol*. 2005;23:8146–8151.
Jemal A, Siegel R, Xu J, et al. Cancer statistics, 2010. *CA Cancer J Clin*. 2010;60:277–300.

Answer 3

The annual rate of prostate cancer specific mortality is lower today than in the prescreening era, though the number of patients needed to treat to reduce one death from prostate cancer is quite large (estimated at 1 death reduced for 48 treatments in the European screening study while a United States study did not find reduction in mortality with screening, though the control group did have a substantial rate of background screening).

Andriole GL, Crawford ED, Grubb RL III, et al. Mortality results from a randomized prostate-cancer screening trial. *N Engl J Med*. 2009;360:1310–1319.
Jemal A, Siegel R, Xu J, et al. Cancer statistics, 2010. *CA Cancer J Clin*. 2010;60:277–300.
Schroder FH, Hugosson J, Roobol MJ, et al. Screening and prostate-cancer mortality in a randomized European study. *N Engl J Med*. 2009;360:1320–1328.

Answer 4

Yes, as part of the Connecticut Tumor Registry over 1,800 biopsy slides originally scored in 1990–1992 were re-reviewed between 2002–2004 and the average Gleason score increased by almost a full point (from 5.95 to 6.8) for the same slides. Gleason score migration over time must be accounted for when comparing treatment results from different time frames across studies.

Albertsen PC, Hanley JA, Barrows GH, et al. Prostate cancer and the Will Rogers phenomenon. *J Natl Cancer Inst*. 2005;97:1248–1253.

Question 5
What did the Prostate Cancer Prevention Trial (PCPT) trial assess?

Question 6
What were the results of the Prostate Cancer Prevention Trial?

Question 7
What is the AUA score, what is its range and what does it measure?

Question 8
What lymph node chains are included in nodal staging for prostate cancer (and covered during targeted pelvic nodal radiation)?

Answer 5

The trial assessed the effectiveness of finasteride (Proscar), a 5-α reductase inhibitor, in preventing prostate cancer compared to placebo in men > 55 years old with PSA ≤ 3 ng/mL, normal DRE, and AUA < 20.

Kaplan SA, Roehrborn CG, Meehan AG, et al. PCPT: evidence that finasteride reduces risk of most frequently detected intermediate- and high-grade (Gleason score 6 and 7) cancer. *Urology.* 2009;73:935–939.

Answer 6

The incidence of prostate cancer was lower in the finasteride arm (18.4% vs 24.4%) – RR reduction of 25%. In the finasteride group, 37% were GS ≥ 7 compared with 22% in placebo group. The results have been controversial due to higher incidence of higher grade disease. One explanation may be greater sampling of prostate due to volume reduction with finasteride though upgrading of disease is also considered. Similar trials using other 5-α reductase agents have demonstrated reduction in incidence of cancer without upstaging.

Andriole GL, Bostwick DG, Brawley OW, et al. Effect of dutasteride on the risk of prostate cancer. *N Engl J Med.* 2010;362:1192–1202.
Kaplan SA, Roehrborn CG, Meehan AG, et al. PCPT: evidence that finasteride reduces risk of most frequently detected intermediate- and high-grade (Gleason score 6 and 7) cancer. *Urology.* 2009;73:935–939.

Answer 7

American Urological Association (AUA) score to assess urinary function was developed for BPH. It was used to assess urinary function in prostate cancer. Scale is out of 35 with a lower score being less symptomatic.

Barry MJ, Fowler FJ Jr, O'Leary MP, et al. The American Urological Association symptom index for benign prostatic hyperplasia. The Measurement Committee of the American Urological Association. *J Urol.* 1992;148:1549–1557; discussion 64.

Answer 8

Internal iliac (hypogastric), External iliac (to junction of common iliac), Obturator, and Presacral (S1-S3).

Lawton CA, Michalski J, El-Naqa I, et al. RTOG GU Radiation oncology specialists reach consensus on pelvic lymph node volumes for high-risk prostate cancer. *Int J Radiat Oncol Biol Phys.* 2009;74:383–387.

Question 9
If a biopsy confirms prostate cancer in a regional lymph node, what stage is the patient?

Question 10
What is the M-staging for adenocarcinoma of the prostate?

Question 11
What are the Roach equations for risk of ECE, seminal vesicle, and pelvic lymph node involvement?

Question 12
Given stage migration of prostate cancer over time and other variables, how reliable are the Roach formulas in modern patients?

Answer 9

The patient would have N1 nodal staging, which makes them stage IV.

Prostate. In: Edge SB, Byrd DR, Compton CC, et al., eds. *AJCC Cancer Staging Manual*. 7th ed. New York, NY: Springer Verlag; 2010:457–468.

Answer 10

As defined by the AJCC 7th edition (2009):

M1a is involvement of non-regional lymph nodes
M1b is metastases to bone
M1c is metastases to other sites

Prostate. In: Edge SB, Byrd DR, Compton CC, et al., eds. *AJCC Cancer Staging Manual*. 7th ed. New York, NY: Springer Verlag; 2010:457–468.

Answer 11

ECE: Risk (%) = 3/2 × PSA + 10 × (Gleason-3)

Seminal Vesicle: Risk (%) = PSA + 10 × (Gleason-6)

Lymph nodes: Risk (%) = 2/3 × PSA + 10 × (Gleason-6)

Diaz A, Roach M III, Marquez C, et al. Indications for and the significance of seminal vesicle irradiation during 3D conformal radiotherapy for localized prostate cancer. *Int J Radiat Oncol Biol Phys*. 1994;30:323–329.

Roach M III, Marquez C, Yuo HS, et al. Predicting the risk of lymph node involvement using the pre-treatment prostate specific antigen and Gleason score in men with clinically localized prostate cancer. *Int J Radiat Oncol Biol Phys*. 1994;28:33–37.

Roach M III, Chen A, Song J, et al. Pretreatment prostate-specific antigen and Gleason score predict the risk of extracapsular extension and the risk of failure following radiotherapy in patients with clinically localized prostate cancer. *Semin Urol Oncol*. 2000;18:108–114.

Answer 12

There has been some suggestion in several reviews of modern surgical pathology that the rates of nodal positivity may be substantially lower than those predicted by the Roach formulas. This may influence treatment decision for today's patients.

Nguyen PL, Chen MH, Hoffman KE, et al. Predicting the risk of pelvic node involvement among men with prostate cancer in the contemporary era. *Int J Radiat Oncol Biol Phys*. 2009;74:104–109.

Question 13 PROSTATE CANCER—LOW RISK

What is the evidence to support treatment of early stage prostate cancer?

Question 14

What are the Epstein criteria for prostate cancer and how are they used?

Answer 13

Swedish study SPCG-4 randomized 695 men to radical prostatectomy vs watchful waiting. The RP arm had improved 15 year CSS compared with watchful waiting (14.6% vs 20.7%).

	DSM 5-yr	DSM 10-yr	DM 5-yr	DM 10-yr	LP 5-yr	LP 10-yr	OM 5-yr	OM 10-yr
WW	4.3%	14.9%	9.8%	25.4%	27.2%	44.3%	9.8%	32.0%
RPR	2.3%	9.6%	8.1%	15.2%	8.1%	19.2%	7.8%	27.0%
p-value		.01		.004		< .001		.04

Abbreviations: DSM, disease specific mortality; DM, Distant mets; LP, local progression; OM, Overall mortality.

In a late-breaking presentation at the 53rd annual ASTRO meeting, Widmark et al showed a reduction in biochemical progression, local progression, and distant metastasis, but not overall survival (non-statistically significant trend) for external beam radiation (low dose, 64–68 Gy) in comparison with observation for Gleason 6 and 7 patients (small study with only 214 pts).

Bill-Axelson A, Holmberg L, Ruutu M, et al. Radical prostatectomy versus watchful waiting in early prostate cancer. *N Engl J Med*. 2011;364:1708–1717.

http://www.abstractsonline.com/Plan/ViewAbstract.aspx?sKey=51e76efe-670c-4e43-9860-05dbbc1d55a8&cKey=d27e5993-148d-4304-ab64-ca3b45b6405a&mKey=%7bCCE7E125-D766-49E6-91B4-0BC792B0063A%7d+. Accessed December 16, 2011.

Widmark A, Tomic R, Modi H, et al. Prospective randomized trial comparing external beam radiotherapy versus watchful waiting in early prostate cancer (T1b-T2, pN0, grade 1-2, M0). ASTRO 2011 Annual Meeting, October 2–6; Florida Miami Beach.

Answer 14

- Cancer not felt on digital rectal examination (stage T1a-c)
- PSA density ≤ 0.1 (see below for definition)
- Gleason score is 6 or less with no Gleason pattern 4 or 5
- No more than 2 cores with cancer, or cancer involving no more than 50% of any core on a prostate biopsy

PSA density defined as total serum PSA divided by ellipsoid volume of prostate gland (length × width × height × 0.52). The Epstein criteria were developed to predict for "clinically insignificant prostate cancer on surgical pathology" (tumor < 0.5 cc), however are informally used as extremely conservative criteria for active surveillance at some centers. Older age (age > 65 years) or medical comorbidities have also been added to the criteria.

Epstein JI, Chan DW, Sokoll LJ, et al. Nonpalpable stage T1c prostate cancer: prediction of insignificant disease using free/total prostate specific antigen levels and needle biopsy findings. *J Urol*. 1998;160:2407–2411.

Question 15

In low risk prostate cancer patients, what are possible treatment recommendations?

Question 16

When evaluating a DVH and dosimetric plan, what normal tissue and target dose constraints are considered acceptable?

Question 17

In the Pollack dose escalation phase III study for prostate cancer, what were the randomized arms and how was radiation treatment delivered?

Answer 15

Active surveillance in select patients (biannual DRE and PSA with prostate biopsy every 1–2 years.)

Radical prostatectomy
Prostate brachytherapy alone
External beam radiation therapy alone

NCCN Guidelines 2011 for prostate cancer.

Answer 16

Cover PTV with at least 98% of the prescribed dose, coldest 0.03 cc's to 95%.
Rectum – V70 < 20–25%, V60 < 50% (if covering nodes), V50 < 50% (without nodes)
Small bowel – max point dose of 52 Gy
Bladder – V70 < 25%, V55 < 50%
Femoral heads – V50 < 5%
Penile bulb – as low as possible, mean dose < 52.5 Gy

http://www.rtog.org/ClinicalTrials/ProtocolTable/StudyDetails.aspx?study=0815
Lawton CA, Michalski J, El-Naqa I, et al. RTOG GU radiation oncology specialists reach consensus on pelvic lymph node volumes for high-risk prostate cancer. *Int J Radiat Oncol Biol Phys.* 2009;74:383–387.

Answer 17

This MD Anderson trial randomized patients to 70 Gy vs 78 Gy EBRT at 2 Gy/fx. Dose prescribed to isocenter with 4-field box technique to 46 Gy followed by a cone down to 70 Gy in arm 1 and a 3D cone down to 78 Gy in arm 2. The CTV included the prostate and seminal vesicles.

Pollack A, Zagars GK, Starkschall G, et al. Prostate cancer radiation dose response: results of the M. D. Anderson phase III randomized trial. *Int J Radiat Oncol Biol Phys.* 2002;53:1097–1105.

Question 18

Which groups benefited from dose escalated radiation in the Pollock dose-escalation phase III trial?

Question 19

Was rectal toxicity increased by high dose radiation in the Pollock dose-escalation phase III trial?

Question 20

On subset analysis of patients in the Pollack dose-escalation phase III trial, was any correlation found between biochemical control and rectal distension at the time of simulation (perhaps as a surrogate for potential interfraction motion)?

Answer 18

Predominantly patients with PSA > 10, though in update bRFS was improved in patients with low-risk disease as well.

	Overall and 5-yr FFF/8-yr FFF	PSA > 10 and 5-yr FFF/8-yr FFF	PSA ≤ 10 and 5-yr FFF/8-yr FFF	Low-Risk and 8-yr FFF	5-yr OS/6-yr OS	Gr 3 Rectal Toxicity (at 6 yrs)
70 Gy	69%/50%	48%/28%	~80%/60%	63%	~90%/83%	17%
78 Gy	79%/73%	75%/72%	~80%/74%	88%	90%/90%	38%
p-value	.058/.004	.011/.001	NS	.042	NS	.006

Kuban DA, Tucker SL, Dong L, et al. Long-term results of the M. D. Anderson randomized dose-escalation trial for prostate cancer. *Int J Radiat Oncol Biol Phys*. 2008;70:67–74.

Pollack A, Zagars GK, Starkschall G, et al. Prostate cancer radiation dose response: results of the M. D. Anderson phase III randomized trial. *Int J Radiat Oncol Biol Phys*. 2002;53:1097–1105.

Answer 19

Yes, grade 3 and higher rectal toxicity was increased in the high-dose group, though this was found to be have a significant correlation with rectal dosimetry in particular:

- When rectal V70 ≤ 25%, there was a 16% Grade 2 or higher toxicity.
- When rectal V70 > 25%, there was a 46% incidence of Grade 2 or higher toxicity.

Kuban DA, Tucker SL, Dong L, et al. Long-term results of the M. D. Anderson randomized dose-escalation trial for prostate cancer. *Int J Radiat Oncol Biol Phys*. 2008;70:67–74.

Pollack A, Zagars GK, Starkschall G, et al. Prostate cancer radiation dose response: results of the M. D. Anderson phase III randomized trial. *Int J Radiat Oncol Biol Phys*. 2002;53:1097–1105.

Answer 20

Yes, patients with rectal distension at the time of simulation were found to have an increase in local failure. The larger the cross-sectional area of the rectum at planning, the greater the likelihood for failure. In addition, patients with distended rectum at planning also had lower toxicity, further suggesting that rectal distension was not maintained during treatment, which resulted in the treatment being targeted too anteriorly. Of note no IGRT was used in this study. This may explain the local failure rate as changes in rectal distension may have caused geographical misses.

de Crevoisier R, Tucker SL, Dong L, et al. Increased risk of biochemical and local failure in patients with distended rectum on the planning CT for prostate cancer radiotherapy. *Int J Radiat Oncol Biol Phys*. 2005;62:965–973.

Question 21

Does the use of IGRT potentially address the concern of increased biochemical failure in patients with distended rectum at the time of simulation?

Question 22

How was radiation delivered in the Zietman PROG 95-09 phase III study on dose escalation for prostate cancer?

Question 23

What were the results and conclusion of the Zietman PROG 95-09 phase III study?

Answer 21

Yes, a review of patients treated with BAT ultrasound guided IGRT at the Cleveland Clinic found no influence of rectal volume on outcome for patients of all risk-groups.

Kupelian PA, Willoughby TR, Reddy CA, et al. Impact of image guidance on outcomes after external beam radiotherapy for localized prostate cancer. *Int J Radiat Oncol Biol Phys*. 2008;70:1146–1150.

Answer 22

Patients received a high, or low-dose proton boost, followed by 3D conformal radiation on the PROG 95-09 trial.

A boost was first delivered via proton beam to 19.8 GyE or 28.8 GyE (applied proton beam dose was corrected to photon equivalent using a RBE of 1.1). CTV was prostate + 5 mm margin with PTV an additional 7–10 mm. All patients then received conformal EBRT to 50.4 Gy with CTV prostate + SVs.

Zietman AL, DeSilvio ML, Slater JD, et al. Comparison of conventional-dose vs high-dose conformal radiation therapy in clinically localized adenocarcinoma of the prostate: a randomized controlled trial. *JAMA*. 2005;294:1233–1239.

Answer 23

The study demonstrated a biochemical advantage to high-dose radiation for patients with clinically localized prostate cancer.

5 year FFF for low risk prostate cancer patients (PSA ≤ 10, < T2a, GS < 6) was 60.1% and 80.5% in the 70.2 GyE and 79.2 GyE arms, respectively. There were also 5 year LC and overall 5 year FFF for all patients included. This was the first randomized trial to demonstrate an advantage to dose-escalation in the low-risk group on subset analysis (though it was not specifically powered for this).

	Overall 5-yr FFF	5-yr LC	5-yr FFF Low Risk: PSA ≤ 10, < T2a, GS < 6	5-yr OS	Acute/Late Gr 2 GI toxicity	
70.2GyE	61.4%	47.6%	60.1%	97%	8%	17%
79.2GyE	80.4%	67.2%	80.5%	96%	41%	57%
p-value	< .001	< .001	< .001	NS	.004	.005

Zietman AL, DeSilvio ML, Slater JD, et al. Comparison of conventional-dose vs high-dose conformal radiation therapy in clinically localized adenocarcinoma of the prostate: a randomized controlled trial. *JAMA*. 2005;294:1233–1239.

Question 24

Is there a benefit to using IMRT over a conventional 4 field box or 3D conformal radiation?

Question 25   PROSTATE CANCER—BRACHYTHERAPY

What are important dose constraints for prostate brachytherapy?

Answer 24

While there has not been evidence for a difference in disease control, toxicity appears to be reduced by the use of IMRT (though this is likely to be simply DVH dependent).

In an MSKCC study, there was a reduction in the rate of Grade 2 or higher GI toxicity comparing IMRT with conventional techniques despite the use of greater radiation dose in the IMRT group – 13% vs 5%, respectively. Analysis of the high-dose arm of RTOG 0126 (a phase III trial comparing high-dose to standard-dose radiation, allowing for either 3D-CRT or IMRT) also seems to suggest lower GI toxicity with the use of IMRT (though tighter margins were used for the IMRT patients).

Zelefsky MJ, Levin EJ, Hunt M, et al. Incidence of late rectal and urinary toxicities after three-dimensional conformal radiotherapy and intensity-modulated radiotherapy for localized prostate cancer. *Int J Radiat Oncol Biol Phys*. 2008;70:1124–1129.

Michalski JM, Yan Y, Watkins-Bruner D, et al. Preliminary analysis of 3DCRT vs IMRT on the high dose arm of the RTOG 0126 prostate cancer trial: toxicity report. *Int J Radiat Oncol Biol Phys*. 2011;81:S2

Answer 25

Pre-plan: For I-125, generally accepted dosimetric parameters to the pre-implant plan planning target volume include:

> D90 110–120% of prescription
> > V100 > 99%
> > V150 < 60%
> > V200 < 20%
> Urethra < 150% of prescription

For Pd-103

> D90 110-120% of prescription
> > V100 > 99%
> > V150 < 70%
> > V200 < 30-40%
> Urethra < 150% of prescription

Post-plan:

> D90 > 130-140 Gy for I-125
> D90 > 110-120 Gy for Pd-103
> V100 > 75%
> 1 cc Rectum < 100% of prescription dose

In a 2002 publication, Stock et al. reported that D90 < 140 Gy associated with decreased biochemical control. D90 > 180 Gy associated with increased long term urinary symptoms.

Nag S, Beyer D, Friedland J, et al. American Brachytherapy Society (ABS) recommendations for transperineal permanent brachytherapy of prostate cancer. *Int J Radiat Oncol Biol Phys*. 1999;44:789–799.

Rosenthal SA, Bittner NH, Beyer DC, et al. American Society for Radiation Oncology (ASTRO) and American College of Radiology (ACR) practice guideline for the transperineal permanent brachytherapy of prostate cancer. *Int J Radiat Oncol Biol Phys*. 2011;79:335–341.

Stock RG, Stone NN, Dahlal M, et al. What is the optimal dose for 125I prostate implants? A dose-response analysis of biochemical control, posttreatment prostate biopsies, and long-term urinary symptoms. *Brachytherapy*. 2002;1:83–89.

Question 26

What is the half-life of I-125 and Pd-103?

Question 27

Is there a difference in outcome between I-125 or Pd-103 for LDR prostate brachytherapy?

Question 28

In what setting is prostate brachytherapy appropriate as monotherapy?

Question 29

In what setting is prostate brachytherapy appropriate with EBRT?

Answer 26
I-125 – 60 days

Pd-103 – 17 days

Rosenthal SA, Bittner NH, Beyer DC, et al. American Society for Radiation Oncology (ASTRO) and American College of Radiology (ACR) practice guideline for the transperineal permanent brachytherapy of prostate cancer. *Int J Radiat Oncol Biol Phys*. 2011;79:335–341.

Answer 27
No, based on a randomized trial of I-125 vs Pd-103 implant. This trial enrolled 126 patients. Patients treated with palladium did have a higher intensity of acute side effects with subsequent faster resolution, likely due to a higher dose rate, but there was no evidence for a difference in outcome.

Herstein A, Wallner K, Merrick G, et al. I-125 vs Pd-103 for low-risk prostate cancer: long-term morbidity outcomes from a prospective randomized multicenter controlled trial. *Cancer J*. 2005;11:385–389.
Wallner K, Merrick G, True L, et al. 125I vs 103Pd for low-risk prostate cancer: preliminary PSA outcomes from a prospective randomized multicenter trial. *Int J Radiat Oncol Biol Phys*. 2003;57:1297–1303.

Answer 28
NCCN low (Gleason 6 with PSA < 10) and intermediate risk disease (Gleason 6 with PSA < 20, or Gleason 7 with PSA < 10). RTOG 0232 was recently completed comparing brachytherapy alone vs brachytherapy + supplemental EBRT for intermediate risk prostate cancer, with results pending (use of brachytherapy alone is controversial in this group).

Nag S, Beyer D, Friedland J, et al. American Brachytherapy Society (ABS) recommendations for transperineal permanent brachytherapy of prostate cancer. *Int J Radiat Oncol Biol Phys*. 1999;44:789–799.
RTOG 0232. http://www.rtog.org/ClinicalTrials/ProtocolTable/StudyDetails.aspx?study=0232

Answer 29
NCCN intermediate risk disease (Gleason 6 with PSA < 20, or Gleason 7 with PSA < 10), or T2b-T3, or Gleason 8-10 or PSA > 20).

Nag S, Beyer D, Friedland J, et al. American Brachytherapy Society (ABS) recommendations for transperineal permanent brachytherapy of prostate cancer. *Int J Radiat Oncol Biol Phys*. 1999;44:789–799.

Question 30

What are American Brachytherapy Society guideline exclusion criteria for brachytherapy?

Question 31

After prostate implant, does any PSA rise represent recurrent tumor?

Question 32

How do prostatectomy, brachytherapy, and external beam radiation compare for disease-specific outcomes in low and intermediate risk prostate cancer?

Question 33   **PROSTATE CANCER—HIGH RISK**

What are the classes of androgen deprivation used for prostate cancer?

Answer 30

Life expectancy < 5 years or distant metastasis are contraindications to definitive local therapy.

Prostate > 60 cc, large or poorly healed TURP defect, T3 disease/gross SV invasion, AUA score ≥ 16, and median lobe hypertrophy are relative contraindications to brachytherapy per ABS guidelines, though institutional phase II data from select centers demonstrates acceptable outcomes for patients beyond size criteria, select patients s/p TURP, and patients with moderate median lobe hypertrophy. Anesthesia risk should also be considered.

Nag S, Beyer D, Friedland J, et al. American Brachytherapy Society (ABS) recommendations for transperineal permanent brachytherapy of prostate cancer. *Int J Radiat Oncol Biol Phys.* 1999;44:789–799.

Rosenthal SA, Bittner NH, Beyer DC, et al. American Society for Radiation Oncology (ASTRO) and American College of Radiology (ACR) practice guideline for the transperineal permanent brachytherapy of prostate cancer. *Int J Radiat Oncol Biol Phys.* 2011;79:335–341.

Answer 31

It is important to look at the pattern of PSA rise after a nadir. If the rise is within 3 years, it may represent a PSA bounce. It could also represent residual untreated prostate cells if the rise is very slow or even residual/recurrent prostate cancer. Most rises within 3 years are due to PSA bounce and resolve spontaneously, while rises beyond 3 years typically portend recurrent/metastatic disease.

Ciezki JP, Reddy CA, Garcia J, et al. PSA kinetics after prostate brachytherapy: PSA bounce phenomenon and its implications for PSA doubling time. *Int J Radiat Oncol Biol Phys.* 2006;64:512–517.

Answer 32

There is no randomized data of sufficient volume comparing these modalities.

Several retrospective series suggest similar outcomes for biochemical and cancer free survival in low and intermediate risk patients with the use of these modalities.

Klein EA, Ciezki J, Kupelian PA, et al. Outcomes for intermediate risk prostate cancer: are there advantages for surgery, external radiation, or brachytherapy? *Urol Oncol.* 2009;27:67–71.

Kupelian PA, Potters L, Khuntia D, et al. Radical prostatectomy, external beam radiotherapy <72 Gy, external beam radiotherapy ≥72 Gy, permanent seed implantation, or combined seeds/external beam radiotherapy for stage T1–T2 prostate cancer. *Int J Radiat Oncol Biol Phys.* 2004;58:25–33.

Answer 33

LHRH agonists, anti-androgens (non-steroidal, steroidal), and 5-α reductase inhibitors

Michalski J, Pisansky TM, Lawton CA, et al. Prostate cancer. In: Gunderson LL, Tepper JE, eds. *Clinical Radiation Oncology.* 3rd ed. Philadelphia, PA: Elsevier; 2011:1037–1098.

Question 34

What are the major short term and long-term side effects of androgen deprivation with an LHRH agonist?

Question 35

What organ(s) are responsible for testosterone production, and approximately what percentage of circulating testosterone do they produce in a normal male?

Question 36

Is there an advantage to radiation in addition to life-long hormones for patients with high-risk prostate cancer?

Answer 34

Short term: fatigue, hot flashes, insomnia, decreased libido, and irritability.

Long term: metabolic side effects (dyslipidemia, coronary artery disease, diabetes, insulin resistance, obesity), decreased bone density, decreased muscle mass, gynecomastia, anemia, mood changes, insomnia, fatigue.

Keating NL, O'Malley AJ, Freedland SJ, et al. Diabetes and cardiovascular disease during androgen deprivation therapy: observational study of veterans with prostate cancer. *J Natl Cancer Inst.* 2010;102:39–46.

Answer 35

Testicles (90%), Adrenals (10%)

Ismail M, Ferroni M, Gomella LG. Androgen suppression strategies for prostate cancer: is there an ideal approach? *Curr Urol Rep.* 2011;12:188–196.

Answer 36

Yes, there is an overall survival advantage demonstrated in two prospective randomized trials.

A randomized Swedish study (Widmark et al.) of lifelong androgen deprivation therapy with or without radiation therapy in patients with palpable disease (78% T3) demonstrated improved 10-year cancer-specific (88.1% vs 76.1%) and overall (70.4% vs 60.6%) survival for the addition of radiotherapy. There were slightly more urinary symptoms and erectile dysfunction but overall quality of life was similar between the two based on patient questionnaires. This has been corroborated in similar smaller series.

Fransson P, Lund JA, Damber JE, et al. Quality of life in patients with locally advanced prostate cancer given endocrine treatment with or without radiotherapy: 4-year follow-up of SPCG-7/SFUO-3, an open-label, randomised, phase III trial. *Lancet Oncol.* 2009;10:370–380.
Widmark A, Klepp O, Solberg A, et al. Endocrine treatment, with or without radiotherapy, in locally advanced prostate cancer (SPCG-7/SFUO-3): an open randomised phase III trial. *Lancet.* 2009;373:301–308.

Question 37

Is there a benefit to the addition of androgen deprivation to EBRT for locally advanced prostate cancer (and if so what is the level of benefit)?

Question 38

Is there evidence for a benefit to the addition of androgen deprivation to EBRT for patients who are high-risk by modern disease parameters (i.e., PSA and Gleason score)?

Answer 37

Randomized trials including mostly patients with T3 disease (plus other subsets of palpable, locally advanced, and node positive patients) have demonstrated improvements in overall survival (10–20%) for some trials (i.e., EORTC 22863 and RTOG 85-31), or at least disease specific survival and distant metastasis in others (RTOG 86-10).

EORTC 22863: 70 Gy EBRT +/− 3 Years Goserelin and 1 Month Cyproterone Acetate

10-Year Data	Overall Survival	Clinical Progression Free Survival	Biochemical Progression Free Survival
EBRT + AD	58.1%	47.7%	37.9%
EBRT alone	39.8%	22.7%	17.6%
p-value	.0004	< .0001	< .0001

RTOG 8As5-31: 64–70 Gy EBRT +/− 2 Years to Lifetime Goserelin (Included 15% Node + Patients and Some Postop as Well)

10-Year Data	Metastasis	PSA < 1.5	Disease Specific Survival	Overall Survival
EBRT + AD	24%	31%	84%	49%
EBRT alone	39%	9%	78%	39%
p-value	< .0001	< .0001	.0052	.002

RTOG 86-10: 64–70 Gy EBRT ± 4 Months Goserelin and Flutamide

10-Year Data	Local Failure	Biochemical Failure	Distant Metastasis	Disease Specific Survival	Overall Survival
EBRT + AD	30%	65%	35%	76%	43%
EBRT alone	42%	80%	47%	64%	34%
p-value	.016	< .001	.006	.01	.12

Bolla M, Van Tienhoven G, Warde P, et al. External irradiation with or without long-term androgen suppression for prostate cancer with high metastatic risk: 10-year results of an EORTC randomised study. *Lancet Oncol.* 2010;11:1066–1073.

Pilepich MV, Winter K, Lawton CA, et al. Androgen suppression adjuvant to definitive radiotherapy in prostate carcinoma—long-term results of phase III RTOG 85-31. *Int J Radiat Oncol Biol Phys.* 2005;61:1285–1290.

Roach M III, Bae K, Speight J, et al. Short-term neoadjuvant androgen deprivation therapy and external-beam radiotherapy for locally advanced prostate cancer: long-term results of RTOG 8610. *J Clin Oncol.* 2008;26:585–591.

Answer 38

Yes, D'Amico et al. randomized patients with prostate cancer (cT1b-T2b and either PSA 10-40 ng/mL or Gleason 7-10 or ECE/SV invasion by MRI) to EBRT (70 Gy) +/−6 months of androgen suppression (goserelin or leuprolide + flutamide) beginning 2 months prior to EBRT.

The addition of androgen suppression improved 8-year overall survival from 61% to 74%, and also improved biochemical control, freedom from salvage hormones, and cancer specific survival.

D'Amico AV, Chen MH, Renshaw AA, et al. Androgen suppression and radiation vs radiation alone for prostate cancer: a randomized trial. *JAMA.* 2008;299:289–295.

Question 39

Is there any randomized evidence to support long-term (vs short-term) androgen deprivation in locally advanced prostate cancer?

Question 40

What is the recommended PSA follow-up for patients after completion of radiation treatment?

Answer 39

Yes, two randomized trials of short (4–6 months) vs long-term (28–36 months) androgen deprivation have demonstrated improved outcomes for locally advanced prostate cancer patients receiving long-term androgen deprivation therapy. RTOG 92-02 demonstrated improvements in biochemical failure, distant metastasis and disease specific survival, however, no significant benefit to overall survival. EORTC 22961 demonstrated improvement in all endpoints for long-term androgen deprivation.

RTOG 92-02

10-yr Data	Disease Free Survival	Biochemical Failure	Local Failure	Distant Metastasis	Disease Specific Survival	Overall Survival
Long-Term AD	17.9	34.8	9.4	17.5	87.3 [95.8]	50.4 (81.0)
Short-Term AD	13.1	55.5	15.9	25.8	80.6 [95]	48.7 (70.7)
p-value	.0001	< .0001	.0002	.0002	.0001 [Gleason 2-7 p = NS]	.25 (GS 8+, p = .044)

EORTC 22961

5-yr Data	Biochemical Progression Free Survival	Clinical Progression Free Survival	Overall Survival
Long-Term AD	78.3%	81.8%	85.3%
Short-Term AD	58.9%	68.9%	80.6%
p-value	< .0001	< .0001	.0191

Bolla M, de Reijke TM, Van Tienhoven G, et al. Duration of androgen suppression in the treatment of prostate cancer. *N Engl J Med*. 2009;360:2516–2527.

Horwitz EM, Bae K, Hanks GE, et al. Ten-year follow-up of radiation therapy oncology group protocol 92-02: a phase III trial of the duration of elective androgen deprivation in locally advanced prostate cancer. *J Clin Oncol*. 2008;26:2497–2504.

Answer 40

PSA blood work every 6 months to optimize sensitivity and specificity of possible biochemical failure. This should take place with follow-up H&P.

Ciezki JP, Reddy CA, Stephenson AJ, et al. The importance of serum prostate-specific antigen testing frequency in assessing biochemical and clinical failure after prostate cancer treatment. *Urology*. 2010;75:467–471.

Question 41

For patients that have biochemical failure after definitive treatment for their prostate cancer, what is the median time to development of a bony metastasis and subsequently death from prostate cancer?

Question 42   PROSTATE CANCER—ADJUVANT AND SALVAGE RADIATION

Where are the most common sites of local recurrence s/p prostatectomy?

Question 43

What are the four most favorable factors from the Stephenson nomogram to predict biochemical outcome of salvage radiation?

Question 44

Which patients appear to derive the greatest benefit in cancer specific survival from salvage radiation?

Answer 41

This is highly variable based on patients, era of treatment (available agents for treatment), and Gleason score + PSA kinetics. A review by Freedland et al. suggested a very large range of 4-15+ years for survival following biochemical failure. Pound et al. suggest a median of 8 years to development of bony metastasis and 5 additional years to death from prostate cancer (though again with a large degree of variability).

Freedland SJ, Humphreys EB, Mangold LA, et al. Risk of prostate cancer-specific mortality following biochemical recurrence after radical prostatectomy. *JAMA*. 2005;294:433–439.

Pound CR, Partin AW, Eisenberger MA, et al. Natural history of progression after PSA elevation following radical prostatectomy. *JAMA*. 1999;281:1591–1597.

Answer 42

Perianastamotic (63%), Bladder neck (10%), Retrovesical (17%) (trigone even slightly higher), 10% other.

Poortmans P, Bossi A, Vandeputte K, et al. Guidelines for target volume definition in post-operative radiotherapy for prostate cancer, on behalf of the EORTC Radiation Oncology Group. *Radiother Oncol*. 2007;84:121–127.

Answer 43

Pre-RT PSA < 2 ng/mL (the lower the better), Surgical margins positive, Gleason score ≤ 7, and PSA doubling time > 10 months.

Stephenson AJ, Scardino PT, Kattan MW, et al. Predicting the outcome of salvage radiation therapy for recurrent prostate cancer after radical prostatectomy. *J Clin Oncol*. 2007;25:2035–2041.

Answer 44

Patients who appear to derive the greatest benefit are those with rapidly progressive disease, though still close to time of initial biochemical failure (i.e., perhaps those with high risk disease caught before metastasis). Benefit to salvage radiation was greatest in men with PSA doubling time ≤ 6 months, and no benefit was seen in those who received salvage RT ≥ 2 years after initial biochemical failure.

Trock BJ, Han M, Freedland SJ, et al. Prostate cancer-specific survival following salvage radiotherapy vs observation in men with biochemical recurrence after radical prostatectomy. *JAMA*. 2008;299:2760–2769.

Question 45

What is the benefit of adjuvant (versus salvage) radiation for prostate cancer s/p prostatectomy with pathological findings of extracapsular extension, positive margins, or involved seminal vesicles?

Question 46

What is the magnitude of the survival benefit for adjuvant radiation in the SWOG study after radical prostatectomy?

Question 47

What was the median PSA at the time of salvage radiation in the SWOG trials?

Answer 45

Improvement in local and biochemical control (from approximately 50 to 75%) was seen consistently in three randomized trials (EORTC 22911, SWOG 8794, and ARO 96-02).

Distant metastasis and overall survival were improved in the 10-year update of the SWOG trial (Thompson et al.), however, no statistically significant difference was seen in the 10-year update of the EORTC trial (Bolla et al.) The German trial has not yet reported 10-year results.

Bolla M, van Poppel H, Collette L, et al. Postoperative radiotherapy after radical prostatectomy: a randomised controlled trial (EORTC trial 22911). *Lancet.* 2005;366:572–578.

Bolla M, VanPoppel H, Tombal B, et al. 10-Year results of adjuvant radiotherapy after radical prostatectomy in pT3N0 prostate cancer (EORTC 22911). *Int J Radiat Oncol Biol Phys.* 2010;78:S29.

Thompson IM, Tangen CM, Paradelo J, et al. Adjuvant radiotherapy for pathological T3N0M0 prostate cancer significantly reduces risk of metastases and improves survival: long-term followup of a randomized clinical trial. *J Urol.* 2009;181:956–962.

Wiegel T, Bottke D, Steiner U, et al. Phase III postoperative adjuvant radiotherapy after radical prostatectomy compared with radical prostatectomy alone in pT3 prostate cancer with postoperative undetectable prostate-specific antigen: ARO 96-02/AUO AP 09/95. *J Clin Oncol.* 2009;27:2924–2930.

Answer 46

10-year overall survival 66% (salvage) vs 75% (adjuvant RT).

Median 13.3 years (salvage) vs 15.2 years (adjuvant).

Thompson IM, Tangen CM, Paradelo J, et al. Adjuvant radiotherapy for pathological T3N0M0 prostate cancer significantly reduces risk of metastases and improves survival: long-term followup of a randomized clinical trial. *J Urol.* 2009;181:956–962.

Answer 47

1.0 (in the 80% of patients with PSA available within 6 months of starting radiation therapy).

Thompson IM, Tangen CM, Paradelo J, et al. Adjuvant radiotherapy for pathological T3N0M0 prostate cancer significantly reduces risk of metastases and improves survival: long-term followup of a randomized clinical trial. *J Urol.* 2009;181:956–962.

Question 48

What evidence exists for hormone treatments in the salvage radiation setting?

Question 49

What dose should be used for adjuvant and salvage radiation?

Question 50

NODE-POSITIVE PROSTATE CANCER

For surgically resected patients found to be lymph node positive, is there evidence for initiation of immediate androgen deprivation?

Answer 48

RTOG 9601 evaluated post-RP pts with pT3N0 or with pT2N0 and positive margins with elevated PSA. Patients were randomized to RT alone (64.8 Gy in 1.8 Gy fractions) vs RT + AAT (24 months of bicalutamide, 150 mg daily) during and after RT. The addition of 24 months of bicalutamide 150 mg daily during and after RT significantly improved FFP (57% vs 40%, $p < .01$) and reduced the incidence of metastatic PC without adding significantly to RT toxicity.

There is no currently reported OS benefit. Evaluation in RTOG 0534, a phase III trial of prostate bed radiation with additional arms of prostate bed radiation + androgen deprivation, and prostate bed and pelvic nodal radiation plus androgen deprivation, is ongoing though the primary endpoint is freedom from progression.

RTOG 0534. http://www.rtog.org/ClinicalTrials/ProtocolTable/StudyDetails.aspx?study=0534

Shipley WU, Hunt D, Lukka H, et al. Initial Report of RTOG 9601: a phase III trial in prostate cancer: anti-androgen therapy (AAT) with bicalutamide during and after radiation therapy (RT) improves freedom from progression and reduces the incidence of metastatic disease in patients following radical prostatectomy (RP) with pT2-3, N0 disease, and elevated PSA levels. *Int J Radiat Oncol Biol Phys*. 2010;78:S58

Answer 49

The radiation doses on the three randomized adjuvant trials were 60-66 Gy and in the salvage setting, a dose of 70 Gy is typically used (and recommended but not standardized in the adjuvant trials).

Bolla M, van Poppel H, Collette L, et al. Postoperative radiotherapy after radical prostatectomy: a randomised controlled trial (EORTC trial 22911). *Lancet*. 2005;366:572–578.

Stephenson AJ, Scardino PT, Kattan MW, et al. Predicting the outcome of salvage radiation therapy for recurrent prostate cancer after radical prostatectomy. *J Clin Oncol*. 2007;25:2035–2041.

Thompson IM, Tangen CM, Paradelo J, et al. Adjuvant radiotherapy for pathological T3N0M0 prostate cancer significantly reduces risk of metastases and improves survival: long-term followup of a randomized clinical trial. *J Urol*. 2009;181:956–962.

Wiegel T, Bottke D, Steiner U, et al. Phase III postoperative adjuvant radiotherapy after radical prostatectomy compared with radical prostatectomy alone in pT3 prostate cancer with postoperative undetectable prostate-specific antigen: ARO 96-02/AUO AP 09/95. *J Clin Oncol*. 2009;27:2924–2930.

Answer 50

Yes, the Messing randomized trial demonstrated a survival advantage to immediate versus delayed lifelong androgen deprivation for histologically proven node-positive patients status post prostatectomy (though is sometimes criticized for extremely late use of hormonal therapy in the observation group).

Messing EM, Manola J, Yao J, et al. Immediate versus deferred androgen deprivation treatment in patients with node-positive prostate cancer after radical prostatectomy and pelvic lymphadenectomy. *Lancet Oncol*. 2006;7:472–479.

Question 51

For histologically proven node positive patients being treated with radiation therapy is there evidence to support the upfront addition of androgen deprivation therapy?

Question 52

Is there evidence to support the addition of radiation following discovery of positive lymph nodes at time of radical prostatectomy?

Question 53   **URETHRAL CANCER**

What is the most common histology for cancer of the urethra?

Question 54

Invasion of what structures would stage a urethral cancer as T3?

Answer 51

Yes, a subset analysis of RTOG 85-31 included 173 histologically node-positive patients treated with EBRT, with or without hormonal therapy. The 5-year progression-free survival was significantly increased (54% vs 33%) by androgen deprivation compared to patients randomized to receive hormonal therapy at the time of relapse.

Lawton CA, Winter K, Grignon D, et al. Androgen suppression plus radiation versus radiation alone for patients with stage D1/pathologic node-positive adenocarcinoma of the prostate: updated results based on national prospective randomized trial Radiation Therapy Oncology Group 85-31. *J Clin Oncol.* 2005;23:800–807.

Answer 52

Several phase II studies of adjuvant prostate bed and pelvic radiation with concurrent androgen deprivation suggest outcomes which appear better than observation or lifelong androgen deprivation, and a European matched pair analysis suggests a potential survival benefit.

Briganti A, Karnes RJ, Da Pozzo LF, et al. Combination of adjuvant hormonal and radiation therapy significantly prolongs survival of patients with pT2-4 pN+ prostate cancer: results of a matched analysis. *Eur Urol.* 2011;59:832–840.

Answer 53

This varies by anatomic site. Transitional cell carcinoma and adenocarcinoma typically arise in the proximal urethra. Although squamous cell carcinoma predominates in the distal (penile) urethra, they can arise in any segment, particularly in patients with a history of chronic inflammation.

Squamous cell carcinoma is thought to be most prevalent (75% of urethral cancer), though some series describe a high percentage of TCC as well. Histology may be related to the underlying risk factors of the population (i.e., chronic inflammation versus HPV).

Dalbagni G, Zhang ZF, Lacombe L, et al. Female urethral carcinoma: an analysis of treatment outcome and a plea for a standardized management strategy. *Br J Urol.* 1998;82:835–841.

Dalbagni G, Zhang ZF, Lacombe L, et al. Male urethral carcinoma: analysis of treatment outcome. *Urology.* 1999;53:1126–1132.

Answer 54

Corpus cavernosum, prostatic capsule, anterior vagina, or bladder neck.

Urethra. In: Edge SB, Byrd DR, Compton CC, et al., eds. *AJCC Cancer Staging Manual.* 7th ed. New York, NY: Springer Verlag; 2010:507–514.

Question 55

What is the N staging for urethral cancer?

Question 56

Which lymph node groups do urethral cancers typically drain to?

Question 57

What is the basic management plan for early versus locally advanced urethral cancer?

Question 58

How could one deliver definitive radiation for a bulbo-membranous urethral lesion?

Answer 55

N0—no nodal metastasis

N1—metastases to single LN ≤ 2 cm

N2—metastases to single LN > 2 cm or multiple positive LNs

Urethra. In: Edge SB, Byrd DR, Compton CC, et al., eds. *AJCC Cancer Staging Manual.* 7th ed. New York, NY: Springer Verlag; 2010:507–514.

Answer 56

Lymphatics from the proximal segment drain into the external and internal iliac, obturator and presacral chains. Distal lesions drain to the superficial and deep inguinal lymph nodes.

Dalbagni G, Zhang ZF, Lacombe L, et al. Female urethral carcinoma: an analysis of treatment outcome and a plea for a standardized management strategy. *Br J Urol.* 1998;82:835–841.

Dalbagni G, Zhang ZF, Lacombe L, et al. Male urethral carcinoma: analysis of treatment outcome. *Urology.* 1999;53:1126–1132.

Answer 57

Early distal lesions are typically treated with surgery, local excision with goal of 2-cm margin.

Early proximal lesions (relatively rare as these are typically locally advanced) require more significant surgical management or definitive radiation.

Locally advanced tumors typically treated with combined modality therapy.

Dalbagni G, Zhang ZF, Lacombe L, et al. Female urethral carcinoma: an analysis of treatment outcome and a plea for a standardized management strategy. *Br J Urol.* 1998;82:835–841.

Dalbagni G, Zhang ZF, Lacombe L, et al. Male urethral carcinoma: analysis of treatment outcome. *Urology.* 1999;53:1126–1132.

Answer 58

Options include external beam radiation to the pelvis, tumor, and inguinal areas to 45 Gy followed by either a brachytherapy or external beam boost to gross disease (final target dose of 60–75 Gy). Alternatively for a localized disease could consider brachytherapy alone (likely using an interstitial implant/Syed template to a total dose of 60–65 Gy).

Dalbagni G, Zhang ZF, Lacombe L, et al. Female urethral carcinoma: an analysis of treatment outcome and a plea for a standardized management strategy. *Br J Urol.* 1998;82:835–841.

Dalbagni G, Zhang ZF, Lacombe L, et al. Male urethral carcinoma: analysis of treatment outcome. *Urology.* 1999;53:1126–1132.

Question 59

How would one deliver radiation for a prostatic urethral cancer?

Question 60   **PENILE CANCER**

What defines T2 penile cancer?

Question 61

What is the risk of nodal disease for T1 and T2 penile cancer?

Question 62

What are the risk factors for the development of penile cancer?

Answer 59

Very similar to treatment of prostate cancer with pelvic nodal coverage to 45 Gy and cone down to tumor to high dose (can safely treat to 70–74 Gy given experience with prostate cancer).

Dalbagni G, Zhang ZF, Lacombe L, et al. Male urethral carcinoma: analysis of treatment outcome. *Urology.* 1999;53:1126–1132.

Answer 60

Invasion of the corpus spongiosum or corpus cavernosum

Penis. In: Edge SB, Byrd DR, Compton CC, et al., eds. *AJCC Cancer Staging Manual.* 7th ed. New York, NY: Springer Verlag; 2010:447–456.

Answer 61

11% for T1, 63% for T2

Solsona E, Iborra I, Rubio J, et al. Prospective validation of the association of local tumor stage and grade as a predictive factor for occult lymph node micrometastasis in patients with penile carcinoma and clinically negative inguinal lymph nodes. *J Urol.* 2001;165:1506–1509.

Answer 62

HPV infection (16 & 18), lack of childhood circumcision, penile lichen sclerosis, age, smoking, phimosis, and poor penile hygiene.

Crook J, Mazeron J-J. Penile cancer. In: Gunderson LL, Tepper JE, eds. *Clinical Radiation Oncology.* 3rd ed. Philadelphia, PA: Elsevier; 2011:1167–1182.

Question 63
What is the most important prognostic factor for patients diagnosed with penile cancer?

Question 64
What is the median survival with localized, regional, and metastatic penile cancer?

Question 65
If considering radiation, what is a potential critical pre-radiation anatomic factor to consider due to treatment related edema/erythema?

Question 66
What is the expected penile preservation rate for a T1–T3 penile cancer treated with brachytherapy to 60 Gy?

Answer 63

LN status is single most important prognostic factor. 5 year OS for LN– is 65%, whereas LN+ is 30%. High grade, sarcomatoid and basaloid subtypes have higher risk of nodal metastasis and poorer survival. Verrucous subtype has an excellent prognosis, though may be minimally responsive to radiation (primary management is surgical).

Crook J, Mazeron J-J. Penile cancer. In: Gunderson LL, Tepper JE, eds. *Clinical Radiation Oncology.* 3rd ed. Philadelphia, PA: Elsevier; 2011:1167–1182.

Answer 64

Localized—4 years
Regional—2.5 years
Metastatic—7 months

Rippentrop JM, Joslyn SA, Konety BR. Squamous cell carcinoma of the penis: evaluation of data from the surveillance, epidemiology, and end results program. *Cancer.* 2004;101:1357–1363.

Answer 65

Circumcision typically recommended prior to treatment (without circumcision skin reaction and lymphedema can be extreme during treatment).

Crook J, Mazeron J-J. Penile cancer. In: Gunderson LL, Tepper JE, eds. *Clinical Radiation Oncology.* 3rd ed. Philadelphia, PA: Elsevier; 2011:1167–1182.

Answer 66

88% at 5 years, 67% at 10 years

Crook JM, Jezioranski J, Grimard L, et al. Penile brachytherapy: results for 49 patients. *Int J Radiat Oncol Biol Phys.* 2005;62:460–467.
Crook J, Ma C, Grimard L. Radiation therapy in the management of the primary penile tumor: an update. *World J Urol.* 2009;27:189–196.

Question 67

RENAL CELL CARCINOMA

What are the subtypes of renal cell carcinoma?

Question 68

Is there any role for radiation in the definitive setting for renal cell carcinoma?

Question 69

Is there an indication for adjuvant radiation for resected T3 or T4 renal cell carcinoma?

Question 70

BLADDER CANCER

What is the TN staging for a muscle invasive tumor (inner half of muscle only) with multiple regional lymph nodes involved that are less than 5 cm each?

Answer 67

Clear cell, chromophilic, chromophobic, and collecting duct. Clear cell is associated with necrosis and is predictive of poorer prognosis. The Fuhrman nuclear grading system is also predictive of outcome.

Wong WW, Buskirk SJ, Tan WW, et al. Kidney and ureteral carcinoma. In: Gunderson LL, Tepper JE, eds. *Clinical Radiation Oncology*. 3rd ed. Philadelphia, PA: Elsevier; 2011:1145–1167.

Answer 68

In general no, particularly given the excellent tolerability of laparoscopic nephrectomy/partial nephrectomy. However, there is a small experience looking at treating renal cell carcinoma definitively. With mild side effects, local control was > 90% with SBRT in a series of 58 lesions including control in 8 out of 8 primary inoperable lesions.

Wersall PJ, Blomgren H, Lax I, et al. Extracranial stereotactic radiotherapy for primary and metastatic renal cell carcinoma. *Radiother Oncol.* 2005;77:88–95.

Answer 69

Typically no. Four randomized trials of neoadjuvant or adjuvant radiation have not revealed a benefit to radiation in combination with surgical resection (in fact some demonstrate a detriment), though these trials are using older radiation treatment techniques and targeting.

Doyle C, Tannock IF. Adjuvant radiation or systemic therapy for renal cell carcinoma: a brief review. *Urol Oncol.* 1995;1:161–165.

Answer 70

T2aN2

Urinary Bladder. In: Edge SB, Byrd DR, Compton CC, et al., eds. *AJCC Cancer Staging Manual*. 7th ed. New York, NY: Springer Verlag; 2010:497–506.

Question 71
What is the most common site for transitional cell carcinoma of the bladder (the most common histology)?

Question 72
What is the most common site for adenocarcinoma of the bladder?

Question 73
What is the general paradigm for treatment planning with radiation to the bladder?

Question 74
What is the 5 year OS for patients treated with chemoRT for bladder cancer?

Answer 71

Trigone, followed by bladder neck.

Efstathiou JA, Zietman AL, Coen JJ, et al. Bladder cancer. In: Gunderson LL, Tepper JE, eds. *Clinical Radiation Oncology*. 3rd ed. Philadelphia, PA: Elsevier; 2011:1099–1124.

Answer 72

Urachus (located at the remnant of the umbilical cord).

Efstathiou JA, Zietman AL, Coen JJ, et al. Bladder cancer. In: Gunderson LL, Tepper JE, eds. *Clinical Radiation Oncology*. 3rd ed. Philadelphia, PA: Elsevier; 2011:1099–1124.

Answer 73

Radiation is targeted to the entire bladder plus pelvic lymph nodes (40-46 Gy), followed by a cone down to the whole bladder (50-54 Gy), and a boost to the tumor + 2 cm (as defined by all available imaging + cystoscopy) to around 64 Gy.

Logue J, McBain CA. Radiation therapy for muscle-invasive bladder cancer: treatment planning and delivery. *Clin Oncol (R Coll Radiol)*. 2005;17:508–513.

Answer 74

~50%, which compares equitably with surgical series—however, this is not the case for all bladder sparing series perhaps due to selection bias in comparison with operative series.

Shipley WU, Winter KA, Kaufman DS, et al. phase III trial of neoadjuvant chemotherapy in patients with invasive bladder cancer treated with selective bladder preservation by combined radiation therapy and chemotherapy: Initial results of Radiation Therapy Oncology Group 89-03. *J Clin Oncol*. 1998;16:3576–3583.

Question 75

What is the CR rate after induction with cisplatinum-based chemoradiation?

Question 76

What are the contraindications (relative or absolute) to bladder conservation treatment with chemoradiation?

Question 77

In patients treated with bladder preservation, what is the rate of grade 3 GI and grade 3 GU toxicity?

Question 78

Is there an advantage to neoadjuvant chemotherapy prior to chemo-radiation for locally advanced bladder cancer?

Answer 75

~70–80% (patients with less than a complete response after induction chemoradiation should go on to salvage cystectomy).

Kaufman DS, Shipley WU, Feldman AS. Bladder cancer. *Lancet*. 2009;374:239–249.

Shipley WU, Winter KA, Kaufman DS, et al. Phase III trial of neoadjuvant chemotherapy in patients with invasive bladder cancer treated with selective bladder preservation by combined radiation therapy and chemotherapy: initial results of Radiation Therapy Oncology Group 89-03. *J Clin Oncol*. 1998;16:3576–3583.

Tester W, Caplan R, Heaney J, et al. Neoadjuvant combined modality program with selective organ preservation for invasive bladder cancer: results of Radiation Therapy Oncology Group phase II trial 8802. *J Clin Oncol*. 1996;14:119–126.

Answer 76

Multifocal tumor/CIS
Tumor size > 5 cm
T4
Ureteral involvement
Hydronephrosis
Chronic cystitis
Poor bladder function
Node positive
Metastatic disease

Kaufman DS, Shipley WU, Feldman AS. Bladder cancer. *Lancet*. 2009;374:239–249.

Answer 77

In a combined analysis of 4 RTOG trials, there is a 6% late grade 3 GU toxicity and 2% late grade 3 GI toxicity. No reported grade 4 or 5 toxicity.

Efstathiou JA, Bae K, Shipley WU, et al. Late pelvic toxicity after bladder-sparing therapy in patients with invasive bladder cancer: RTOG 89-03, 95-06, 97-06, 99-06. *J Clin Oncol*. 2009;27:4055–4061.

Answer 78

No per RTOG 8903. Patients were randomized to +/− neoadjuvant chemotherapy with methotrexate, cisplatin, and vinblastine followed by chemo-radiation to 64.8 Gy total.

Shipley WU, Winter KA, Kaufman DS, et al. Phase III trial of neoadjuvant chemotherapy in patients with invasive bladder cancer treated with selective bladder preservation by combined radiation therapy and chemotherapy: initial results of Radiation Therapy Oncology Group 89-03. *J Clin Oncol*. 1998;16:3576–3583.

Question 79

What are common risk factors for testicular cancer?

Question 80

What are the subtypes of germ cell tumors, and what are the associated tumor markers?

Question 81

What is the half-life of β-HCG and AFP?

Answer 79

CIS (50%), Cryptorchidism (35 × baseline), undescended testis, previous testicular cancer within 5 years (2–5%), infertility, family history (father – 4× baseline, brother 8–10× baseline). Klinefelter's associated with risk of mediastinal germ cell tumors.

Warde PR, Hogg D, Gospodarowicz MK. Testicular cancer. In: Gunderson LL, Tepper JE, eds. *Clinical Radiation Oncology*. 3rd ed. Philadelphia, PA: Elsevier; 2011:1125–1144.

Answer 80

Seminoma – may express β-HCG modestly (< 100 ng/ml) in 15% of pure seminomas (due to syncytio-trophoblastic cells, no difference in treatment or prognosis from non-β-HCG expressing seminoma), if other markers expressed pure seminoma is ruled out (though AFP can occasionally be from a liver source).

Classic Seminoma – most common

Anaplastic – more mitosis per high-power field than classic, in older series suggestion of worse prognosis, modern series suggest similar outcomes and treatment is the same as Classic Seminoma.

Spermatocytic – rare subtype, seen predominately in men over 45 y/o, not associated w CIS, almost never spreads to nodes therefore typically adjuvant treatment is not indicated.

Non-seminoma

Yolk Sack Tumor +AFP, −β-HCG

Choriocarcinoma −AFP, +β-HCG (typically extremely high)

Embryonal +AFP, +β-HCG

Teratoma variable, typically marker negative

Warde PR, Hogg D, Gospodarowicz MK. Testicular cancer. In: Gunderson LL, Tepper JE, eds. *Clinical Radiation Oncology*. 3rd ed. Philadelphia, PA: Elsevier; 2011:1125–1144.

Answer 81

β-HCG – 1.5–2 days
AFP – 5–7 days

Warde PR, Hogg D, Gospodarowicz MK. Testicular cancer. In: Gunderson LL, Tepper JE, eds. *Clinical Radiation Oncology*. 3rd ed. Philadelphia, PA: Elsevier; 2011:1125–1144.

Question 82

What is the risk of recurrence with observation for a stage I seminoma patient choosing to undergo observation with a:

a. 2-cm tumor, no LVSI or rete-testis invasion?
b. 5-cm tumor, no LVSI or rete-testis invasion?
c. 5-cm tumor, with LVSI and rete-testis invasion?

Question 83

For a patient with stage I seminoma undergoing adjuvant radiation, what is the 5-year relapse free and overall survival, and for those patients who do suffer relapse where does relapse typically occur?

Question 84

What are the relative advantages of treating 20 vs 30 Gy for adjuvant radiation for stage I seminoma with respect to tumor control and toxicity (based on the best available randomized evidence)?

Question 85

What are the relative advantages of treating a para-aortic strip versus dogleg field for adjuvant radiation for stage I seminoma with respect to tumor control, and toxicity (based on the best available randomized evidence)?

Answer 82

a. 6–12%
b. 16%
c. 32%

Aparicio J, Garcia del Muro X, Maroto P, et al. Multicenter study evaluating a dual policy of postorchiectomy surveillance and selective adjuvant single-agent carboplatin for patients with clinical stage I seminoma. *Ann Oncol.* 2003;14:867–872.

Aparicio J, Germa JR, Garcia del Muro X, et al. Risk-adapted management for patients with clinical stage I seminoma: the Second Spanish Germ Cell Cancer Cooperative Group Study. *J Clin Oncol.* 2005;23:8717–8723.

Warde P, Specht L, Horwich A, et al. Prognostic factors for relapse in stage I seminoma managed by surveillance: a pooled analysis. *J Clin Oncol.* 2002;20:4448–4452.

Answer 83

5-year OS 99%, 5-year RFS 97%

Patterns of failure: 1% in pelvis, 1% in mediastinum/SCV, 1% distant (typically pulmonary).

Fossa SD, Horwich A, Russell JM, et al. Optimal planning target volume for stage I testicular seminoma: a Medical Research Council randomized trial. Medical Research Council Testicular Tumor Working Group. *J Clin Oncol.* 1999;17:1146

Jones WG, Fossa SD, Mead GM, et al. Randomized trial of 30 vs 20 Gy in the adjuvant treatment of stage I testicular seminoma: a report on Medical Research Council Trial TE18, European Organisation for the Research and Treatment of Cancer Trial 30942 (ISRCTN18525328). *J Clin Oncol.* 2005;23:1200–1208.

Oliver RT, Mason MD, Mead GM, et al. Radiotherapy versus single-dose carboplatin in adjuvant treatment of stage I seminoma: a randomised trial. *Lancet.* 2005;366:293–300.

Answer 84

On the MRC TE18/EORTC 30942 randomized trial of over 600 patients, there was no evidence of any difference in disease control (relapse free survival of 97% on both arms), while toxicity was less for patients receiving 20 Gy (moderate to severe lethargy 5% vs 20%, and inability to work 28% vs 46%).

Jones WG, Fossa SD, Mead GM, et al. Randomized trial of 30 vs 20 Gy in the adjuvant treatment of stage I testicular seminoma: a report on Medical Research Council Trial TE18, European Organisation for the Research and Treatment of Cancer Trial 30942 (ISRCTN18525328). *J Clin Oncol.* 2005;23:1200–1208.

Answer 85

On the MRC TE10 randomized trial of over 475 patients, there was no significant difference in 3-year disease free (96.6% for dogleg vs 96.0% for PA strip), or overall survival (100% vs 99.3%), though there were 4 pelvic failures in the PA strip alone group. The PA strip patients did experience less toxicity (lower rates of nausea and vomiting, diarrhea, leukopenia, and azoospermia) compared to patients in the dogleg arm.

Fossa SD, Horwich A, Russell JM, et al. Optimal planning target volume for stage I testicular seminoma: a Medical Research Council randomized trial. Medical Research Council Testicular Tumor Working Group. *J Clin Oncol.* 1999;17:1146–1154.

Question 86

The MRCTE19/EORTC 30982 study by Oliver and colleagues tested a single cycle of carboplatinum; is there a potential advantage to more cycles?

Question 87

What is the standard of care for management of stage IIA or IIB seminoma with pelvic adenopathy ≤ 5 cm?

Question 88

What is the standard of care for management of stage IIC or higher seminoma, or non-seminomatous germ cell tumors?

Question 89

What is the rate of second malignancies in long-term survivors of seminoma treated with radiation, chemotherapy, or both?

Answer 86

Yes, the recurrence rate appears to be perhaps numerically lower with 2 cycles of carboplatinum (though without a head-to-head randomized comparison).

In combination of trials recurrences in patients given 2 cycles of carboplatin was 2–3%.

Aparicio J, Germa JR, Garcia del Muro X, et al. Risk-adapted management for patients with clinical stage I seminoma: the Second Spanish Germ Cell Cancer Cooperative Group study. *J Clin Oncol.* 2005;23:8717–8723.
Dieckmann KP, Bruggeboes B, Pichlmeier U, et al. Adjuvant treatment of clinical stage I seminoma: is a single course of carboplatin sufficient? *Urology.* 2000;55:102–106.
Steiner H, Scheiber K, Berger AP, et al. Retrospective multicentre study of carboplatin monotherapy for clinical stage I seminoma. *BJU Int.* 2011;107:1074–1079.

Answer 87

The standard of care for stage IIA or IIB seminoma is radiation to a dogleg field (PA strip is not appropriate for stage II disease as these patients were excluded from the Fossa trial), with a boost to the involved lymph node if greater than 2 cm.

Warde PR, Hogg D, Gospodarowicz MK. Testicular cancer. In: Gunderson LL, Tepper JE, eds. *Clinical Radiation Oncology.* 3rd ed. Philadelphia, PA: Elsevier; 2011:1125–1144.

Answer 88

The standard of care for management of stage IIC or higher seminoma, or non-seminomatous germ cell tumors is chemotherapy with BEP (bleomycin, etoposide, and cisplatinum). Both advanced seminomatous tumors as well as non-seminomatous germ cell tumors are radiation responsive, and in-field recurrence rates are low with radiation, however distant failure rates are high without systemic therapy in these patients.

Warde PR, Hogg D, Gospodarowicz MK. Testicular cancer. In: Gunderson LL, Tepper JE, eds. *Clinical Radiation Oncology.* 3rd ed. Philadelphia, PA: Elsevier; 2011:1125–1144.

Answer 89

Elevated risk documented in 10 year survivors and remains above baseline for 35 years.

Radiation: Relative Risk = 2.0, 36% incidence (23% general population)
Chemotherapy: Relative Risk = 1.8, 31% incidence (23% general population)
Both: Relative Risk = 2.9

Travis LB, Fossa SD, Schonfeld SJ, et al. Second cancers among 40,576 testicular cancer patients: focus on long-term survivors. *J Natl Cancer Inst.* 2005;97:1354–1365.

Question 90

Special Situations in Testicular Cancer:

a. How would you handle radiation for a patient with trans-scrotal orchiectomy, or trans-scrotal biopsy?
b. When would you cover the inguinal scar?
c. What is the role of prophylactic mediastinal irradiation?
d. Treatment options for a patient with a horseshoe kidney, difficulty sparing kidney, or inflammatory bowel disease?

Answer 90

a. Classically the inguinal nodes and scrotum were often covered in treatment fields for these patients, however, this dramatically increases contralateral testicular dose and a Royal Marsden/Princess Margaret series also describes 15% of patients having had scrotal violation without any patient suffering scrotal or inguinal recurrence. Recommend treatment of scrotum + inguinals for gross tumor spillage with scrotal violation, or primary invasion of the scrotum by tumor.

b. Only for gross tumor spillage during surgery. At Cleveland Clinic, we encourage the scar to be wired for all cases as a double check on laterality of surgery/radiation.

c. There is no longer a role as the increased risk of cardiac death exceeds any potential benefit.

d. These patients should be treated with observation (if stage I), or chemotherapy (1–2 cycles of carboplatinum for stage I patients, or BEP for stage II patients).

Warde PR, Hogg D, Gospodarowicz MK. Testicular cancer. In: Gunderson LL, Tepper JE, eds. Clinical Radiation Oncology. 3rd ed. Philadelphia, PA: Elsevier; 2011:1125–1144.

7

GYNECOLOGIC CANCERS

HENRY BLAIR

Question 1

What are the FIGO approved evaluation procedures for staging cervix cancer?

Question 2

What are the FIGO allowed imaging procedures for cervix cancer?

Question 3

How does twice daily radiation therapy (BID) + standard brachytherapy compare with once daily radiation therapy + standard brachytherapy with respect to OS, DFS and toxicity in patients with IB2-IVA cancer of the cervix who are not receiving chemotherapy?

Answer 1

The FIGO-approved evaluation procedures are physical exam including pelvic exam, colposcopy, biopsy, conization of the cervix, cystoscopy and proctosigmoidoscopy.

NCCN Clinical Practice Guidelines in Oncology: Cervical Cancer Version 1.2012. Fort Washington, PA: National Comprehensive Cancer Network, 2011. http://www.nccn.org/professionals/physician. Accessed October 14, 2011.

Answer 2

FIGO staging of cervix cancer is clinically based not surgically based.

FIGO allowed imaging procedures for cervix cancer include plain film xrays of the lungs and skeleton, IVP, and barium enema. CT and MRI scans are not allowed imaging procedures per FIGO, although they are often obtained for treatment planning.

NCCN Clinical Practice Guidelines in Oncology: Cervical Cancer Version 1.2012. Fort Washington, PA: National Comprehensive Cancer Network, 2011. http://www.nccn.org/professionals/physician. Accessed October 14, 2011.
Edge SB, Byrd DR, Compton CC, et al., eds. *AJCC Cancer Staging Handbook: From the AJCC Cancer Staging Manual.* Cervix Uteri. 7th ed. New York, NY: Springer; 2010: 475.

Answer 3

RTOG 88-05 compared BID to once-a-day radiation therapy. Comparing the survival and late effects of RTOG 88-05 with the control arms of RTOG 80-05 and RTOG 79-20, BID radiation showed no advantage to once-a-day radiation.

- Trial Info (phase I/II): 1.2 Gy BID to pelvis followed by one or two low-dose-rate intracavitary implants. Total minimum dose 85 Gy to Point A and 65 Gy to the lateral pelvic lymph nodes.
- Eligible clinical stages: clinical stage IB2, IIA, IIB, IIIA, IIIB, or IVA
- 81 patients enrolled and 73 patients completed EBRT + brachytherapy.
- DFS rate: 43% at 3 years, 38% at 5 years, and 33% at 8 years.
- The pelvic failure rate was 41%.
- Grade 3 and 4 late effects:
  stages IB2, IIA, IIB: 7% at 3 years, 7% at 5 years, and 10% at 8 years.
  stages III, IVA disease: 7% at 3 years and 12% at 5 years.

Grigsby P, Winter K, Komaki R, et al. Long-term follow-up of RTOG 88-05: Twice-daily external irradiation with brachytherapy for carcinoma. *Int J Radiat Oncol Biol Phys.* 2002;54:51–57.

Question 4

How does twice daily radiation therapy (BID) + standard brachytherapy compare with once daily radiation therapy + standard brachytherapy with respect to OS, DFS, and toxicity in patients with IB2-IVA cancer of the cervix, biopsy-proven para-aortic LN metastasis who receive chemotherapy?

Question 5

What is the role for amifostine to reduce acute toxicity in patients with cervix cancer and para-aortic LN metastasis treated with extended field radiation therapy, brachytherapy, and concurrent chemotherapy?

Answer 4

RTOG 92-10: Concluded no significant increase in OS compared with daily EBRT + chemotherapy; unacceptable increase in Grade 3 and higher toxicity. Survival estimates seemed no better than standard fractionation irradiation without chemotherapy.

Trial Info: phase II trial in stage I–IV with biopsy-proven para-aortic LN metastasis received chemotherapy (cisplatin + 5FU) + EBRT: 1.2 Gy BID (pelvis and para-aortic LNs). 29 patients were enrolled, 20 completed radiation therapy (EBRT + brachytherapy) + chemotherapy.

Results:

- 4-yr OS: 29%
- Probability LR failure @ 3-yr: 50%
- Probability of disease failure at any site @ 3-yr: 63%
- Grade 5 (death) 1 patient died < 90 days completion RT

Grigsby P, Lu J, Mutch D, et al. Twice-daily fractionation of external irradiation with brachytherapy and chemotherapy in carcinoma of the cervix with positive para-aortic lymph nodes: phase II study of the Radiation Therapy Oncology Group 92-10. *Int J Radiat Oncol Biol Phys*. 1998;41:817–822.

Grigsby P, Heydon K, Mutch D, et al. Long-term follow-up of RTOG 92-10: cervical cancer with positive para-aortic lymph nodes. *Int J Radiat Oncol Biol Phys*. 2001;51:982–987.

Answer 5

Conclusion: RTOG 0116: extended field and intracavitary irradiation with cisplatin for para-aortic or high common iliac metastasis from cervical cancer is associated with significant acute and late toxicity. Amifostine did not reduce acute toxicity in this patient population.

Trial Info: Concurrent weekly cisplatin-based chemotherapy and extended field (pelvis and para-aortic region) radiotherapy and intracavitary brachytherapy in patients with high-common iliac or para-aortic metastasis from cervical cancer. RT Dose: 45 Gy/25 fx with intracavitary brachytherapy. IMRT was not allowed. The final point A dose was 85 Gy low-dose rate equivalent. HDR techniques were allowed. The positive para-aortic and iliac nodes were to be boosted to 54 to 59.4 Gy. Amifostine (Arm 2) at 500 mg was to be delivered with every fraction of radiotherapy (8/1/00 – 3/3/07). There were no treatment related deaths. Due to GI acute toxicity the study was amended August 1, 2003, to mandate use of proton-pump inhibitors during radiotherapy. The estimated median survival was 34.8 months.

	Arm 1 ($n = 21$)	Arm 2 ($n = 15$) (Amifostine)
Med f/u	17.1 mos	22.9 mos
Acute Grade 3/4 toxicity excluding grade 3 leukopenia	81	87
Late Grade 3/4 toxicity	20	20

Small W, Winter K, Levenback C, et al. Extended-field irradiation and intracavitary brachytherapy with cisplatin chemotherapy for cervical cancer with positive para-aortic or high common iliac lymph nodes: results of arm 1 of RTOG 0116. *Int J Radiat Oncol Biol Phys*. 2007;68:1081–1087.

Small W, Winter K, Levenback C, et al. Extended-field irradiation and intracavitary brachytherapy combined with cisplatin and amifostine for cervical cancer with positive para-aortic or high common iliac lymph nodes: results of arm II of Radiation Therapy Oncology Group (RTOG) 0116. *Int J Gynecol Cancer*. 2011;7:1266–1275.

Question 6

What are the high risk factors for patients with clinical stage IA2, IB, IIA cervix cancer treated with radical hysterectomy (type 3) with pelvic lymphadenectomy that warrant the use of adjuvant chemotherapy and radiation therapy?

Question 7

Which clinical stages of cervix cancer, based on most recent FIGO revision published in 2009, are suitable for surgery as the definitive treatment?

Question 8

When treating IB2–IVA cancer of the cervix with RT + concurrent chemotherapy, what is the recommended dose of RT and type of chemotherapy?

Answer 6

(1) Positive pelvic lymph nodes *and/or* (2) Positive margins *and/or* (3) Microscopic involvement of the parametrium.

Published results of an intergroup trial (SWOG, RTOG, GOG) randomizing patients between post-op RT vs RT + CT. Chemotherapy = Cisplatin and 5 FU. Between 1991 and 1996, 243 out of 268 patients enrolled were: 127 RT + CT and 116 RT. No brachytherapy was allowed.

- HR for PFS and OS for RT vs RT + CT: 2.01 ($p = .003$) and 1.96 ($p = .007$), respectively.
- Projected PFS at 4 years was 63% with RT and 80% with RT + CT.
- Projected overall survival rate at 4 years was 71% with RT and 81% with RT + CT.
- Grades 3 and 4 hematologic and gastrointestinal toxicity were more frequent in the RT + CT group.

Peters III WA, Liu PY, Barrett II J, et al. Concurrent chemotherapy and pelvic radiation therapy compared with pelvic radiation therapy alone as adjuvant therapy after radical surgery in high-risk early-stage cancer of the cervix. *J Clin Oncol.* 2000;18:1606–1613.

Benedet JL, ed. *Staging Classifications and Clinical Practice Guidelines for Gynecological Cancers.* 3rd ed. http://www.figo.org/publications/staging_classifications. Accessed Novembre 26, 2011.

Answer 7

IA1: Extrafascial hysterectomy *or* observe if patient desires fertility or inoperable (only if cone biopsy has negative margins), *or* modified radical hysterectomy *or* trachelectomy + pelvic lymph node dissection if lymphovascular invasion

IA2: Radical hysterectomy + pelvic lymph node dissection (+/−) para-aortic lymph node sampling, *or* radical trachelectomy + pelvic lymph node dissection (+/−) para-aortic lymph node sampling

IB1: Radical trachelectomy for tumors ≤ 2 cm + pelvic LND (+/−) para-aortic lymph node sampling
   Selected IIA: Radical hysterectomy + pelvic LND (+/−) para-aortic lymph node sampling

NCCN Clinical Practice Guidelines in Oncology: Cervical Cancer Version 1.2012. Fort Washington, PA: National Comprehensive Cancer Network, 2011. http://www.nccn.org/professionals/physician. Accessed October 14, 2011.

Answer 8

Chemoradiation therapy: Pelvic RT (45 Gy/25 fx) + brachytherapy to the cervix + cisplatin chemotherapy, or cisplatin + 5-FU. To follow with HDR to bring Pt A dose to 75–85 Gy.

NCCN practice guidelines in: Cervical cancer version 1.2012. Fort Washington, PA: National Comprehensive Cancer Network, 2011. http://www.nccn.org/professionals/physician. Accessed October 14, 2011.

Question 9

What structures should be covered via pelvic fields when definitive treatment with chemoradiation therapy is used?

Question 10

What lymph nodes should be included in the PTV for patients with negative lymph node metastasis on surgical or radiological imaging?

Question 11

What nodal volumes should be included in the PTV for patients with bulky (> 4 cm) primary or suspected or confirmed lymph node metastasis confined to the low true pelvis?

Question 12

What nodal volume should be included when patients have common iliac and/or para-aortic lymph node metastasis?

What is the typical superior border with respect to bony landmarks for the para-aortic fields?

What is the typical lateral border bony landmark for para-aortic fields?

Answer 9

Gross disease (if present)

Parametrial tissues

Uterosacral ligaments

Sufficient vaginal margin from the gross disease (at least 3 cm)

Presacral nodes

NCCN Practice Guidelines in : Cervical Cancer Version 1.2012. Fort Washington, PA: National Comprehensive Cancer Network, 2011. http://www.nccn.org/professionals/physician. Accessed October 14, 2011.

Answer 10

Include: External iliac, internal iliac, and obturator nodal basins

NCCN Practice Guidelines in : Cervical Cancer Version 1.2012. Fort Washington, PA: National Comprehensive Cancer Network, 2011. http://www.nccn.org/professionals/physician. Accessed October 14, 2011.

Answer 11

Include: Common iliac, external iliac, internal iliac, and obturator nodal basins

NCCN Practice Guidelines in Cervical Cancer Version 1.2012. Fort Washington, PA: National Comprehensive Cancer Network, 2011. http://www.nccn.org/professionals/physician. Accessed October 14, 2011.

Answer 12

Include: Common iliac, external iliac, internal iliac and obturator nodal basins

Extend PTV to include: Para-aortic lymph nodes up to the level of the renal vessels (or more cephalad as dictated by level of known involvement). Typical superior border for the para-aortic fields is L1–L2 interspace, reasonable to extend superiorly by 1–2 vertebra heights if necessary to encompass known disease. The lateral border for the para-aortic region covered known para-aortic disease with a 2-cm margin at least to the tips of the transverse processes of the lumbar vertebrae.

NCCN Practice Guidelines in Cervical Cancer Version 1.2012. Fort Washington, PA: National Comprehensive Cancer Network, 2011. http://www.nccn.org/professionals/physician. Accessed October 14, 2011.

Walker JL, Morrison A, DiSilvestro P, et al. A phase I/II study of extended field radiation therapy with concomitant paclitaxel and cisplatin chemotherapy in patients with cervical carcinoma metastatic to para-aortic lymph nodes: a gynecologic group study. *Gynecol Oncol.* 2009;112:78–84.

Question 13

What are the typical chemotherapy agents used for concurrent chemoradiation therapy for definitive cancer of the cervix?

What is the usual weekly dose of chemotherapy for concurrent chemoradiation for cervix cancer in mg/m² and what is the typical maximum weekly dose?

Question 14

What is the typical percentage of patients with metastasis to para-aortic lymph nodes in cervix cancer by clinical stage?

Question 15

What is the typical EBRT dose for definitive concurrent chemoradiation therapy of cervix cancer?

Question 16

What is the typical reference point to calculate the limiting dose for brachytherapy for cancer of the cervix as described by Tod in 1938?

What is the current description of this point with respect to the cervical os?

What anatomical structure does this reference point refer to?

What is the typical brachytherapy dose for definitive concurrent chemoradiation therapy?

Answer 13

- Cisplatin or Cisplatin + 5-FU
- Cisplatin: 40 mg/m² once weekly, or 70 mg maximum weekly dose.
- Cisplatin + 5FU: Cisplatin (50 mg/m²) given by intravenous infusion on day 1 and day 29 of the external beam radiation therapy. 5-FU (1000 mg/m²/24 hours) given by continuous intravenous infusion over 96 hours on days 2–5 and repeated on days 30–33.

NCCN Practice Guidelines in Cervical Cancer Version 1.2012. Fort Washington, PA: National Comprehensive Cancer Network, 2011. http://www.nccn.org/professionals/physician. Accessed October 14, 2011.

Varia MA, Bundy BN, Deppe G, et al. Cervical carcinoma metastatic to para-aortic nodes: extended field radiation therapy with concomitant 5-fluorouracil and cisplatin chemotherapy: a Gynecologic Oncology Group study. *Int J Radiat Oncol Biol Phys*. 1998;42:1015–1023.

Answer 14

- Stage IB: 5%
- Stage II: 16%
- Stage III: 25%

98 of 621 evaluable patients (16%) with cervical cancer enrolled into Gynecologic Oncology Group protocols were found to have para-aortic lymph node metastases at staging laparotomy or at exploration for definitive operative management. 5% of 150 patients with stage IB, 16% of 222 patients with stage II, and 25% of 135 patients with stage III. Para-aortic lymph node metastases in the absence of pelvic lymph node metastases was an infrequent occurrence in patients who were evaluated. This study reported a median survival of 15.2 months and a probability of survival of 25% at 3 years.

Berman ML, Keys H, Creasman W, et al. Survival and patterns of recurrence in cervical cancer metastatic to periaortic lymph nodes: a Gynecologic Oncology Group Study. *Gynecol Oncol*. 1984;19:8–16.

Answer 15

EBRT: 1.8 Gy × 25 fx = 45 Gy

NCCN Practice Guidelines in Cervical Cancer Version 1.2012. Fort Washington, PA: National Comprehensive Cancer Network, 2011. http://www.nccn.org/professionals/physician. Accessed October 14, 2011.

Answer 16

Point A is the reference point to calculate the limiting dose and represents an average figure for the dose received in the paracervical triangle. This is where the ureter crosses the uterine artery.

Current description is 2 cm cephalad to the cervical os and 2 cm lateral to the endometrial canal. Typically, this is represented by the tandem of the applicator.

Typical brachytherapy dose as part of definitive chemoradiation therapy treatment for cervix cancer is 40 Gy for LDR and × 30 Gy in 5 fx @ 6 Gy/fx for HDR.

Tod MC, Meredith WJ. A dosage system for use in the treatment of cancer of the uterine cervix. *Br J Radiol*. 1938;11:809–824.

Question 17

What is the description of Point B with respect to the cervical os?

What anatomical structure does Point B refer to?

What is the intended percent of dose to Pt A that should be delivered to Pt B?

Question 18

What percent of patients eventually diagnosed with invasive cervix cancer have a false-negative Pap smear and what percent of patients eventually diagnosed with invasive cervix cancer failed to follow-up (includes failure to notify as well as patient inaction) after abnormal Pap smear?

Question 19

Based on SEER database for cases diagnosed in 2004-2008:

Which racial/ethnic group has the highest incidence of cervical cancer?

Which racial/ethnic group has the highest death rate from cervical cancer?

Question 20

What percent of cervix cancers is caused by persistent HPV infection?

What are the two most common HPV subtypes?

Answer 17

Point B: located 2 cm superior to the os and 5 cm from the midline of the uterine canal.

It refers to the dose delivered to the main lymphatic pathway from the cervix along the base of the broad ligament, and the first lymph node usually occupies the upper end of the inner surface of the obturator membrane, obturator lymph node.

25% of the dose to Point A should be delivered to Point B.

NCCN Practice Guidelines in Cervical Cancer Version 1.2012. Fort Washington, PA: National Comprehensive Cancer Network, 2011. http://www.nccn.org/professionals/physician. Accessed October 14, 2011.

Tod MC, Meredith WJ. A dosage system for use in the treatment of cancer of the uterine cervix. *Br J Radiol.* 1938;11:809–824.

Answer 18

An estimated 29.3% of failures to prevent invasive cervical cancer can be attributed to false-negative Pap smears and 11.9% to poor follow-up of abnormal results.

Spence AR, Goggin P, Franco EL, et al. Process of care failures in invasive cervical cancer: systematic review and meta-analysis. *Prev Med.* 2007;93–106.

Answer 19

Highest incidence is Hispanic race/ethnicity: 12.2 per 100,000 women

All races: 8.1 per 100,000 women
Black: 10.0 per 100,000 women
White: 8.0 per 100,000 women

Highest death rate is black race/ethnicity: 4.3 per 100,000 women

All races: 2.4 per 100,000 women
White: 2.2 per 100,000 women

seer.cancer.gov/statfacts/html/cervix.html. Accessed Novembre 12, 2011.

Answer 20

99.7 % (squamous cell and adenocarcinoma) have HPV infection.

Approximately 15 subtypes are known to be oncogenic.

HPV 16 and HPV 18 are found in over 70 percent of all cervical cancers.

The International Biological Study on Cervical Cancer (IBSCC) study of invasive cervical cancers collected from 22 countries: the worldwide HPV prevalence in cervical carcinomas is 99.7%.

IARC. Monographs on the Evaluation of Carcinogenic Risks to Humans. Human Papillomaviruses, Vol 64. Lyon: International Agency for Research on Cancer; 1995.

Walboomers JM, Jacobs MV, Manos MM, et al. Human papillomavirus is a necessary cause of invasive cervical cancer worldwide. *J Pathol.* 1999;189:12–19.

http://www.uptodate.com/contents/invasive-cervical-cancer-epidemiology-clinical-features-and-diagnosis?source=search_result&search=Cervix+cancer&selectedTitle=1%7E150. Accessed November 11, 2011.

Question 21

What are the four major steps in cervical cancer development?

Question 22

What is the relative rank based on the relative incidence (most frequent to least frequent) of these histologies in cervix cancer: squamous cell carcinoma, adenocarcinoma, and adenosquamous carcinoma in the U.S.?

Question 23

What is the most important determinant of outcome in stage I–II cervix cancer?

Question 24

Which histology of cervix cancer exhibits the highest percentage of EGFR amplification and what is the correlation with survival?

Answer 21

1. Oncogenic HPV infection of the metaplastic epithelium at the transformation zone.
2. Persistence of the HPV infection.
3. Progression of a clone of epithelial cells from persistent viral infection to precancer
4. Development of carcinoma and invasion through the basement membrane.

Schiffman M, Castle PE, Jeronimo J, et al. Human papillomavirus and cervical cancer. *Lancet.* 2007;370:890–907.

Answer 22

Squamous cell cancer > adenocarcinoma > adenosquamous carcinoma

Based on SEER data, in the US: Squamous cell carcinomas (SCCs) account for approximately 67% of cervical cancers. Adenocarcinomas account for 27%. Adenosquamous carcinomas account for 4%.

http://seer.cancer.gov/csr/1975_2008/results_merged/sect_05_cervix_uteri.pdf. Accessed October 21, 2011.

Answer 23

Tumor size (T: category in AJCC staging system) is the most important determinant of outcome in cervix cancer.

Edge SB, Byrd DR, Compton CC, et al., eds. *AJCC Cancer Staging Handbook: From the AJCC Cancer Staging Manual.* Cervix Uteri. 7th ed. New York, NY: Springer; 2010:475.
Eifel PJ, Berek JS, Markman MA. Cancer of the cervix, vagina, and vulva. In DeVita VT, Lawrence TS, Rosenberg SA, eds. *Cancer Principles & Practice of.* 9th ed. New York, NY: Wolters Kluwer/Lippincott Williams & Wilkins; 2011:1317–1318.

Answer 24

Squamous cell cancer (10%) and EGFR amplification significantly correlated with shorter overall survival in squamous cell carcinomas of the cervix.

Retrospective review by Iida et al., 6 (10.2%) of 59 cervical squamous cell carcinomas, showed significant amplification of EGFR. None of the 52 adeno/adenosquamous cell carcinomas showed detectable EGFR amplification ($p < .05$). Multivariate analysis showed EGFR amplification significantly correlated with shorter overall survival ($p = .001$) for squamous cell carcinoma of the cervix.

Iida K, Nakayama K, Rahman MT, et al. EGFR gene amplification is related to adverse outcomes in cervical squamous cell carcinoma, making the EGFR pathway a novel therapeutic target. *Br J Cancer.* 2010;105:420–427.

Question 25

What treatment choices are recommended for early adenocarcinoma of the uterine cervix?

Question 26

Which MRI sequence is most accurate to determine local tumor invasion in cervical cancer?

Question 27

Which shows better progression free survival (PFS) and overall survival (OS) for locally advanced cervical cancer, surgery or neoadjuvant chemotherapy plus surgery?

What did the 2010 Cochrane review of the role of neoadjuvant chemotherapy plus surgery vs surgery in women with early or locally advanced cervical cancer demonstrate in terms of progression free survival (PFS) and overall survival (OS)?

Question 28

What percentage of cervical cancer is squamous cell cancer and adenocarcinoma?

Answer 25

Surgery for early stage adenocarcinoma of the uterine cervix in carefully staged patients is recommended. Primary chemoradiation remains a second best alternative for patients unfit for surgery; chemoradiation is probably first choice in patients with (MRI or PET-CT-suspected) positive lymph nodes.

Baalbergen A, Veenstra Y, Stalpers LL, et al. Primary surgery versus primary radiation therapy with or without chemotherapy for early adenocarcinoma of the uterine cervix (Review). *Cochrane Database Syst Rev.* 2010;1:1–30.

Answer 26

T2-weighted sequence is the best sequence to determine local tumor invasion. In the 1993 study by Sironi, 53 patients with FIGO clinical Stage IB (squamous cell: 45 pts; adenocarcinoma: 7 pts, and clear cell: 1 pt), < 3 cm diameter underwent MRI followed by radical hysterectomy. Overall accuracy for depth of invasion was 85% for non-enhanced T2-weighted and 57% ($p < .05$) for enhanced T1-weighted imaging.

Sironi S, DeCobelli F, Scarfone G, et al. Carcinoma of the cervix: value of plain and gadolinium-enhanced MR imaging in assessing degree of invasiveness. *Radiology.* 1993;188:797–801.
Sala E, Wakely S, Senior E, et al. MRI of malignant neoplasms of the uterine corpus and cervix. *AJR.* 2007;188:1577–1587.

Answer 27

A Cochrane systemic review of randomized controlled trials comparing neoadjuvant chemotherapy with surgery in women with early or locally advanced cervical cancer.

PFS was significantly improved with neoadjuvant chemotherapy (HR = 0.76; $p = .01$),

No OS benefit was observed (HR = 0.85; $p = .17$).

Estimates for both local (OR = 0.76; $p = .21$) and distant (OR = 0.68; $p = .13$) recurrence and rates of resection (OR = 1.55; $p = .07$) only tended to favor neoadjuvant chemotherapy.

Rydzewska L, Tierney J, Vale CL, et al. Neoadjuvant chemotherapy plus surgery versus surgery for cervical cancer (Review). *Cochrane Database Syst Rev.* 2010;1:1–46.

Answer 28

Squamous cell cancer accounts for 80% of cervical cancer and adenocarcinoma accounts for 20% of cervical cancer.

NCCN Practice Guidelines in Cervical Cancer Version 1.2012. Fort Washington, PA: National Comprehensive Cancer Network, 2011. http://www.nccn.org/professionals/physician. Accessed October 14, 2011.

Question 29

Which histology of cancer of the cervix has increased worldwide over the past 30 years?

What is the most likely explanation for this increase?

Which HPV subtype is more frequently found in adenocarcinoma of the cervix versus squamous cell cancer of the cervix?

Question 30

How accurate is clinical staging compared to surgical staging in determining the extent of disease in cervix cancer?

Question 31

What is the risk of metastatic disease to the para-aortic lymph nodes in patients with IIB and IIIB cervix cancer?

Answer 29

Adenocarcinoma of the cervix has increased worldwide over the past 30 years.

More adenocarcinomas start in the endocervical canal, which may not be sampled during routine Pap smear.

HPV-18 is more frequently found in adenocarcinoma.

HPV-16 is more frequently found in squamous cell.

NCCN Practice Guidelines in Cervical Cancer Version 1.2012. Fort Washington, PA: National Comprehensive Cancer Network, 2011. http://www.nccn.org/professionals/physician. Accessed October 14, 2011.

Sasieni P, Castanon A, Cuzick J. Screening and adenocarcinoma of the cervix. *Int J Cancer*. 2009;125:525–529.

Bosch FX, Burchell AN, Schiffman M, et al. Epidemiology and natural history of human papillomavirus infections and type-specific implications in cervical neoplasia. *Vaccine*. 2008;26 (Suppl 10):K1–k16.

Answer 30

Clinical staging is 60% accurate compared with surgical staging, most often lymph node metastasis.

Based on a retrospective review of three GOG randomized phase III protocols involving para-aortic LN sampling versus radiologic staging (no PET scans), the benefit to surgical staging was greatest in the stage III/IV patients: estimated 4-year OS was 40% (radiographic staging) and 54.3% (surgical staging), ($p = .38$).

Differences in PFS and OS between the two groups was not significant in patients with stage II disease ($p = .143$).

1. GOG 85: RT + Hydroxyurea or cisplatin plus 5FU
2. GOG 120: RT and either cisplatin alone, hydroxyurea alone, or cisplatin plus 5-FU and hydroxyurea
3. GOG 165: RT and either cisplatin or protracted venous infusion 5-FU

Gold MA, Tian C, Whitney CW, et al. Surgical versus radiographic determination of para-aortic lymph node metastases before chemoradiation for locally advanced cervical carcinoma: a Gynecologic Group Study. *Cancer*. 2008;112:1954–1963.

Whitney CW, Sause W, Bundy BN, et al. Randomized comparison of fluorouracil plus cisplatin versus hydroxyurea as an adjunct to radiation therapy in stage IIB-IVA carcinoma of the cervix with negative para-aortic lymph nodes: a Gynecologic Oncology Group and Southwest Oncology Group study. *J Clin Oncol*. 1999;17:1339–1348.

Rose PG, Bundy BN, Watkins EB, et al. Concurrent cisplatin-based radiotherapy and chemotherapy for locally advanced cervical cancer. *N Engl J Med*. 1999;340:1144–1153.

Lanciano R, Calkins A, Bundy BN, et al. Randomized comparison of weekly cisplatin or protracted venous infusion of fluorouracil in combination with pelvic radiation in advanced cervix cancer: a Gynecologic Group study. *J Clin Oncol*. 2005;23:8289–8295.

Answer 31

Stage IIB has para-aortic LN involvement in 16–21% of patients.

Stage IIIB has para-aortic LN involvement in 25–31% of patients.

Heller PB, Maletano JH, Bundy BN, et al. Pathologic study of stage IIB, III, and IVA carcinoma of the cervix: extended diagnostic evaluation for paraaortic node metastasis—a Gynecologic Oncology Group study. *Gynecol Oncol*. 1990;38:425–430.

Berman ML, Keys H, Creasman W, et al. Survival and patterns of recurrence in cervical cancer metastatic to periaortic lymph nodes (A Gynecologic Oncology Group study). *Gynecol Oncol*. 1984;19:8–16.

Petereit DG, Hartenbach EM, Thomas GM. Para-aortic lymph node evaluation in cervical cancer: the impact of staging upon treatment decisions and outcome. *Int J Gynecol Cancer*. 1998;8:353–364.

Question 32

What are the results of the review by Havrilesky et al. with respect to sensitivity and specificity of PET for pelvic and para-aortic lymph node metastasis in patients with newly diagnosed cervix cancer?

Question 33

What was the benefit from the five trials referenced in the NCI February 1999 release that formed the basis for the recommendation of concurrent chemoradiation therapy for cervix cancer over radiation therapy alone?

Answer 32

15 studies on PET in cervical cancer met inclusion criteria for review.

Pooled sensitivity and specificity for pelvic lymph node metastasis are:

- PET: 0.79, and 0.99, respectively (both within 95% CI)
- MRI: 0.72 and 0.96, respectively (both within 95% CI)

Pooled sensitivity and specificity of PET for para-aortic metastasis are 0.84, and 0.95 (both within 95% CI).

Havrilesky LJ, Kulasingam SL, Matchar DB, et al. FDG-PET for management of cervical and ovarian cancer. *Gynecol Oncol.* 2005;97:183–191.

Answer 33

The 5 trials combined treated FIGO stages: IB2, II, III, IVA cervix cancer and the benefit was a reduction in the relative risk of death.

Table of Estimates of the Relative Risk of Death in Five Clinical Trials of Concurrent Chemotherapy and Radiotherapy

Study	FIGO Stage	Control Group	Comparison Group	Relative Risk of Death in Comparison Group
Keys et al.	IB2	RT	RT + weekly Cisplatin	0.54
Rose et al.	IIB-IVA	RT + Hydroxyurea	RT + weekly cisplatinRT + cisplatin, fluorouracil and hydroxyurea	0.610.58
Morris et al.	IB2-IVA	Extended-field RT	RT + cisplatin + fluorouracil	0.52
Whitney et al.	IIB-IVA	RT + Hydroxyurea	RT + cisplatin + fluorouracil	0.72
Peters et al.	IB or IIA (selected postop)	RT	RT + cisplatin + fluorouracil	0.50

RT = radiotherapy

NIH News Advisory Febrary 22, 1999. http://www.nih.gov/news/pr/feb99/nci-22.htm

Thomas GM. Improved treatment for cervical cancer-concurrent chemotherapy and radiotherapy. *N Engl J Med.* 1999;340:1198–200.

Question 34

What were the treatment arms for the phase III trial by Keys et al. (GOG 123)?

Question 35

What were the treatment arms and results (PFS and OS) for the phase III trial by Rose et al. (GOG 120)?

Answer 34
GOG 123 randomized patients to:

1. Radiation therapy (EBRT + brachytherapy: 75 Gy Pt A (cervical parametrium) and 55 Gy to Pt B (pelvic wall) with cisplatin (40 mg/m^2 weekly x 6 weeks, maximal weekly dose 70 mg) (n = 183) vs.
2. Radiation alone (same treatment scheme) (n = 186)

369 patients with stage IB bulky (tumor ≥ 4 cm in diameter) were enrolled from 1992–1997 followed by total hysterectomy. The EBRT fields extended 3 cm beyond known disease and included iliac and lower common iliac lymph nodes.

Results:

- 4-yr PFS was higher in combined therapy group (80%) versus radiation therapy alone group (62%) ($p < .001$).
- 3-yr OS was higher in combined therapy group (83%) versus radiation therapy alone group (74%) ($p = .008$)

Keys HM, Bundy BN, Stehman FB, et al. Cisplatin, radiation, and adjuvant hysterectomy compared with radiation and adjuvant hysterectomy for bulky stage IB cervical carcinoma. *Lancet*. 1999;340:1154–1161.

Answer 35
GOG 120

1. Radiation therapy with cisplatin vs.
2. Radiation therapy with cisplatin, 5-FU, and hydroxyurea versus
3. Radiation therapy with hydroxyurea.

526 patients with stages IIB, III, IVA were enrolled from 1992–1997.

Results:

- PFS @ 2-yr was higher for both groups that received cisplatin versus hydoxyurea alone ($p < .001$)
- RT + Cisplatin: 67%
- RT + Cisplatin / 5FU / hydroxyurea: 64%
- RT + Hydroxyurea: 47%

4-yr OS was significantly higher in groups receiving cisplatin versus hydroxyurea

- RT + Cisplatin: 66% ($p = .004$)
- RT + Cisplatin / 5FU / hydroxyurea: 67% ($p = .002$)
- RT + Hydroxyurea: 50%
- In both groups receiving radiation and cisplatin, the three-year survival rate was 65% compared to 47% for women receiving radiation and hydroxyurea.

Rose PG, Bundy BN, Watkins EB, et al. Concurrent cisplatin-based radiotherapy and chemotherapy for locally advanced cervical cancer. *N Engl J Med*. 1999;340:1144–1153.

Question 36

What were the treatment arms and results (OS and DFS) for the phase III trial by Morris et al. (RTOG 9001)?

Question 37

What were the treatment arms and results (PFS and OS) for the phase III trial by Whitney et al. (GOG 85)?

Question 38

What were the treatment arms and results (PFS and OS) for the phase III trial by Peters et al. (SWOG 8797)?

Answer 36
RTOG 9001

1. Radiation therapy (EBRT: 45 Gy/ 25 fx to pelvis/ Brachy = LDR; Pt A cumulative dose at least 85 Gy) with 5-FU and cisplatin (n =195) vs.
2. Radiation therapy (EBRT: 45 Gy / 25 fx to pelvis + PA LN's / Brachy = LDR; Pt A cumulative dose at least 85 Gy) alone (n = 193)

389 patients, stages IIB, III, and IVA, enrolled 1990–1997

Results:

- Estimated OS at 5 yrs: 73% for women receiving cisplatin and 5-FU + radiotherapy vs 58% receiving radiation alone, ($p = .004$).
- Estimated DFS at 5 yrs: 67% for cisplatin / 5FU + RT vs 40% for RT alone ($p < .001$)

Morris M, Eifel PJ, Jiandong L, et al. Pelvic radiation with concurrent chemotherapy compared with pelvic and para-aortic radiation for high-risk cervical cancer. *Lancet*. 1999;340:1137–1143.

Answer 37
GOG 85

1. Radiation therapy together with the drugs cisplatin and 5-fluorouracil (5-FU) (CF group) vs.
2. Radiation therapy with the drug hydroxyurea (HU group).

   N = 386 patients, stages IIB, III, and IVA, enrolled 1986–1990.

   PA LN sampling in all patients. PALN (+) or peritoneal cytology (+) were excluded.

Results:

- Three years from the time of diagnosis, 67% of women receiving radiation with cisplatin and 5FU were alive compared to 57% of those receiving radiation therapy and hydroxyurea.
- Median f/u = 8.7 yrs
- PFS: CF group: 43% versus HU group: 53% ($p = .033$)

OS: CF group: 55% versus HU group: 43% ($p = .018$)

Whitney CW, Sause W, Bundy BN, et al. Randomized comparison of fluorouracil plus cisplatin versus hydroxyurea as an adjunct to radiation therapy in stage IIB-IVA carcinoma of the cervix with negative para-aortic lymph nodes: a Gynecologic Oncology Group and Southwest Oncology Group study. *J Clin Oncol*. 1999;17:1339–1348.

Answer 38
SWOG 8797

Surgery: Type 3 radical hysterectomy and pelvic lymphadenectomy

Arms:

1. Radiation therapy with 5-FU and cisplatin (n = 127) vs.
2. Radiation therapy alone (n = 116)
   243 patients with stages IA2, IB, IIA, with adverse pathology found at time of surgery, (LN + or parametrial extension + or margin +) were enrolled from 1992–1996.

Results:

- 4-yr projected PFS: RT: 63% versus RT + chemotherapy: 80% ($p = .003$)
- 4-yr projected OS: RT: 71% versus RT + chemo: 81% ($p = .007$)

Peters III WA, Liu PY, Barrett II, RJ, et al. Concurrent chemotherapy and pelvic radiation therapy compared with pelvic radiation therapy alone as adjuvant therapy after radical surgery in high-risk early-stage cancer of the cervix. *J Clin Oncol*. 2000;18:1606–1613.

Question 39

What is the more likely histology (squamous cell versus adenocarcinoma) based on each epidemiologic factors?

- Younger age versus older age
- Barrel-shaped cervix
- Less likely to be detected by Pap smear

Question 40

What is the effect on survival of correcting hydronephrosis in patients with stage IIIB cervical cancer and hydronephrosis prior to starting treatment?

Question 41

What is the effect on 5-year survival from chemoradiation therapy in advanced cervix cancer?

Question 42

FIGO staging guidelines allow physical exam to determine tumor diameter which helps determine clinical stage. What is the accuracy of clinical exam on determining tumor diameter?

Answer 39

Adenocarcinoma is the correct answer for all the questions. Adenocarcinoma occurs more frequently in younger women, barrel shaped cervix, and less likely to be detected via Pap smear.

Answer 40

Rose et al. published a retrospective review of patients with stage IIIB cervical cancer and hydronephrosis treated with radiation and concurrent chemotherapy drawn from 4 GOG trials (56,85,120,165). 539 stage IIIB patients were studied. Hydronephrosis was present in 238 (44.2%). Ureteral obstruction relief occurred for 88% of patients and was associated with improved survival.

Rose PG, Ali S, Whitney CW, et al. Impact of hydronephrosis on outcome of stage IIIB cervical cancer patients with disease limited to the pelvis, treated with radiation and concurrent chemotherapy: a Gynecologic Oncology Group Study. *Gynecol Oncol.* 2010;117:270–275.

Answer 41

The Chemoradiotherapy for Cervical Cancer Meta-analysis Collaboration described a 6% improvement in 5-yr survival with chemoradiation therapy based on 18 trials. (HR = 0.81, $p < .001$). Use of platinum-based (HR 0.83, $p = .017$) and non-platinum-based (HR = 0.77, $p = .009$) chemoradiation therapy showed a significant survival benefit.

Chemoradiotherapy for Cervical Cancer Meta-Analysis Collaboration. Reducing uncertainties about the effects of chemoradiotherapy for cervical cancer: a systematic review and meta-analysis of individual patient data from 18 randomized trials. *J Clin Oncol.* 2008;26:5802–5812.

Answer 42

Accuracy of tumor diameter is 50%.

Hoffman et al. observed 50% (±25%) accuracy between tumor diameter as measured during pelvic exam for 67 patients with clinical IB-IIA cancer of the cervix and tumor diameter as measured in the operating room after radical hysterectomy.

Alvarez et al. found clinical and pathologic correlation in tumor diameter in 50% of 178 patients undergoing radical hysterectomy.

Hoffman MS, Cardosi RJ, Roberts WS, et al. Accuracy of pelvic examination in the assessment of patients with operable cervical cancer. *Am J Obstet Gynecol.* 2004;190:986–993.
Alvarez RD, Potter ME, Soong SJ, et al. Rationale for using pathologic tumor dimensions and nodal status to subclassify surgically treated stage IB cervical cancer patients. *Gynecol Oncol.* 1991;43:108–112.

Question 43

What is the recommended "not to exceed" completion time for chemoradiation therapy for cervix cancer?

Question 44

What is the maximum recommended HDR fraction size for cancer of the cervix?

When is it recommended to administer chemotherapy concomitantly with HDR brachytherapy for cancer of the cervix?

Question 45

During EBRT, HDR brachytherapy and concurrent chemotherapy for cancer of the cervix, does the greatest decrease in tumor volume occur during EBRT or HDR?

Question 46

What were the radiation therapy fields and brachytherapy dosing for the phase III trial by Rose et al. (GOG 120)?

Answer 43

American Brachytherapy Society recommended completing all chemoradiation therapy for cancer of the cervix within 56 days.

Nag S, Chao C, Erickson B, et al. The American Brachytherapy Society recommendations for low-dose-rate brachytherapy for carcinoma of the cervix. *Int J Radiat Oncol Biol Phys*. 2002;52:33–48.

Answer 44

ABS recommends 7.5 Gy/fx due to reported higher toxicity with larger fraction sizes.

Outside of a protocol, ABS recommends not administering chemotherapy concomitantly with HDR brachytherapy due to reports of increased complications. Clark et al. reported 26% Grade 3 and 4 late rectal complications in their patients in phase I/II trial. 43 patients treated with EBRT (46 Gy) + ICBT HDR (10 Gy × 3 applications to Pt A) + weekly cisplatin 30 mg/m^2. Brachytherapy is given during last 3 weeks of pelvic RT.

Nag S, Erickson B, Thomadsen B, et al. The American Brachytherapy Society recommendations for high-dose-rate brachytherapy for carcinoma of the cervix. *Int J Radiat Oncol Biol Phys*. 2000;48:201–211.

Clark BG, Souhami L, Roman TN, et al. The prediction of late rectal complications in patients treated with high dose-rate brachytherapy for carcinoma of the cervix. *Int J Radiat Oncol Biol Phys*. 1997;38:989–993.

Answer 45

In a prospective trial of 49 patients with cervix cancer treated with EBRT and MRI-assisted brachytherapy (+/−) cisplatin, the patients underwent MRI at diagnosis and during HDR fractions. They found the greatest decrease in tumor volume occurs during EBRT (75%) and tumor regression during brachytherapy is 10%.

Dimopoulos JC, Schirl G, Baldinger A, et al. MRI assessment of cervical cancer for adaptive radiotherapy. *Strahlenther Onkol*. 2009;185:282–287.

Answer 46

RT: whole pelvis : 40.8–51.0 Gy / 24–30 fx followed by intracavitary brachytherapy (ICBT) (1-2 implants)

ICBT dose: stage IIB 40 Gy and stage III/IVA: 30 Gy

Interstitial brachytherapy and HDR brachytherapy were not allowed.

Total (EBRT + ICBT) dose: Pt A total dose: stage IIB: 80.8 Gy and stage IIIA/IV: 81.0 Gy. Pt B: stage IIB: 55.0 Gy and stage IIIA/IV: 60 Gy

Pelvic field borders: AP/PA fields: Superior: superior border of L5, Inferior border: midportion of the obturator foramen or lowest level of disease with 3-cm margin, Lateral borders: > 7 cm from the midline, Lat field: (modified to include areas of known tumor) but at least: Anterior border: anterior border of pubic symphysis, Posterior border: space between S2 and S3.

Rose PG, Bundy BN, Watkins EB, et al. Concurrent cisplatin-based radiotherapy and chemotherapy for locally advanced cervical cancer. *N Eng J Med*. 1999;340:1144–1153.

Question 47

What were the radiation therapy fields and doses and brachytherapy dosing used in the phase III trial by Whitney et al. (GOG 85)?

Question 48

What was the radiation therapy dose for pelvic RT versus pelvic + PA RT for the phase III trial by Peters et al. (SWOG 8797)?

What was the brachytherapy dose for SWOG 8797?

Question 49   UTERINE CANCER

In 2009, the revised FIGO staging system for uterus cancer was published, replacing the 1988 FIGO staging system.

What stage is endocervical glandular only involvement?

Answer 47

RT description: IIB: EBRT: 40.8Gy/24 fx whole pelvis, external-beam therapy. ICBT: Pt A: 40 Gy via one or two intracavitary applications (tandem and colpostats) of radium or its equivalent. If necessary, a parametrial boost was given to bring the point B dose to 55 Gy. III/IVA: EBRT: 51 Gy/30 fractions if an intracavitary implant was not possible. Point A received 30 Gy from one or two intracavitary implants. Pt B received 60 Gy from both sources with or without a parametria boost.

Those patients treated solely with external beam therapy received 61.2 Gy.

RT fields included whole uterus, the paracervical, parametrial and uterosacral regions, as well as the external iliac, hypogastric, and obturator lymph nodes.

AP/PA: Superior border: Upper margin of L-5, Inferior border: midportion of the obturator foramen or the lowest extension of the disease. Lateral margins: 1 cm beyond the lateral margins of the bony pelvis and its widest plane

Lat fields: Anterior margin: anterior edge of the symphysis or 3 cm in front of the sacral promontory. Posterior margin: S2-S3 interspace.

Whitney CW, Sause W, Bundy BN, et al. Randomized comparison of fluorouracil plus cisplatin versus hydroxyurea as an adjunct to radiation therapy in stage IIB-IVA carcinoma of the cervix with negative para-aortic lymph nodes: a Gynecologic Oncology Group and Southwest Oncology Group Study. *J Clin Oncol*. 1999;17:1339–1348.

Answer 48

RT description: 49.3 Gy / 29 fx using 1.7 Gy/fx to whole pelvis.
Patients with positive high common iliac lymph nodes: PA field: 45 Gy / 30 fx using 1.5 Gy/fx to PA LN's. Brachytherapy was not permitted.

Peters III WA, Liu PY, Barrett II RJ, et al. Concurrent chemotherapy and pelvic radiation therapy compared with pelvic radiation therapy alone as adjuvant therapy after radical surgery in high-risk early-stage cancer of the cervix. *J Clin Oncol*. 2000;18:1606–1613.

Answer 49

Endocervical glandular involvement is considered stage I and no longer as stage II.

Pecorelli S. Revised FIGO staging for carcinoma of the vulva, cervix, and endometrium. *Int J Gynaecol Obstet*. 2009;105:103–104.
Mutch DG. The new FIGO staging system for cancers of the vulva, cervix, endometrium and sarcomas. *Gynecol Oncol*. 2009;115:325–328.
Creasman W. Revised FIGO staging for carcinoma of the endometrium. *Int J Gynaecol Obstet*. 2009;105:109.

Question 50

What was the trial design of the Aalders phase III trial?

Question 51

What were the results of the Aalders phase III trial of postoperative pelvic irradiation in stage I endometrial cancer patients with respect to locoregional recurrence and distant metastases?

What is the main criticism of this trial?

Question 52

What was the high risk subgroup identified in the Aalders phase III trial that showed benefit from postoperative pelvic irradiation?

Question 53

What was the trial design of the PORTEC-1 phase III trial for endometrial cancer?

Answer 50

Trial description: Aalders et al. randomized 540 stage I adenocarcinoma endometrial cancer patients.

All patients received intravaginal radium irradiation: 6000 rads to the vaginal surface.

At the time vaginal radium was given, randomization was performed:

Group A: no further treatment (control)

Group B: 4000 rads to the pelvis to treat the pelvic lymph nodes

Aalders J, Abeler V, Kolstad P, et al. Postoperative external irradiation and prognostic parameters in stage I endometrial carcinoma; clinical and histopathologic study of 540 patients. *Obstet Gynecol*. 1980;56:419–427.

Answer 51

With a follow-up of 3–10 years, this trial showed a significant reduction in vaginal and pelvic recurrences in group B (pelvic irradiation) vs group A (observation) (1.9% versus 6.9%, $p < .01$).

More patients in group B developed distant metastases than those in group A (9.9% versus 5.4%).

5-yr OS (NS different) between Group A (91%) versus Group B (89%)

Criticism: Complete surgical staging not done and patients enrolled between 1968 and 1974, prior to use of FIGO staging.

Aalders J, Abeler V, Kolstad P, et al. Postoperative external irradiation and prognostic parameters in stage I endometrial carcinoma; clinical and histopathologic study of 540 patients. *Obstet Gynecol*. 1980;56:419–427.

Answer 52

High risk subgroup: Stage IC (FIGO 1988), grade 3.

Locoregional recurrence decreased from 20% (vaginal brachytherapy) to 5% (vaginal brachytherapy followed by pelvic irradiation) in this high-risk subgroup, and there was a trend toward improved survival.

Aalders J, Abeler V, Kolstad P, et al. Postoperative external irradiation and prognostic parameters in stage I endometrial carcinoma; clinical and histopathologic study of 540 patients. *Obstet Gynecol*. 1980;56:419–427.

Answer 53

PORTEC-1 (Postoperative Radiation Therapy in Endometrial Cancer) enrolled patients from 1990–1997.

714 patients with:
1. grade I lesions with ≥ 50% myometrial invasion (FIGO 1988 IC)
2. grade II lesions with any amount of myometrial invasion (FIGO 1988 IB, IC)
3. grade III lesions with < 50% invasion (superficial) (FIGO 1988 IB)

Randomized postoperatively (TAH/BSO, cytology optional, no lymphadenectomy) between two treatment arms:

I: external beam pelvic radiotherapy (EBRT): 46 Gy/23 fx using 2 Gy/fx (354 pts)
II: no additional treatment (NAT) (351 pts)

Creutzberg CL, vanPutten WL, Koper PC, et al. Surgery and postoperative radiotherapy versus surgery alone for patients with stage-1 endometrial carcinoma: multicentre randomized trial. PORTEC Study Group. Post Operative Radiation Therapy in Endometrial Carcinoma. *Lancet*. 2000;355:1404–1411.

Question 54

What were the results of the PORTEC-1 trial in stage I endometrial cancer patients with respect to locoregional recurrence and survival advantage?

What is the main criticism of this trial?

Question 55

PORTEC-1 identified which subset of patients as being at high intermediate risk (> 15% risk) for locoregional recurrence?

GOG-33 identified which subset of patients as being at high intermediate risk (25% risk) for recurrence?

How did these risk factors inform the stratification of patients as being at high intermediate risk recurrence for patients enrolled on GOG-99?

Answer 54

Locoregional recurrence was significantly decreased from 14% to 5% in patients with pelvic irradiation ($p < .001$).

No overall survival benefit was seen between pelvic radiation therapy (81%) versus no additional treatment (NAT) 85% ($p = .31$).

Criticism: Lack of complete surgical staging for patients.

Creutzberg CL, vanPutten WL, Koper PC, et al. Surgery and postoperative radiotherapy versus surgery alone for patients with stage-1 endometrial carcinoma: multicentre randomized trial. PORTEC Study Group. Post Operative Radiation Therapy in Endometrial Carcinoma. *Lancet*. 2000;355:1404–1411.

Answer 55

A. Patients with ≥ 2 of the following risk factors:

   a. Grade 3 histology

   b. Age ≥ 60 years

   b. Deep (> 50%) myometrial invasion

Risk factors for increased local recurrence (25% risk) on GOG-33 included:

A. Moderately-to-poorly differentiated tumor grade

B. Presence of lymphovascular invasion

C. Outer one-third myometrial involvement

D. Increasing age

As such, GOG-99 considered patients with the following parameters to be at high intermediate risk for recurrence:

A. ≥ 70 years of age with ≥ 1 additional risk factor (A–C, above)

B. ≥ 50 years of age with ≥ 2 additional risk factors (A–C, above)

C. Any age with all 3 additional risk factors (A–C, above)

Creutzberg CL, van Putten MLJ, Koper PC, et al. Survival after relapse in patients with endometrial cancer: results from a randomized trial. *Gynecol Oncol*. 2003;89: 201–209.

Keys HM, Roberts JA, Brunetto VL, et al. A phase III trial of surgery with or without adjunctive external pelvic radiation therapy in intermediate risk endometrial adenocarcinoma: a Gynecologic Oncology Group study. *Gynecol Oncol*. 2004;92:744–751.

Question 56

What was the trial design of the GOG-99 phase III study?

Question 57

What trial was used to define "intermediate risk" of recurrence for patients with uterine cancer?

Question 58

What did the phase III GOG-99 trial of adjuvant pelvic radiation in uterine cancer show with respect to locoregional recurrence versus survival benefit?

Question 59

What was the trial design of the PORTEC-2 trial?

What was the primary endpoint in PORTEC-2?

Answer 56

GOG-99 randomized 392 patients between June 1987 and July 1995 with intermediate risk of recurrence (stages IB, IC, IIA (occult), and IIB [occult] endometrial cancer,) and complete surgical staging (total abdominal hysterectomy, bilateral salpingo-oophorectomy, selective bilateral pelvic, and para-aortic lymphadenectomy) between 50.4 Gy pelvic irradiation versus observation (NAT = no adjuvant therapy) to study the benefit of postoperative radiation therapy in this group of patients.

Keys HM, Roberts JA, Brunetto VL, et al. A phase III trial of surgery with or without adjunctive external pelvic radiation therapy in intermediate risk endometrial adenocarcinoma: a Gynecologic Oncology Group study. *Gynecol Oncol*. 2004;92:744–751.

Answer 57

GOG-33 enrolled patients from June 1977 to February 1983, to determine the incidence of pelvic and aortic lymph node metastases associated with stage I and II adenocarcinoma of the uterus and the relationship of these node metastases to other important prognostic factors. 895 patients with stage I or II (occult) endometrial cancer were enrolled into a surgical-pathologic staging study. Greatest determinant of recurrence was grade 3 histology. Of 48 patients with histologically documented aortic LN mets, 47 had one or more of the following features: 1) grossly positive pelvic nodes, 2) grossly positive adnexal mets, or 3) outer one-third myometrial invasion.

Morrow CP, Bundy BN, Kurman RJ. Relationship between surgical-pathological risk factors and outcome in clinical stage I and II carcinoma of the endometrium: a Gynecologic Oncology Group study. *Gynecol Oncol*. 1991;40:55–65.
Keys HM, Roberts JA, Brunetto VL, et al. A phase III trial of surgery with or without adjunctive external pelvic radiation therapy in intermediate risk endometrial adenocarcinoma: a Gynecologic Oncology Group study. *Gynecol Oncol*. 2004;92:744–751.

Answer 58

Locoregional recurrence was significantly decreased. Estimated 2-year cumulative incidence of any recurrence (CIR) was 12% in the no RT arm versus 3% in the RT arm ($p = .007$).

No survival advantage was noted for adjuvant radiation therapy ($p = .557$).

Keys HM, Roberts JA, Brunetto VL, et al. A phase III trial of surgery with or without adjunctive external pelvic radiation therapy in intermediate risk endometrial adenocarcinoma: a Gynecologic Oncology Group study. *Gynecol Oncol*. 2004;92:744–751.

Answer 59

PORTEC-2 was a multicenter randomized phase III trial, in which 19 of the 21 Dutch radiation oncology centers participated between 5/27/02 to 9/25/06. 427 high-intermediate-risk patients with stage I/IIA endometrial cancer were randomized between pelvic EBRT (46 Gy/23 fx) versus vaginal brachytherapy (VBT 21 Gy HDR / 3 fx or 30 Gy LDR) to determine whether VBT would be equally effective as EBRT in reduction of vaginal recurrence with improved QOL.

Primary endpoint was vaginal recurrence.

Nout RA, Smit VT, Putter H, et al. Vaginal brachytherapy versus pelvic external beam radiotherapy for patients with endometrial cancer of high-intermediate risk (PORTEC-2): an open-label, non-inferiority, randomized trial. *Lancet*. 2010;375:816–823.

Question 60

What staging procedures were allowed in PORTEC-2?

What surgical procedures were allowed in PORTEC-2?

Question 61

What were the eligible stage/FIGO/age combinations for high intermediate risk for PORTEC-2?

Question 62

What was the CTV and PTV for external beam radiation therapy (EBRT) for PORTEC-2?

Answer 60

Staging procedures allowed in PORTEC-2 included: pelvic examination, endometrial tissue biopsy, chest radiography, hematology and chemistry tests

Surgery: peritoneal cytology specimen, abdominal exploration, TAH/BSO, clinically suspicious pelvic or periaortic lymph nodes were removed, but no routine lymphadenectomy was done.

FIGO 1988 staging was assigned

Nout RA, Smit VT, Putter H, et al. Vaginal brachytherapy versus pelvic external beam radiotherapy for patients with endometrial cancer of high-intermediate risk (PORTEC-2): an open-label, non-inferiority, randomized trial. *Lancet*. 2010;375:816–823.

Answer 61

High-intermediate risk:

1. age > 60 years old and stage 1C grade 1 or 2 disease, or stage 1B grade 3 disease;
2. stage IIA disease, any age (apart from grade 3 with greater than 50% myometrial invasion).

Nout RA, Smit VT, Putter H, et al. Vaginal brachytherapy versus pelvic external beam radiotherapy for patients with endometrial cancer of high-intermediate risk (PORTEC-2): an open-label, non-inferiority, randomized trial. *Lancet*. 2010;375:816–823.

Answer 62

EBRT CTV: proximal half of the vagina, the parametrial tissues, the internal and proximal external iliac lymph node region, caudal part of the common iliac lymph node chain (up to 1 cm below the level of the promontory).

EBRT PTV = CTV + 1 cm three-dimensional margin.

Nout RA, Smit VT, Putter H, et al. Vaginal brachytherapy versus pelvic external beam radiotherapy for patients with endometrial cancer of high-intermediate risk (PORTEC-2): an open-label, non-inferiority, randomized trial. *Lancet*. 2010;375:816–823.

Question 63

What was the brachytherapy applicator and treatment volume for brachytherapy and dose fractionation for high dose rate brachytherapy (HDR), medium dose rate brachytherapy (MDR) and low dose rate brachytherapy (LDR) for PORTEC-2?

Question 64

What were the estimated 5-year results of PORTEC-2 regarding vaginal recurrence, pelvic recurrence, overall survival, and DFS?

Question 65

What is the definition of a patient with low risk of recurrence?

What is the definition of a patient with intermediate risk of recurrence?

What is the definition of a patient with high-intermediate risk of recurrence?

What is the definition of a patient with high risk of recurrence?

Answer 63

Brachytherapy applicator = vaginal cylinder.

Reference isodose covered the proximal half of the vagina. The dose was specified at 5 mm distance from the surface of the cylinder. The dose at 5 mm cranially from the vaginal vault along the axis of the cylinder could not vary more than plus or minus 10% of the specified dose.

- Brachytherapy Dose: equivalent to 45–50 Gy to the vaginal mucosa
- LDR schedule: 30 Gy at 50–70 cGy/h
- MDR schedule: 28 Gy at 100 cGy/h in one session.
- HDR schedule: 21 Gy in 3 fractions of 7 Gy separated 1 week apart

Doses in the bladder and rectum reference points (according to ICRU-38 criteria) and vaginal mucosal surface were documented.

Nout RA, Smit VT, Putter H, et al. Vaginal brachytherapy versus pelvic external beam radiotherapy for patients with endometrial cancer of high-intermediate risk (PORTEC-2): an open-label, non-inferiority, randomized trial. *Lancet*. 2010;375:816–823.

Answer 64

Estimated 5-year rates of vaginal recurrence:

VBT: 1.8% vs EBRT: 1.6% (HR 0.78; $p = .74$).

Estimated 5-year rate of pelvic recurrence: sig. lower with EBRT

VBT: 3.8% vs EBRT: 0.5% (HR 8.29; $p = .02$)

Estimated 5-year OS: No difference.

VBT: 84.8% vs EBRT: 79.6% (HR 1·17; $p = .57$)

Estimated 5-year DFS: No difference:

VBT: 82.7% vs EBRT: 78.1% (HR 1.09; $p = .74$).

Nout RA, Smit VT, Putter H, et al. Vaginal brachytherapy versus pelvic external beam radiotherapy for patients with endometrial cancer of high-intermediate risk (PORTEC-2): an open-label, non-inferiority, randomized trial. *Lancet*. 2010;375:816–823.

Answer 65

Risk Level	Definition
Low risk	Confined to the endometrium, or with < 50% myometrial invasion, grade 1 or 2 (stage IA)
Intermediate risk	Confined to the uterus but with invasion into the outer 1/3rd myometrium, or demonstrates occult cervical involvement. Other poor prognostic factors include: grade 2/3 and LVSI.
High intermediate risk	High-intermediate risk: Patients of any age with all three adverse prognostic factors: outer third myometrial invasion, grade 2 or 3 and LVSI. Patients 50–69 yo with two adverse prognostic factors: outer third myometrial invasion, grade 2 or 3 and LVSI. Patients > 70 with any one of the adverse prognostic factors: outer third myometrial invasion, grade 2 or 3 and LVSI.
High risk	High risk: Gross involvement of the cervix, stage III/IV, papillary serous or clear cell histologies, LVSI,

Dewdney SB, Mutch DG. Evidence-based review of the utility of radiation therapy in the treatment of endometrial cancer. *Women's Health*. 2010;6:695–704.

Question 66

What is the role for adjuvant radiation therapy in patients with low risk disease in endometrial cancer?

Question 67

Describe the design of the MRC ASTEC trial of systematic pelvic lymphadenectomy in endometrial cancer.

What was the outcome with respect to OS, recurrence-free survival?

Question 68

What event resulted in the National Cancer Institute of Canada Clinical Trials Group (NCIC CTG EN.5) merging with MRC ASTEC trial?

Answer 66

No role for adjuvant radiation therapy in patients with low risk disease in endometrial cancer. Low risk disease is confined to the endometrium or with < 50% myometrial invasion, grade 1 and 2. (Stage IA)

Dewdney SB, Mutch DG. Evidence-based review of the utility of radiation therapy in the treatment of endometrial cancer. *Women's Health*. 2010;6:695–704.

Answer 67

ASTEC (A Study in the Treatment of Endometrial Cancer) enrolled patients from July 1998 to March 2005. These patients were preoperatively thought to have disease confined to the uterus.

Two separate trials:

1. Surgical: TAH/BSO and pelvic lymphadenectomy (iliac and obturator nodes; para-aortic node sampling optional) versus TAH/BSO.
2. Radiation therapy: intermediate-risk and high-risk early-stage endometrial cancer, comparing EBRT and observation with no EBRT or systematic treatment until recurrence.

Low-risk: FIGO IA, IB and G1, G2

Intermediate-risk/high-risk: FIGO IA or IB with high-grade pathology [G3, papillary serous or clear cell], FIGO IC or IIA

Advanced: spread beyond the uterine corpus (FIGO stage IIB, IIIA, IIIB, and IV

FIGO stage IIIC (pelvic LN) not included.

Primary outcome measure was overall survival. No benefit in overall survival or recurrence-free survival for pelvic lymphadenectomy.

The writing committee on behalf of the ASTEC study group, Kitchener H, Swart AMC, Qian W et al. Efficacy of systemic pelvic lymphadenectomy in endometrial cancer (MRC ASTEC trial): a randomized study. *Lancet*. 2009;373:125–136.

Answer 68

The EN.5 trial of the National Cancer Institute of Canada (NCIC) Clinical Trials Group started in 1996, but could not recruit sufficient patient numbers to complete the study.

In 1998, the UK Medical Research Council (MRC) launched ASTEC, and invited the NCIC Clinical Trials Group to plan a prospective combination of the EN.5 data with those of ASTEC. ASTEC/EN.5 therefore consists of two trials with separate randomizations, which were combined to make one intergroup trial.

The ASTEC/EN.5 writing committee on behalf of the ASTEC/EN.5 Study Group. Adjuvant external beam radiotherapy in the treatment of endometrial cancer (MRC ASTEC and NCIC CTG EN.5 randomised trials): pooled trial results, systematic review, and meta-analysis. *Lancet*. 2009;373:137–146.

Question 69

What was the design of phase III ASTEC/EN.5 trial?

Question 70

What was the benefit of EBRT with respect to OS and local recurrence in the ASTEC/EN.5 trial?

What percent of patients had positive lymph nodes in observation vs EBRT arms recurrence in the ASTEC/EN.5 trial?

Question 71

What are the main criticisms of ASTEC/EN.5 phase III trial?

Question 72

What are radiation treatment options for early endometrial cancer versus patients with more aggressive stage I or stage II endometrial cancer patients who are inoperable due to medical comorbidities?

What are results for these options?

Answer 69

Between July 1996 and March 2005, 905 (789 ASTEC, 116 EN.5) patients with intermediate-risk for high-risk early stage uterus cancer were randomly assigned postoperatively to observation or EBRT (40-46 Gy/20-25 fx) to the pelvis.

The ASTEC/EN.5 writing committee on behalf of the ASTEC/EN.5 Study Group. Adjuvant external beam radiotherapy in the treatment of endometrial cancer (MRC ASTEC and NCIC CTG EN.5 randomised trials): pooled trial results, systematic review, and meta-analysis. *Lancet*. 2009;373:137–146.

Answer 70

The 5-yr OS was 84% in both groups ($p = .77$).

Brachytherapy used in 53% of women in ASTEC/EN.5. The local recurrence rate in the observation group at 5 years was 6.1%.

96% patients in each group were N0.

The ASTEC/EN.5 writing committee on behalf of the ASTEC/EN.5 Study Group. Adjuvant external beam radiotherapy in the treatment of endometrial cancer (MRC ASTEC and NCIC CTG EN.5 randomised trials): pooled trial results, systematic review,and meta-analysis. *Lancet*. 2009;373:137–146.

Answer 71

1. Para-aortic LN sampling was not included, which understaged 50% of patients.
2. Positive LN patients were randomized to no treatment arm.
3. Approximately 50% patients in both arms received vaginal brachytherapy.

The ASTEC/EN.5 writing committee on behalf of the ASTEC/EN.5 Study Group. Adjuvant external beam radiotherapy in the treatment of endometrial cancer (MRC ASTEC and NCIC CTG EN.5 randomised trials): pooled trial results, systematic review, and meta-analysis. *Lancet*. 2009;373:137–146.

Answer 72

For patients with superficial disease (MRI-determined) or grade 1–2 disease based on biopsy can be treated with HDR brachytherapy alone (35 Gy/5 fractions) given BID, using Rötte-Y intrauterine HDR applicator. For more aggressive stage I or II endometrial cancer, one can use EBRT to 45 Gy/25 fx followed by Rötte-Y intrauterine HDR applicator with 20 Gy/5 fx.

Coon D, Beriwal S, Heron DE, et al. High Dose Rate Rotte "Y" applicator brachytherapy for definitive treatment of medically inoperable endometrial cancer: 10-year results. *Int J Radiat Oncol Biol Phys*. 2008;71:779–783.

Wegner RE, Beriwal S, Heron DE, et al. Definitive radiation therapy for endometrial cancer in medically inoperable elderly patients. *Brachytherapy*. 2010;9:260–265.

Question 73
What distinguishes between FIGO IA and and FIGO IB for patients with leiomyosarcomas and endometrial stromal sarcoma?

Question 74
What is the FIGO stage of a uterine sarcoma with metastasis to regional lymph nodes?

Question 75
What is the difference in FIGO staging for a uterine sarcoma between FIGO IIA and FIGO IIB?

Question 76
What histologies are grouped as uterine sarcomas?

Answer 73

FIGO IA: Tumor 5 cm or less in greatest dimension

FIGO IB: Tumor > 5 cm

NCCN clinical practice guidelines in oncology: uterine neoplasms version 2.2012. Fort Washington, PA: National Comprehensive Cancer Network, 2011. http://www.nccn.org/professionals/physician. Accessed October 14, 2011.

Edge SB, Byrd DR, Compton CC, et al., eds. *AJCC Cancer Staging Handbook: From the AJCC Cancer Staging Manual.* Corpus Uteri. 7th ed. New York, NY: Springer, 2010;488.

Answer 74

FIGO IIIC: Regional lymph node metastasis

NCCN clinical practice guidelines in oncology: uterine neoplasms version 2.2012. Fort Washington, PA: National Comprehensive Cancer Network, 2011. http://www.nccn.org/professionals/physician. Accessed October 14, 2011.

Edge SB, Byrd DR, Compton CC, et al., eds. *AJCC Cancer Staging Handbook: From the AJCC Cancer Staging Manual.* Corpus Uteri. 7th ed. New York, NY: Springer, 2010:488–489.

Answer 75

FIGO IIA: Tumor involves adnexa

FIGO IIB: Tumor involves other pelvic tissues

NCCN Clinical Practice Guidelines in Oncology: Uterine Neoplasms Version 2.2012. Fort Washington, PA: National Comprehensive Cancer Network, 2011. http://www.nccn.org/professionals/physician. Accessed October 14, 2011.

Answer 76

Endometrial stromal sarcoma

Leiomyosarcoma

Undifferentiated sarcoma

NCCN clinical practice guidelines in oncology: uterine neoplasms version 2.2012. Fort Washington, PA: National Comprehensive Cancer Network, 2011. http://www.nccn.org/professionals/physician. Accessed October 14, 2011.

Question 77

What are clinicopathologic prognostic factors for leiomyosarcomas?

Question 78

What stages of endometrial stromal sarcoma is adjuvant radiation therapy recommended for, based on NCCN guidelines?

Question 79

What did the 10-year update of PORTEC-1 show with respect to locoregional relapse rate between EBRT arm versus observation arm and 10-yr OS?

Question 80

What did the 15-year update of PORTEC-1 show with respect to locoregional recurrence, OS and failure-free survival?

For the subgroup of high-intermediate risk, what is the OS and endometrial cancer (EC) related death rate?

What was the prognostic significance of the high-intermediate risk factors with respect to LRR andendometrial cancer death rate?

Answer 77

Size: < or > 5 cm

Mitotic activity: < or equal to 10 mitotic figures / 10 high power fields

Age: < or > 50 years

Vascular invasion: present or absent

NCCN clinical practice guidelines in oncology: uterine neoplasms version 2.2012. Fort Washington, PA: National Comprehensive Cancer Network, 2011. http://www.nccn.org/professionals/physician. Accessed October 14, 2011.

Answer 78

Stages II, III, IVA. For stage IVB, palliative RT is recommended.

NCCN clinical practice guidelines in oncology: uterine neoplasms version 2.2012. Fort Washington, PA: National Comprehensive Cancer Network, 2011. http://www.nccn.org/professionals/physician. Accessed October 14, 2011.

Answer 79

Scholten et al. published 10-year update of PORTEC-1 in 2005.

Locoregional relapse rates were 5% (EBRT) and 14% (no EBRT) ($p < .0001$),

10-year overall survival was 66% (EBRT) and 73%, (no EBRT) ($p = .09$).

Endometrial cancer related death rates were 11% (EBRT) and 9% (no EBRT) ($p = .47$).

5-yr survival after any relapse was 13% for EBRT versus 48% for no EBRT ($p < .001$).

Scholten AN, vanPutten W, Beerman H, et al. Postoperative radiotherapy for Stage I endometrial carcinoma: long-term outcome of the randomized PORTEC trial with central pathology review. *Int J Radiat Oncol Biol Phys*. 2005;63:834–838.

Answer 80

Creutzberg et al. reported median follow-up time of 13.3 years.

15-yr OS EBRT (52%) vs no-EBRT (60%) ($p = .14$)

For high-intermediate risk: 15-yr OS EBRT (41%) vs no-EBRT (48%) ($p = .51$) 15-yr endometrial cancer related death: EBRT (14%) vs no-EBRT (13%).

High-intermediate risk factors: LRR for Grade 3: (HR 3.4, $p = .0003$), EC death for Grade 3: (HR 7.3, $p < .0001$), LRR for age > 60: (HR 3.9, $p = .002$), EC death for age > 60: (HR 2.7, $p = .01$), LRR for myometrial invasion > 50%: (HR 1.9, $p = .03$), EC for myometrial invasion > 50%: (HR 1.9, $p = .02$).

Creutzberg CL, Nout RA, Lybeert MLM, et al. Fifteen-year radiotherapy outcomes of the randomized PORTEC-1 trial for endometrial carcinoma. Int J Radiat Oncol Biol Phys 2011;81:e631–e639.

Question 81

What histologies, grade and FIGO stage were included in the intermediate-risk subgroup and the high-risk subgroup for the ASTEC and EN.5 trials?

Question 82

What type of surgical and pathologic findings were allowed for ASTEC/EN.5 trial?

Question 83

What was the EBRT dose for ASTEC/EN.5?

Was brachytherapy allowed for ASTEC/EN.5?

Question 84

A Cochrane systematic review and meta-analysis published in 2007, authored by Kong et al. of adjuvant radiation therapy for stage I endometrial cancer included Aalders 1980, GOG-99 (Keys 2004), PORTEC-1 (Schoten 2005), and an unpublished study by Solderini 2003.

1. What was the distribution of patients?
2. What was the primary outcome measure?
3. What was the effect of pelvic external beam radiotherapy after surgery on locoregional recurrence?
4. What was the number needed to treat (NNT) to prevent one locoregional recurrence (LR)?
5. What was the reduction in risk of distant recurrence?

Answer 81

Intermediate risk subgroup: FIGO stage IA grade 3, IC (grade 1, 2), stage IIA (grade 1, 2)

High risk subgroup: Papillary serous / clear cell, FIGO IC, grade 3, IIA grade 3

The ASTEC/EN.5 Writing Committee on Behalf of the ASTEC/EN.5 Study Group. Adjuvant external beam radiotherapy in the treatment of endometrial cancer (MRC ASTEC and NCIC CTG EN.5 randomised trials): pooled trial results, systematic review, and meta-analysis. *Lancet.* 2009;373:137–146.

Answer 82

Lymphadenectomy was not a requirement. Women with positive pelvic lymph nodes were eligible for ASTEC, but not for EN.5. Peritoneal cytology could be negative, positive or not done.

The ASTEC/EN.5 writing committee on behalf of the ASTEC/EN.5 Study Group. Adjuvant external beam radiotherapy in the treatment of endometrial cancer (MRC ASTEC and NCIC CTG EN.5 randomised trials): pooled trial results, systematic review, and meta-analysis. *Lancet.* 2009;373:137–146.

Answer 83

EBRT: ASTEC: 40-46 Gy/ 20-25 fx, EN.5: 45 Gy/25 fx

Brachytherapy was allowed.

ASTEC: two fractions of 4 Gy, HDR at 0.5 cm over 3-7 days, or 15 Gy at LDR (50 cGy/hr) to upper 1/3rd vagina.

EN.5, brachytherapy was allowed and given according to local practice

235 (52%) in the observation group and 242 (54%) in the external beam radiotherapy group received brachytherapy.

The ASTEC/EN.5 Writing Committee on Behalf of the ASTEC/EN.5 Study Group. Adjuvant external beam radiotherapy in the treatment of endometrial cancer (MRC ASTEC and NCIC CTG EN.5 randomised trials): pooled trial results, systematic review, and meta-analysis. *Lancet.* 2009;373:137–146.

Answer 84

1. Distribution of 1770 patients were 870 in the treatment group and 900 patients in the control group.
2. Primary outcome measure was overall survival.
3. Pelvic radiation led to a relative risk (RR) of 0.28 ($p < .00001$). This was a 72% reduction in the risk of pelvic relapse and an absolute risk reduction of 6%.
4. The number needed to treat to prevent one locoregional recurrence is 16.7 patients.
5. This reduction in the risk of locoregional recurrence did not translate into either a reduction in the risk of distant recurrence or death from all causes or endometrial cancer death.

Kong AA, Johnson N, Cornes P, et al. Adjuvant radiotherapy for stage I endometrial cancer (Review). *Cochrane Database Syst. Rev.* 2007;2:1–30.

Question 85

Typically the dose from HDR vaginal cuff brachytherapy is prescribed either to surface or 5-mm depth.

What is the presumed target and what did Choo et al. demonstrate in vaginal autopsy specimens?

Question 86

What is the most common site of relapse of stage I uterus cancer within the vaginal canal after TAH/BSO?

What are the indications to treat the distal 1/3rd of the vaginal canal?

Question 87

Based on SEER database (2004-2008):

Which race/ethnicity has the highest incidence of uterus cancer?

Which race/ethnicity has the highest death rate from uterus cancer?

Question 88

In 2009, the revised FIGO staging system for uterus cancer was published replacing the 1988 FIGO staging system.

FIGO 2009 stage IA consists of which FIGO 1988 stages?

FIGO 1988 stage IC is classified as which stage in FIGO 2009?

Answer 85

The presumed target when performing vaginal cuff brachytherapy is the vaginal lymphatics.

Choo et al. showed approximately 95% of vaginal lymphatic channels are located within 3-mm depth from the vaginal surface.

Choo JJ, Scudiere J, Bitterman P, et al. Vaginal lymphatic channel location and its implication for intracavitary brachytherapy radiation treatment. *Brachytherapy*. 2005;4:236–240.

Answer 86

The most common site of relapse of stage I uterus cancer after TAH/BSO is within the proximal one-half of the vaginal canal.

Indications to include the distal third of the vagina include: unfavorable histology when treating with chemo + brachy only and vaginal recurrence.

Chadha M. Early stage endometrial cancer; Role of vaginal brachytherapy. ABS Brachytherapy School; July 2011, Chicago IL

Answer 87

Highest incidence of uterine cancer: White: 24.8 per 100,000 women
All Races: 23.9 per 100,000 women
Black: 20.9 per 100,000 women
Hispanic: 18.9 per 100,000 women

Incidence Rates by Race
Highest death rate of uterine cancer: Black: 7.2 per 100,000 women
All Races: 4.2 per 100,000 women
White: 3.9 per 100,000 women
Hispanic: 3.2 per 100,000 women

Seer.cancer.gov/statfacts/html/corp.html. Accessed November 12, 2011.

Answer 88

FIGO 1988 stage IA and IB have been grouped together in FIGO 2009 as stage IA.

FIGO 1988 stage IC is IB in FIGO 2009.

Pecorelli S. Revised FIGO staging for carcinoma of the vulva, cervix, and endometrium. *Int J Gynaecol Obstet*. 2009;105:103–104.
Mutch DG. The new FIGO staging system for cancers of the vulva, cervix, endometrium and sarcomas. *Gynecol Oncol*. 2009;115:325–328.
Creasman W. Revised FIGO staging for carcinoma of the endometrium. *Int J Gynaecol Obstet*. 2009;105:109.

Question 89

In 2009, the revised FIGO staging system for uterus cancer was published replacing the 1988 FIGO staging system.

What was the change for FIGO 1988 stage IIA and stage IIB?

What was the change for FIGO 1988 peritoneal cytology?

Question 90

In 2009, the revised FIGO staging system for uterus cancer was published, replacing the 1988 FIGO staging system.

What stage is parametrial involvement?

How was FIGO stage III 1988 modified?

Question 91

What is role for adjuvant radiation therapy in women with intermediate risk endometrial cancer for recurrence?

Question 92

What is the role for adjuvant radiation therapy in high risk for recurrence endometrial cancer?

Answer 89

FIGO 1988 IIA and IIB have been grouped together in FIGO 2009 as stage II.

FIGO 1988 peritoneal cytology is not included in FIGO 2009, but should be reported without changing the stage.

Pecorelli S. Revised FIGO staging for carcinoma of the vulva, cervix, and endometrium. *Int J Gynaecol Obstet.* 2009;105:103–104.

Mutch DG. The new FIGO staging system for cancers of the vulva, cervix, endometrium and sarcomas *Gynecol Oncol.* 2009;115:325-328.

Creasman W. Revised FIGO staging for carcinoma of the endometrium. *Int J Gynaecol Obstet.* 2009;105:109.

Answer 90

FIGO 1988 did not describe parametrial involvement. It is stage IIIB in the FIGO 2009 staging system. FIGO 1988 IIIC is subdivided into IIIC1 and IIIC2 in FIGO 2009 staging system.

Pecorelli S. Revised FIGO staging for carcinoma of the vulva, cervix, and endometrium. *Int J Gynaecol Obstet.* 2009;105:103–104.

Mutch DG. The new FIGO staging system for cancers of the vulva, cervix, endometrium and sarcomas. *Gynecol Oncol.* 2009;115:325–328.

Creasman W. Revised FIGO staging for carcinoma of the endometrium. *Int J Gynaecol Obstet.* 2009;105:109.

Answer 91

Consensus is external beam radiotherapy does not improve overall survival but provides a small but real improvement in local control for patients with intermediate-risk disease.

Vaginal brachytherapy is equally effective to external beam radiation therapy (EBRT) to the pelvis and proximal vagina with an improved quality of life compared with EBRT in the high intermediate-risk group as described in the PORTEC-2 trial.

Dewdney SB, Mutch DG. Evidence-based review of the utility of radiation therapy in the treatment of endometrial cancer. *Women's Health.* 2010;6:695–704.

Answer 92

Adjuvant radiation therapy is recommended for patients in the high-risk group. Although this was shown in a randomized controlled trial, it was not adequately powered (GOG 99). In addition, these patients may benefit from both chemotherapy and radiotherapy. Additional trials are in progress.

Dewdney SB, Mutch DG. Evidence-based review of the utility of radiation therapy in the treatment of endometrial cancer. *Women's Health.* 2010;6:695–704.

Question 93

What is the role for adjuvant radiation therapy in advanced stage endometrial cancer?

Question 94

What were the radiation therapy fields for the phase III trial by Morris et al. (RTOG 9001)?

Question 95

Which of the following imaging modalities, MRI vs CT vs US, is more accurate for assessing lymph node metastasis?

Answer 93

Most patients with advanced-stage disease should receive chemotherapy and may benefit from adjuvant radiation therapy, although the optimal combination of chemotherapy and radiation therapy remains to be determined.

Dewdney SB, Mutch DG. Evidence-based review of the utility of radiation therapy in the treatment of endometrial cancer. *Women's Health*. 2010;6:695–704.

Answer 94

Radiation therapy fields for pelvic radiation therapy: Superior border: space between L4 and L5 to the mid-pubis or to a line 4 cm below the most distal vaginal or cervical site of disease. Lateral fields: encompass S3 posteriorly, with a margin of at least 3 cm from the primary cervical tumor. Custom shielding was designed to treat the pelvic lymph nodes, with a margin of at least 1 to 1.5 cm.

ICBT (or interstitial) was LDR.

Radiation therapy alone: Pelvic and paraaortic areas were treated as a continuous area, with a superior field. border at the space between L1 and L2. The radiation dose was keyed to the central ray at the patient's midplane (for AP/PA fields) or to the isocenter of the beams. ICBT (or interstitial) was LDR.

Morris M, Eifel PJ, Jiandong L, et al. Pelvic radiation with concurrent chemotherapy compared with pelvic and para-aortic radiation for high-risk cervical cancer. *Lancet*. 1999;340:1137–1143.

Answer 95

MRI and CT are superior to US; but overall neither is sufficiently sensitive to include as routine workup especially in clinical stage I patients, unless it is done to evaluate symptoms.

Among 56 women who had preoperative CT scans and lymph node samplings, positive and negative predictive values for nodal involvement were 50% and 94%, respectively, and sensitivity and specificity were 57% and 92%, respectively. The authors recommended CT scanning of any woman with endometrial cancer should be discouraged unless it is to evaluate symptoms.

Evaluation of pelvic and para-aortic lymph nodes can be performed concurrently with accuracy comparable to CT with sensitivity of 44% to 66% and specificity of 73% to 98%

Connor JP, Andrews JI, Anderson B, et al. Computed tomography in endometrial cancer. *Obstet Gynecol*. 2000;95:692–696.

Rockall AG, Meroni R, Sohaib SA, et al. Evaluation of endometrial carcinoma on magnetic resonance imaging. *Int J Gynecol Cancer*. 2007;17:188–196.

Lee JH, Dubinsky T, Andreotti RF, et al. ACR appropriateness criteria pretreatment evaluation and follow-up of endometrial cancer of the uterus. *Ultrasound Quarterly*. 2011;27:139–145.

Question 96

What percent of uterine cancers are due to uterine papillary serous cancer (UPSC)?

What percent of deaths due to uterine cancer are due to uterine papillary serous cancer?

Question 97

Based on SEER database (2004–2008):

Which race/ethnicity has the highest incidence of vulva cancer?

Which race/ethnicity has the highest death rate from vulva cancer?

Question 98

What percent of all gynecologic cancers is invasive vulvar carcinoma?

Answer 96

UPSC represents 10% uterine cancers and 40% of deaths due to uterine cancer based on a Medline search of literature published between January 1966 and June 2009 from Boruta et al.

Boruta DM, Paola A, Fader AN, et al. Management of women with uterine papillary serous cancer: a Society of Gynecology (SGO) review. *Gynecol Oncol.* 2009;115:142–153.

Answer 97

Highest incidence of vulva cancer: White: 2.4 per 100,000 women

All Races: 2.3 per 100,000 women

Black: 1.8 per 100,000 women

Hispanic: 1.7 per 100,000 women

Highest death rate for vulva cancer: White: 0.5 per 100,000 women

All Races: 0.5 per 100,000 women

Black: 0.3 per 100,000 women

Hispanic: 0.3 per 100,000 women

Seer.cancer.gov/statfacts/html/vulva.html. Last Accessed November 12, 2011.

Answer 98

Invasive vulvar carcinoma accounts for 4% gynecologic cancers.

Eifel PJ, Berek JS, Markman M. Cancer of the cervix, vagina and vulva. In: DeVita VT, Lawrence TS, Rosenberg SA, eds. *DeVita, Hellman, and Rosenberg's Cancer: Principles & Practice of Oncology.* 9th ed. Philadelphia, PA: Lippincott Williams & Wilkins, 2011:1335.

Question 99

What are the anatomical structures in the vulva?

Which is the most common site of primary cancer of the vulva?

Question 100

What is the incidence of lymph node metastasis when the primary vulvar lesion is 2.1–3.0 mm versus 3.1–5.0 mm?

Which lymph node group is the most common site of metastasis from vulvar cancer?

What is the most common distant metastatic site for vulvar cancer?

Question 101

What are is the most common precursor lesion for vulvar cancer?

Answer 99

Mons pubis

Labia majora

Labia minora

Clitoris

Vestibular bulb

Vestibular glands

Vestibule of the vagina

Labia majora

Labia majora and labia majora: Site of 70% of vulvar squamous cancers

Eifel PJ, Berek JS, Markman M. Cancer of the cervix, vagina and vulva. In: DeVita VT, Lawrence TS, Rosenberg SA, eds. *DeVita, Hellman, and Rosenberg's Cancer: Principles & Practice of Oncology.* 9th ed. Philadelphia, PA: Lippincott Williams & Wilkins, 2011:1335–1336.

Answer 100

15% of patients with 2.1–3.0 mm primary thickness have positive lymph nodes versus 26% of patients with 3.1–5.0 mm primary thickness.

Initial regional metastasis is to the inguinal lymph nodes superficial to Camper fascia.

Lung is the most common distant metastatic site for vulvar cancer.

Eifel PJ, Berek JS, Markman M. Cancer of the cervix, vagina and vulva. In: DeVita VT, Lawrence TS, Rosenberg SA, eds. *DeVita, Hellman, and Rosenberg's Cancer: Principles & Practice of Oncology.* 9th ed. Philadelphia, PA: Lippincott Williams & Wilkins, 2011:1336.

Answer 101

HPV-associated vulvar intraepithelial neoplasia (VIN) is the most common precursor lesion for vulvar cancer.

Eifel PJ, Berek JS, Markman M. Cancer of the cervix, vagina and vulva. In: DeVita VT, Lawrence TS, Rosenberg SA, eds. *DeVita, Hellman, and Rosenberg's Cancer: Principles & Practice of Oncology.* 9th ed. Philadelphia, PA: Lippincott Williams & Wilkins, 2011:1335.

Question 102

FIGO Staging for vulvar cancer revised most recently in 2009.

What is the FIGO 2009 stage for vulvar cancer with one lymph node metastasis at least 5 mm in size?

What is the FIGO 2009 stage for vulvar cancer with positive lymph nodes with extracapsular spread?

What percent of patients with LVSI in the primary vulvar cancer have positive inguinal lymph node metastasis?

What imaging tests are required for FIGO staging vulvar cancer?

Question 103

What size of primary vulvar cancer is resection appropriate?

How deep should the incision extend?

What is the minimum margin of normal tissue around the tumor?

Lesions < 4 cm that do not invade beyond what distance can be managed with local resection alone?

Question 104

What is role for radiation therapy in positive or close margins after radical vulvectomy for vulvar cancer?

Answer 102

FIGO 2009 stage with one lymph node metastasis at least 5 mm in size is stage IIIA

FIGO 2009 stage with positive lymph nodes with extracapsular spread is stage IIIC

75% of patients with LVSI have positive inguinal lymph nodes. ($p < .0001$) independent of tumor thickness.

No imaging tests are included in FIGO Staging.

Hacker NF. Revised FIGO staging for carcinoma of the vulva. *Int J Gynaecol Obstet.* 2009;105:105–106.

Homesley HD, Bundy BN, Sedlis A, et al. Prognostic factors for groin node metastasis in squamous cell carcinoma of the vulva (A Gynecologic Oncology Group study). *Gynecol Oncol.* 1993;49:279–283.

Answer 103

Radical resection for tumor < 4 cm that does not involve urethra, anus or other adjacent structure.

Depth of incision should extend to the inferior fascia of the urogenital diaphragm.

Minimum margin = 1 cm.

Lesions that invade ≤ 1 mm can be managed by local resection alone.

Eifel PJ, Berek JS, Markman M. Cancer of the cervix, vagina and vulva. In: DeVita VT, Lawrence TS, Rosenberg SA, eds. *DeVita, Hellman, and Rosenberg's Cancer: Principles & Practice of Oncology.* 9th ed. Philadelphia, PA: Lippincott Williams & Wilkins, 2011:1339.

Answer 104

Retrospective review of 62 patients with close (< 8 mm) or positive margins after radical vulvectomy or wide local excision examined the role of radiation therapy. Patients were treated from 1980-1994: 31 observed and 31 treated with adjuvant radiation.

Radiation treatment fields included the vulva, bilateral inguinal nodal regions and low pelvis and prescribed to 3-cm depth to the inguinal nodes, mean dose 56.64 Gy using 1.8 Gy/fx.

Local recurrence in 58% observed patients versus 16% in irradiated patients.

Adjuvant RT reduced local recurrence rate in both close margin ($p = .036$) and positive margin ($p = .0048$).

2-yr actuarial survival after local recurrence was 25%, local recurrence was a significant predictor for death from vulvar carcinoma (RR 3.54, 95% CI not given).

On subgroup analysis, radiation therapy significantly improved survival for patients with positive margins ($p = .001$), but not close margins ($p = .63$).

Faul CM, Mirmow D, Huang Q, et al. Adjuvant radiation for vulvar carcinoma: improved local control. *Int J Radiat Oncol Biol Phys.* 1997;38:381–389.

Question 105

Why did GOG 37, which was a randomized trial for patients with squamous cell cancer of the vulva found to have positive inguinal lymph nodes after radical vulvectomy and bilateral groin lymphadenectomy, close two years earlier than planned?

Question 106

What were the treatment arms for GOG 37?

What was the OS?

What were the two major poor prognostic factors?

Question 107

What is the 6-year overall survival and cancer-related death rate when results from GOG 37 were updated?

What is the HR for the two major prognostic factors (clinically suspected or fixed ulcerated LN) and two or more positive groin LN metastasis?

What ratio of number positive/number resected groin lymph nodes was significantly associated with contralateral lymph node metastasis, relapse and cancer-related death?

Answer 105

This phase III trial randomized patients in the operating room after groin dissection. Patients were enrolled from 1977–1984. Interim analysis showed statistically significant survival difference. Since the estimated 2-yr survival rate (68% versus 54%, respectively; $p = .03$) favored the adjuvant radiation therapy arm over the pelvic node resection group, the trial was closed early.

Homesley HD, Bundy BN, Sedlis A, et al. Radiation therapy versus pelvic node resection for carcinoma of the vulva with positive groin nodes. *J Am Coll Obstet and Gynecol.* 1986;68:733–740.

Answer 106

114 patients, FIGO I–IV, were randomized after radical vulvectomy and bilateral groin lymphadenectomy to radiation therapy or pelvic node resection for the GOG 37 trial.

Pelvic lymphadenectomy arm: Ipsilateral pelvic node dissection to resect external iliac, internal iliac, obturator and common iliac lymph nodes.

Randomization occurred in operating room at time of initial vulvectomy and pelvic node dissection was ipsilateral and included: external iliac, internal iliac, obturator and common iliac lymph nodes.

EBRT arm: 45–50 Gy in 5–6.5 weeks to bilateral groin and pelvis (including obturator, external iliac, internal iliac lymph nodes) even if only unilateral positive groin node; no RT to central vulvar area.

Field borders: extending from L5/ S1 to border of obturator foramina.

Dose calculated to 2–3 cm depth over inguinal and femoral LN areas, otherwise calculated to mid-depth in mid-pelvis.

Two major poor prognostic factors: clinically suspicious or fixed ulcerated groin nodes and two or more positive groin nodes.

Estimated 2-yr OS 68% for EBRT vs 54% for pelvic lymphadenectomy ($p = .03$).

Homesley HD, Bundy BN, Sedlis A, et al. Radiation therapy versus pelvic node resection for carcinoma of the vulva with positive groin nodes. *J Am Coll Obstet and Gynecol.* 1986;68:733–740.

Answer 107

6-year OS was 51% for EBRT arm compared with 41% for pelvic lymphadenectomy (HR 0.61; $p = .18$)

Cancer related death rate: pelvic node resection (51%) versus radiation therapy (29%) at 6 years.

6-yr OS for radiation in patients with clinically suspected or fixed ulcerated groin lymph nodes ($p = .004$) and two or more positive groin nodes ($p < .001$).

Ratio [(+) ipsilateral groin LN / number groin LN resected] > 20% was significantly associated with contralateral lymph node metastasis, relapse and cancer-related death

Kunos C, Simpkins F, Gibbons H, et al. Radiation therapy compared with pelvic node resection for node-positive vulvar cancer: a randomized controlled trial. *Obstet Gynecol.* 2009;114:537–546.

Question 108

What percent of patients who are cN0 on palpation will have histopathologically determined lymph node metastasis?

What percent of patients who have palpable lymph nodes (N2/N3) with have pN0 lymph nodes after lymphadenectomy?

Question 109

The objective of a recent Cochrane Database review of groin irradiation in vulvar cancer was to determine whether the effectiveness and safety of primary radiotherapy to the inguinofemoral lymph nodes in early vulvar cancer is comparable with surgery.

What were the main results?

Question 110

What is the role for neoadjuvant chemoradiation therapy in locally advanced vulvar cancer?

Answer 108

25% patients with cN0/cN1 on clinical palpation will have lymph node metastasis at histopathologic exam.

25% patients with clinically suspicious LN's (N2/N3) will have negative lymph nodes at lymphadenectomy.

Stehman, FB, Look KY. Carcinoma of the vulva. *Obstet Gynecol*. 2006;107:719–133.

Answer 109

Out of twelve identified papers only one met the selection criteria.

A randomized controlled trial of 52 women:
- Trend towards increased groin recurrence rates (relative risk (RR) 10.21
- Lower disease-specific survival rates (RR 3.70)
- Less lymphedema (RR 0.06)
- Fewer life-threatening cardiovascular complications (RR 0.08) in the radiotherapy group

Primary surgery was associated with a longer hospital stay than primary groin irradiation (RR 0.28).

van der Velden J, Fons G, Lawrie TA. Primary groin irradiation versus primary groin surgery for early vulvar cancer. *Cochrane Database Syst Rev*. 2011;(5):CD002224. doi: 10.1002/14651858.CD002224.pub2.

Answer 110

GOG 101 was a phase II trial of 73 patients with clinical III/IV squamous cell cancer of the vulva consisting of planned split course of concurrent cisplatin and 5-FU and RT followed by surgical excision of the residual primary tumor plus bilateral inguinal-femoral LND and enrolled patients from 8/89 to 2/94. EBRT was BID (1.7 Gy BID) for half of each split course during cisplatin.

EBRT: 47.6 Gy at 1.7 Gy/fx. Patients with inoperable groin nodes received chemoRT to primary vulvar tumor, inguinal femoral and lower pelvic lymph nodes.

Results

Only 2/71 (2.8%) had unresectable disease. 46.5% had no visible vulvar cancer at time of surgery.

Moore DH, Thomas GM, Montana GS, et al. Preoperative chemoradiation for advanced vulvar cancer: a phase II study of the gynecologic oncology group. *Int J Radiat Oncol Biol Phys*. 1998;42:79–85.

Question 111

What is the effectiveness and safety of neoadjuvant and primary chemoradiation for locally advanced primary vulva cancer compared to other primary treatment modalities such as primary surgery or primary radiation?

Question 112   VAGINAL CANCER

What percent of all gynecologic malignancies does vaginal cancer account for?

What are the two most common histologies by percent incidence?

Which gynecologic cancer primary is most common source of metastasis to the vagina?

Question 113

What is the leading risk factor for developing vagina cancer?

What are the FIGO defined anatomical limits for vagina cancer?

What is the most frequent location for primary vagina cancer?

What is the most frequent location for primary vaginal melanoma?

Answer 111

The Cochrane Database conducted a review of one RCT and two non-randomized studies (total of 141 women).

One RCT found that neoadjuvant chemoradiation did not appear to offer longer survival compared to primary surgery in advanced vulvar tumors (RR = 1.29). There was also no statistically significant difference in survival between primary chemoradiation and primary surgery in a study that included 63 women (pooled adjusted HR = 1.09) and in another study that only included 12 eligible women and compared the same interventions (HR was non-informative when statistical adjustment was made).

Shylasree TS, Bryant A, Howells REJ. Chemoradiation for advanced primary vulvar cancer. *Cochrane Database Syst Rev.* 2011;(4):CD003752. doi: 10.1002/14651858.CD003752.pub3.

Answer 112

Primary vagina cancer accounts for 2% of all gynecologic malignancies.

The two most common histologies are squamous cell (80–90%) and adenocarcinoma (4–10%). Cancer in the vagina is more likely to be due to metastasis versus primary.

Cervix (32%) is most common source of metastasis to the vagina.

Eifel PJ, Berek JS, Markman M. Cancer of the cervix, vagina and vulva. In: DeVita VT, Lawrence TS, Rosenberg SA, eds. *DeVita, Hellman, and Rosenberg's Cancer: Principles & Practice of Oncology.* 9th ed. Philadelphia, PA: Lippincott Williams & Wilkins, 2011:1330–1331.
Lilic V, Lilic G, Filipovic S, et al. Primary carcinoma of the vagina. *J BUON.* 2000;15:241–247.

Answer 113

Infection with HPV-16 (60–65% in women with vaginal cancer) is the leading risk factor for developing vagina cancer.

Proximally: Any tumor extension to the cervical portio and the area of the external os should be classified as a cervix cancer.

Distally: Any tumor extension from the vulva to involve the vagina should be classified as a primary vulvar cancer.

Upper third: 50% arise in the upper third of the vagina.

Primary vaginal melanoma most common site of origin is distal third of the vagina.

International Agency for Research on Cancer (IARC). Monographs on the evaluation of carcinogenic risks to humans. *Human Papillomaviruses.* Vol 64, Lyon (France): IARC;1995.
Eifel PJ, Berek JS, Markman M. Cancer of the cervix, vagina and vulva. In: DeVita VT, Lawrence TS, Rosenberg SA, eds. *DeVita, Hellman, and Rosenberg's Cancer: Principles & Practice of Oncology.* 9th ed. Philadelphia, PA: Lippincott Williams & Wilkins, 2011:1330–1332.
Buchanan DJ, Schlaerth J, Kurosaki T. Primary vaginal melanoma: thirteen-year disease-free survival after wide local excision and review of the recent literature. *Am J Obstet Gynecol.* 1998;178:1177–1184.

Question 114

What are the lymphatic pathways for the vagina?

What is the likelihood of lymph node involvement in stage II vaginal cancer?

Question 115

What are the radiation therapy doses based on the FIGO stage for primary cancer of the vagina?

Question 116

BRACHYTHERAPY

Low Dose Rate (LDR) brachytherapy vs Medium Dose Rate (MDR) brachytherapy vs High Dose Rate (HDR) brachytherapy.

1. What is the dose rate range for LDR?
2. What is the minimum dose rate for MDR?
3. What is the minimum dose rate for HDR?

What is the LDR tolerance limit for the total dose to the rectum / sigmoid, vagina, bladder?

Answer 114

Vaginal vault: drain to lower cervix, then laterally to obturator and hypogastric lymph nodes.

Posterior wall: anastamose with anterior rectal wall, then to the superior and inferior gluteal lymph nodes.

Lower 1/3rd vagina: drain to vulva then either pelvic lymph nodes or inguinofemoral lymph nodes.

Incidence of positive pelvic lymph node metastasis with stage II vaginal cancer is 25–30%.

Eifel PJ, Berek JS, Markman M. Cancer of the cervix, vagina and vulva. In: DeVita VT, Lawrence TS, Rosenberg SA, eds. *DeVita, Hellman, and Rosenberg's Cancer: Principles & Practice of Oncology*. 9th ed. Philadelphia, PA: Lippincott Williams & Wilkins, 2011:1331.

Davis KP, Stanhope CR, Garton GR, et al. Invasive vaginal carcinoma: analysis of early-stage disease. *Gynecol Oncol*. 1991;42:131–136.

Answer 115

For stage 0–I when tumor thickness < 5 mm: HDR can be used, prescribing to 5 mm depth and treating to 42 Gy at 7 Gy/fx. (Mock et al.).

For stage I (tumor thicker that 5 mm) or stage II: EBRT (40–50 Gy) to the pelvic lymph nodes and HDR boost total dose to 70–75 Gy or boost with 50–60 Gy prescribed to the surface (Frank et al.).

For stage III and IV cancers treatment ranges from EBRT alone (median dose 77 Gy with shrinking field technique after 45 Gy to lymph nodes) to concurrent chemoradiation therapy and HDR reserved to boost residual disease. Inguinal lymphatics typically included when primary tumor site is lower 1/3rd of the vagina.

Mock U, Kucera H, Fellner C. High-Dose-Rate (HDR) brachytherapy with or without external beam radiotherapy in the treatment of primary vaginal carcinoma: long-term results and side effects. *Int J Radiat Oncol Biol Phys*. 2003;56:950-7.

Frank SJ, Jhingran A, Levenback C, et al. Definitive radiation therapy for squamous cell carcinoma of the vagina. *Int J Radiat Oncol Biol Phys*. 2005;62:138-47.

Eifel PJ, Berek JS, Markman M. Cancer of the cervix, vagina and vulva. In: DeVita VT, Lawrence TS, Rosenberg SA, eds. *DeVita, Hellman, and Rosenberg's Cancer: Principles & Practice of Oncology*. 9th ed. Philadelphia: Lippincott Williams & Wilkins, 2011:1333–1334.

Answer 116

1. 0.4 Gy/hr – 2 Gy/hr
2. > 2 Gy/hr – < 12 Gy/hr
3. > 12 Gy/hr

LDR tolerance limits: Rectum and Sigmoid: 70–75 Gy, Vagina: 130 Gy, Bladder: < 90% Pt A, Total dose limit: 80 Gy

Stewart AJ, Viswanathan AN. Current controversies in high-dose-rate versus low-dose-rate brachytherapy for cervical cancer. *Cancer*. 2006;107:908–915.

Wang X, Liu R, Ma B, et al. High dose rate versus low dose rate intracavity brachytherapy for locally advanced uterine cervix cancer. *Cochrane Database Syst Rev*. 2010;(7):CD007563. doi: 10.1002/14651858.CD007563.pub2.

Nag S, Chao C, Erickson B, et al. The American Brachytherapy Society recommendations for low-dose-rate brachytherapy for carcinoma of the cervix. *Int J Radiat Oncol Biol Phys*. 2002;52:33–48.

Question 117

Has HDR-ICBT for patients with histologically proven locally advanced cervical cancer, stage I–III (IGO staging) improved local control rates, survival and complications related to treatment compared to LDR?

Question 118

What are the definitions for the bladder and rectal points for absorbed dose from ICRU Report 38?

Answer 117

A Cochrane Database meta-analysis compared HDR to LDR, using 4 studies involving 1265 patients with histologically proven locally advanced cervical cancer, stage I–III (FIGO staging)

This review showed no significant differences between HDR- and LDR-ICBT when considering OS, DSS, RFS, local control rate, recurrence, and metastasis. There was an increase in small bowel complications with HDR-ICBT ($p = .04$), no other increase in treatment-related complications. Due to some potential advantages of HDR-ICBT (rigid immobilization, outpatient treatment, patient convenience, accuracy of source and applicator positioning, individualized treatment) they recommend the use of HDR-ICBT for all clinical stages of cervix cancer.

Wang X, Liu R, Ma B, et al. High dose rate versus low dose rate intracavity brachytherapy for locally advanced uterine cervix cancer. *Cochrane Database Syst Rev.* 2010;(7):1–41, CD007563. doi: 10.1002/14651858.CD007563.pub2.

Answer 118

Relies on AP/Lateral perpendicular radiographs.

Bladder reference point: Foley catheter balloon filled with 7 cm³ radio-opaque fluid, pull downward to bring balloon against urethra. Lat radiograph: reference point is on anterior-posterior line drawn through the center of the balloon at posterior surface of the balloon. AP radiograph: center of balloon is reference point.

Rectal reference point: Localized posterior vaginal wall (relies on intravaginal mould or opacification of vaginal cavity with radio-opaque gauze for packing). Lat radiograph: anterior-posterior line from lower end of intrauterine source (or middle of intravaginal source). Reference point on this line, 5 mm posterior to the posterior vaginal wall. AP radiograph: reference point at lower end of the intrauterine source (middle of the intravaginal source).

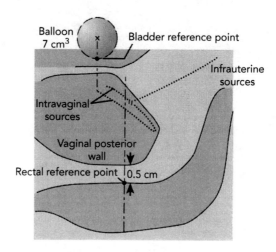

http://health-7.com/imgs/520/7734.jpg. Accessed November 14, 2011.

Question 119

What are the GEC-ESTRO guidelines for the dose to organs at risk when considering irradiated tissue volumes?

Question 120   **GYNECOLOGIC ONCOLOGY—GENERAL**

What is the risk for femoral neck fracture after 50 Gy external beam radiation therapy to the groin, AP/PA approach?

Question 121   **SIDE EFFECTS**

What are effective interventions for psychosexual dysfunction in women treated for gynecological cancer (uterine cervix, uterine corpus, ovary, vulva)?

Answer 119

The dose to organs at risk should be recorded for volumes: 0.1, 1, 2 cm³, optional for 5 and 10 cm³

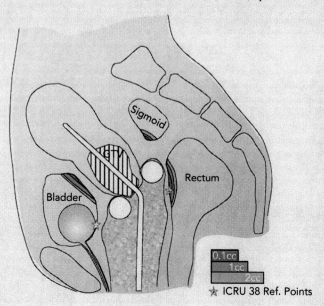

Schematic anatomical diagram (sagittal view) indicating the most irradiated tissue volumes adjacent to the applicator for rectum, sigmoid, bladder: 0.1, 1, 2 cm3

Answer 120

Grigsby et al. reviewed radiation therapy records of patients at Mallinckrodt Institute of Radiology. They identified 207 patients treated with 50 Gy to the groin, AP/PA technique and found cumulative actuarial incidence of fracture in the femoral neck was 11% at 5 yrs and 15% at 10 yrs.

Grigsby PW, Roberts HL, Perez CA, et al. Femoral neck fracture following groin irradiation. *Int J Radiat Oncol Biol Phys*. 1995;32:63–67.

Answer 121

A Cochrane Review included data from 5 studies comprising a total of 413 patients that examined 5 different interventions. One trial suggested a short-term benefit for the use of vaginal Dienoestrol in women after pelvic radiotherapy (NNT = 4). Another trial suggested a short term benefit for one regime of low dose-rate brachytherapy over another but this modality is not in widespread use. Studies of a clinical nurse specialist intervention, psychoeducational group therapy and a couple-coping intervention, did not show any significant benefit. All the studies were of poor methodological quality.

Flynn P, Kew F, Kisely SR. Interventions for psychosexual dysfunction in women treated for gynaecological malignancy. *Cochrane Database Syst Rev*. 2009;(2):CD004708. doi: 10.1002/14651858.CD004708.pub2.
Varela VS, Nelson CJ, Bober SL. Sexual problems. In: DeVita VT, Lawrence TS, Rosenberg SA, eds. *DeVita, Hellman, and Rosenberg's Cancer: Principles & Practice of Oncology*. 9th ed. Philadelphia, PA: Lippincott Williams & Wilkins, 2011:2462–2463.

8

LYMPHOMAS

VINCENT LEE

Question 1

What features constitute the International Prognostic Index (IPI) for non-Hodgkin lymphoma?

How is risk stratified based upon IPI?

Question 2

What are the associated 3-year OS rates—stratified by risk—for patients receiving rituximab in treatment for NHL?

Question 3

The following cytogenetic translocations and their associated oncogenes are seen in which histologic subtypes of lymphoma?

t(14:18) → bcl-2
t(8:14) → c-myc
t(11:14) → bcl-1

Answer 1

LDH > normal
Age > 60
Performance status (ECOG) ≥ 2
Stage III, IV
Extranodal sites > 1

mnemonic: "LAPSE"

Low risk: IPI 0–1
Low-intermediate: IPI 2
High-intermediate: IPI 3
High risk: IPI 4–5

Shipp MA, Harrington DP, Anderson JR, et al. A predictive model for aggressive non-Hodgkin's lymphoma. *N Engl J Med*. 1993;329:987–994.
Ziepert M, Hasenclever D, Kuhnt E, et al. Standard International Prognostic Index remains a valid predictor of outcome for patients with aggressive CD20+ B-cell lymphoma in the rituximab era. *J Clin Oncol*. 2010;28:2373–2380.

Answer 2

3 prospective trials utilizing rituximab + CHOP-based regimen were analyzed; IPI score was found to remain a significant prognostic factor in the rituximab era and remains valid for risk stratification.

IPI 0–1 – 91% 3-yr OS
IPI 2 – 81% 3-yr OS
IPI 3 – 65% 3-yr OS
IPI 4–5 – 59% 3-yr OS

Ziepert M, Hasenclever D, Kuhnt E, et al. Standard International Prognostic Index remains a valid predictor of outcome for patients with aggressive CD20+ B-cell lymphoma in the rituximab era. *J Clin Oncol*. 2010;28:2373–2380.

Answer 3

t(14:18) → bcl-2 → Follicular (85%) (also 30% DLBCL)

t(8:14) → c-myc → Burkitt (> 90%)

t(11:14) → bcl-1 → Mantle cell (> 90%)

Friedberg JW, Mauch PM, Rimsza LM, et al. Non-Hodgkin's lymphomas. In: DeVita VT, Lawrence TS, Rosenberg SA, eds. *DeVita, Hellman, and Rosenberg's Cancer: Principles & Practice of Oncology*. 8th ed. Philadelphia: Lippincott Williams & Wilkins; 2008:2098–2142.

Question 4

What laboratory studies are essential in the workup for a patient with newly diagnosed NHL by tissue biopsy?

Question 5

What were the eligibility criteria and treatment arms for the phase III SWOG 8736 trial?

Question 6

Which stage I/II DLBCL study compared the addition of Rituxan to CHOPx3 followed by IFRT against a historical control of the same treatment without Rituxan?

What was the outcome?

Answer 4

CBC with WBC differential, platelet count

peripheral smear examination

LDH

comprehensive metabolic panel

Hepatitis B serology if rituximab contemplated

Under select circumstances:

Hepatitis C and HIV serology

Beta-2-microglobulin (indolent lymphomas)

Immunoglobulin studies (CLL/SLL, Waldenstrom's)

Uric acid

NCCN Clinical Practice Guidelines in Oncology: Non-Hodgkin's Lymphomas. Fort Washington, PA: National Comprehensive Cancer Network; 2011. http://www.nccn.org/professionals/physician_gls/pdf/nhl.pdf. Accessed October 18, 2011.

Answer 5

Patients enrolled March 1988–June 1995

Intermediate or high grade NHL (excl. lymphoblastic)

(75% were DLBCL)

Stage I, IE (including bulky)

Stage II, IIE (non-bulky only)

RANDOMIZE

→ CHOP × 8

→ CHOP × 3 + IFRT

(40 Gy ± boost → up to 55 Gy)

Miller TP, Dahlberg S, Cassady JR, et al. Chemotherapy alone compared with chemotherapy plus radiotherapy for localized intermediate- and high-grade non-Hodgkin's lymphoma. *N Engl J Med*. 1998;339:21–26.

Answer 6

SWOG 0014

Enrolled 71 patients from April 2000–January 2002

R-CHOP × 3 + IFRT (40–46 Gy)

4-year PFS 88%, 4-year OS 92%

Superior findings in comparison to SWOG 8736 (4-year PFS 78%, 4-year OS 88%).

Persky DO, Unger JM, Spier CM, et al. Phase II study of rituximab plus three cycles of CHOP and involved-field radiotherapy for patients with limited-stage aggressive B-cell lymphoma: Southwest Oncology Group study 0014. *J Clin Oncol*. 2008;26:2258–2263.

Question 7

What are the current (ver 4.2011) NCCN recommendations for the treatment of stage I–II diffuse large B-cell lymphoma?

Question 8

What demographic and cytogenetic features help to distinguish primary mediastinal large B-cell lymphoma from diffuse large B-cell?

Question 9

What is the most common site of involvement for NK/T-cell lymphoma?

Which part of the world has the highest frequency?

Question 10

Is concurrent chemoradiation an appropriate treatment option for stage I/II nasal NK/T-cell lymphoma?

Answer 7

R-CHOP × 3 cycles with IFRT, or

R-CHOP × 6 cycles +/− IFRT.

Strongly consider R-CHOP × 6 cycles + IFRT for patients with adverse risk factors, including bulky disease.

Consolidation dose in DLBCL:

after CR to chemo: 30–36 Gy

for residual disease (PR) : 40–50 Gy

NCCN Clinical Practice Guidelines in Oncology: Non-Hodgkin's Lymphomas. Fort Washington, PA: National Comprehensive Cancer Network; 2011. http://www.nccn.org/professionals/physician_gls/pdf/nhl.pdf. Accessed October 18, 2011.

Answer 8

Primary Mediastinal Large B-Cell Lymphoma:

Median age 35; females > males

Arise from thymic B-cells

Sites of possible locoregional spread:
mediastinum, supraclavicular, cervical, hilar nodes

Genetic expression similar to Classic Hodgkin

B-cell antigen, CD19, CD20, CD22, CD30 positive

Cazals-Hatem D, Lepage E, Brice P, et al. Primary mediastinal large B-cell lymphoma. A clinicopathologic study of 141 cases compared with 916 nonmediastinal large B-cell lymphomas, a GELA ("Groupe d'Etude des Lymphomes de l'Adulte") study. *Am J Surg Pathol.* 1996;20:877–888.

Answer 9

NK/T-cell lymphomas are predominantly extranodal. The majority are nasal. Frequency is higher in Asian countries. EBV infection is involved in its pathogenesis. It is classified as an aggressive lymphoma where relapses are common; cumulative 5-year OS has been reported at 45%.

Au WY, Weisenburger DD, Intragumtornchai T, et al. Clinical differences between nasal and extranasal natural killer/T-cell lymphoma: a study of 136 cases from the International Peripheral T-Cell Lymphoma Project. *Blood.* 2009;113:3931–3937.

Lee J, Park YH, Kim WS, et al. Extranodal nasal type NK/T-cell lymphoma: elucidating clinical prognostic factors for risk-based stratification of therapy. *Eur J Cancer.* 2005;41:1402–1408.

Answer 10

Yes, particularly for high risk disease (lymph node involvement, B symptoms, elevated LDH.) In a comparison of concurrent chemo/RT with dexamethasone, etoposide, ifosfamide, and carboplatin, an improvement in 2-year OS was seen over a historical control of RT alone (78% vs 45%). RT dose of 50 Gy is recommended.

Yamaguchi M, Tobinai K, Oguchi M, et al. Phase I/II study of concurrent chemoradiotherapy for localized nasal natural killer/T-cell lymphoma: Japan Clinical Oncology Group Study JCOG0211. *J Clin Oncol.* 2009;27:5594–5600.

Question 11

What delineates an "involved field" for lymphoma involving a unilateral cervical lymph node, with or without supraclavicular involvement?

Question 12

What delineates an "involved field" for lymphoma involving the mediastinum?

Question 13

What was the effect of Rituximab on 3-yr EFS and OS in the MabThera International Trial (MInT)?

Answer 11

Upper border:

1–2 cm above the lower tip of the mastoid; mid-point through the chin.

Lower border:

2 cm below the bottom of the clavicle.

Lateral border:

Include medial 2/3 of clavicle.

Medial border:

Supraclav not involved—ipsilateral tranverse process; if medial nodes involved, include enitre vertebral body.

Supraclav involved—contralateral transverse process.

Other considerations:

Laryngeal block if nodes not involved in that location

Posterior cervical cord block if cord dose > 40 Gy

Yahalom J, Mauch P. The involved field is back: issues in delineating the radiation field in Hodgkin's disease. *Ann Oncol.* 2002;13(Suppl 1):79–83.

Answer 12

Medial supraclavicular LNs are included

Upper border

C5–C6 interspace

Lower border

The lower of a) 5 cm below the carina or b) 2 cm below the pre-chemo inferior border.

Lateral border

The post-chemo volume with 1.5 cm margin

Hilar area

To be included with 1 cm margin (1.5 cm if involved)

Yahalom J, Mauch P. The involved field is back: issues in delineating the radiation field in Hodgkin's disease. *Ann Oncol.* 2002;13(Suppl 1):79–83.

Answer 13

Low/low-intermediate risk age-adjusted IPI patients

Diffuse large B-cell lymphoma

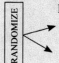

RANDOMIZE

CHOP-like chemo × 6 cycles ± RT

CHOP-like chemo × 6 cycles + rituximab ± RT

RT: Bulky and extranodal sites received RT (30–40 Gy)

R-CHOP arm had significantly higher EFS and OS

3-yr EFS: (79% vs 59%)

3-yr OS: (93% vs 84%)

Pfreundschuh M, Trumper L, Osterborg A, et al. CHOP-like chemotherapy plus rituximab versus CHOP-like chemotherapy alone in young patients with good-prognosis diffuse large-B-cell lymphoma: a randomized controlled trial by the MabThera International Trial (MInT) Group. *Lancet Oncol.* 2006;7:379–391.

Question 14

What was the effect of RT following complete response to CHOP × 8 on DFS and OS in ECOG 1484, a phase III cooperative group clinical trial for early stage non-Hodgkin lymphoma?

Question 15

What features constitute the Follicular Lymphoma International Prognostic Index (FLIPI?)

What are the associated 5-year OS rates, stratified by risk?

Question 16

When treating stage I, II follicular lymphoma with radiation therapy, what is an appropriate dose to administer?

Answer 14

Diffuse aggressive NHL (Working Formulation)

   (80% were DLBCL)

Stage I bulky, IE

Stage II bulky, IIE

CR patients received 30 Gy to initial disease sites

RT arm had significantly higher DFS;

OS difference not significant

6-yr DFS: (73% vs 56%) $p = .05$

15-yr OS: (60% vs 44%) $p = .24$

Horning SJ, Weller E, Kim K, et al. Chemotherapy with or without radiotherapy in limited-stage diffuse aggressive non-Hodgkin's lymphoma: Eastern Cooperative Oncology Group study 1484. *J Clin Oncol*. 2004;22:3032–3038.

Answer 15

LDH > normal

Age > 60

Stage III, IV

Extranodal sites > 4

Hemoglobin level < 12.0 g/dL

Low risk: FLIPI 0–1 – 91% 5-yr OS

Intermediate: FLIPI 2 – 78% 5-yr OS

High: FLIPI 3+ – 52% 5-yr OS

Solal-Celigny P, Roy P, Colombat P, et al. Follicular lymphoma international prognostic index. *Blood*. 2004;104:1258–1265.

Answer 16

   24–36 Gy

In a prospective randomized trial, overall response rate was 92–93% for both the 40–45 Gy arm as well as the 24 Gy arm.

Lowry L, Smith P, Qian W, et al. Reduced dose radiotherapy for local control in non-Hodgkin lymphoma: a randomised phase III trial. *Radiother Oncol*. 2011;100:86–92.

Question 17
Which patients have the greatest benefit from involved field radiation therapy (IFRT) in the treatment of gastric MALT?

Question 18
What is appropriate management for stage I small lymphocytic lymphoma (SLL)?

Question 19
What is appropriate therapy for stage IB/IIA mycosis fungoides (excluding those with > 5% Sezary cells, large cell transformed, or folliculotropic variants)?

Answer 17

H. pylori negative

disease with t(11;18) translocation

extension to the muscularis or serosa (T2 or T3)

disease extending from GI tract to adjacent organs (IIE)

Schechter NR, Portlock CS, Yahalom J. Treatment of mucosa-associated lymphoid tissue lymphoma of the stomach with radiation alone. *J Clin Oncol.* 1998;16:1916–1921.

Answer 18

Small lymphocytic lymphoma is the third most common histologic subtype of NHL. Chronic lymphocytic leukemia (CLL) and SLL are considered different manifestations of the same disease; a significant number of the abnormal lymphocytes are in the bone marrow and blood in CLL, versus in the lymph nodes in SLL.

Stage I SLL can be treated with 30–40 Gy involved field radiation therapy; 10-year freedom from relapse with radiation is: 80%.

Stage II treated with RT alone: 10-yr FFR: 62%.

Morrison WH, Hoppe RT, Weiss LM, et al. Small lymphocytic lymphoma. *J Clin Oncol.* 1989;7:598–606.

Answer 19

Topical chemotherapy (mechlorethamine, carmustine)

Topical corticosteroids

Total skin electron beam therapy (30–36 Gy)

Phototherapy (UVB or PUVA-thicker plaques)

Stage IB—patch, plaque, or papule involvement involving 10% or more of total skin surface with no lymph node or viscera involvement.

Stage IIA—any size patch, plaque, or papule involvement with reactive palpable lymph nodes (N1) or with isolated and scattered neoplastic cells in the lymph nodes (N2) on histology, but preservation of the nodal architecture, and no involvement of the viscera.

Poor prognostic features: > 5% Sezary cells, large cell transformed, or folliculotropic variants

NCCN Clinical Practice Guidelines in Oncology: Non-Hodgkin's Lymphomas. Fort Washington, PA: National Comprehensive Cancer Network; 2011. http://www.nccn.org/professionals/physician_gls/pdf/nhl.pdf. Accessed October 18, 2011.

Question 20

How is Total Skin Electron Beam Therapy administered for mycosis fungoides?

What dose is given, and in what fashion?

Question 21

What is an appropriate dose to administer for mantle cell lymphoma, either for local control following chemotherapy or for palliation?

Question 22

What is appropriate management for stage IE primary breast lymphoma, diffuse large B-cell type?

Question 23

What immunophenotype is associated with marginal zone lymphoma?

Answer 20

36 Gy, 2 Gy/fx

Six patient positions, resulting in AP, LAO, RAO, PA, LPO, RPO treatment fields

Extended SSD, typically 380 cm

Sequential 2-day treatment cycle, 3 fields per day

Lucite scatterer/energy degrader panel to improve uniformity

One week break after 18 Gy if significant skin erythema seen

American Association of Physicists in Medicine report no. 23. Total skin electron therapy: technique and dosimetry. In: *AAPM Radiotherapy Task Group 30*. Woodbury, NY: American Institute of Physics, Inc.; 1987:1–55.
Hoppe RT. Total skin electron beam therapy in the management of mycosis fungoides. *Front Radiat Ther Oncol.* 1991;25:80–89.

Answer 21

24–36 Gy

Although mantle cell lymphoma frequently presents in advanced stage, its radiosensitivity make radiation therapy a useful modality, even in the palliative setting.

Rosenbluth BD, Yahalom J. Highly effective local control and palliation of mantle cell lymphoma with involved-field radiation therapy (IFRT). *Int J Radiat Oncol Biol Phys.* 2006;65:1185–1191.

Answer 22

Primary breast lymphoma contributes to about 2% of all extranodal NHL. The most common subtype is diffuse large B-cell.

R-CHOP × 3 cycles plus IFRT (30–36 Gy)

Or R-CHOP × 6–8 cycles +/– IFRT (30 Gy)

Avilés A, Delgado S, Nambo MJ, et al. Primary breast lymphoma: results of a controlled clinical trial. *Oncology.* 2005;69:256–260.

Answer 23

CD19, CD20, CD22 positive

CD3, CD10 negative

Friedberg JW, Mauch PM, Rimsza LM, et al. Non-Hodgkin's lymphomas. In: DeVita VT, Lawrence TS, Rosenberg SA, eds. *DeVita, Hellman, and Rosenberg's Cancer: Principles & Practice of Oncology.* 8th ed. Philadelphia: Lippincott Williams & Wilkins; 2008:2098–2142.

Question 24
What immunophenotype is associated with follicular cell lymphoma?

Question 25
What are considered B symptoms?

Question 26
What is the Ann Arbor stage of a patient with biopsy-proven liver involvement by lymphoma and no additional sites of disease?

Question 27
Using prospective data, another prognostic index was developed in 2009 by the International Follicular Lymphoma Prognostic Factor Project—the FLIPI2. What five parameters comprise the FLIPI2?

Answer 24

CD10, CD19, CD20, CD22 positive

CD3, CD5 negative

Friedberg JW, Mauch PM, Rimsza LM, et al. Non-Hodgkin's lymphomas. In: DeVita VT, Lawrence TS, Rosenberg SA, eds. *DeVita, Hellman, and Rosenberg's Cancer: Principles & Practice of Oncology*. 8th ed. Philadelphia: Lippincott Williams & Wilkins; 2008:2098–2142.

Answer 25

Fever > 38 degrees C, night sweats, or > 10% weight loss over the past 6 months

B symptoms occur with greater frequency in aggressive NHL (Diffuse large B-cell: 33%; Follicular: 28%).

Armitage JO, Weisenburger DD. New approach to classifying non-Hodgkin's lymphomas: clinical features of the major histologic subtypes. Non-Hodgkin's Lymphoma Classification Project. *J Clin Oncol*. 1998;16:2780–2795.

Answer 26

Stage IV.

Liver, bone marrow, CSF, or lung involvement (other than direct extension from another site) is considered stage IV disease.

Lymphoma, Edge SB, Byrd DR, Compton CC, et al., eds. *AJCC Cancer Staging Handbook*. 7th ed. New York, NY: Springer; 2010:661–687.

Answer 27

New parameters not in FLIPI: Bone marrow involvement, serum beta-2 microglobulin level greater than the upper limit of normal, and longest diameter of largest node > 6 cm. Two from FLIPI also in FLIPI2: Age > 60 yrs and Hgb < 12 g/dL.

Federico M, Bellei M, Marcheselli L, et al. Follicular lymphoma international prognostic index 2: a new prognostic index for follicular lymphoma developed by the international follicular lymphoma prognostic factor project. *J Clin Oncol*. 2009;27:4555–4562.

Question 28

When should a lumbar puncture be considered as part of the workup for NHL?

Question 29

What are the subtypes of marginal zone lymphoma, ranked from most common to least common?

Which ones have the potential to transform to diffuse large B-cell?

Question 30

What is the most common stage of presentation for marginal zone B-cell lymphoma?

Answer 28

When the following sites are involved:

    paranasal sinus
    parameningeal
    testicular
    periorbital
    paravertebral
    bone marrow

Also consider if patient is HIV positive.

NCCN Clinical Practice Guidelines in Oncology: Non-Hodgkin's Lymphomas. Fort Washington, PA: National Comprehensive Cancer Network; 2011. http://www.nccn.org/professionals/physician_gls/pdf/nhl.pdf. Accessed October 18, 2011.

Answer 29

Extranodal (including MALT) – 50–70%

Splenic (associated with Hepatitis C) – 20%

Nodal – 10%

Nodal and splenic can transform to DLBCL.

Friedberg JW, Mauch PM, Rimsza LM, et al. Non-Hodgkin's lymphomas. In: DeVita VT, Lawrence TS, Rosenberg SA, eds. *DeVita, Hellman, and Rosenberg's Cancer: Principles & Practice of Oncology*. 8th ed. Philadelphia: Lippincott Williams & Wilkins; 2008:2098–2142.

Answer 30

    Stage IE or IIE (70%);
    Stomach is the most common extranodal site
    50% of gastric lymphoma is MALT
    Nodal and splenic can transform to DLBCL.

Extranodal marginal zone B-cell lymphoma is also referred to as MALT lymphoma. Extranodal marginal zone B-cell lymphoma comprises 5% of all NHL.

Friedberg JW, Mauch PM, Rimsza LM, et al. Non-Hodgkin's lymphomas. In: DeVita VT, Lawrence TS, Rosenberg SA, eds. *DeVita, Hellman, and Rosenberg's Cancer: Principles & Practice of Oncology*. 8th ed. Philadelphia: Lippincott Williams & Wilkins; 2008:2098–2142.

Question 31

Besides stomach, what are some other extranodal sites for MALT lymphoma involvement?

Question 32

What should the treatment volume include in radiation therapy for stage IE gastric MALT?

What is the recommended dose?

Question 33

What is conventional treatment for splenic marginal zone B-cell lymphoma?

What is conventional treatment for localized nodal marginal zone B-cell lymphoma?

Answer 31

Salivary glands (associated with Sjogren's syndrome), thyroid (associated with Hashimoto's thyroiditis), Waldeyer's ring, large/small intestine, orbit, lung, conjunctiva, breast, skin.

Friedberg JW, Mauch PM, Rimsza LM, et al. Non-Hodgkin's lymphomas. In: DeVita VT, Lawrence TS, Rosenberg SA, eds. *DeVita, Hellman, and Rosenberg's Cancer: Principles & Practice of Oncology.* 8th ed. Philadelphia: Lippincott Williams & Wilkins; 2008:2098–2142.

Answer 32

Include the entire stomach, perigastric, and celiac lymph nodes to 30–35 Gy.

Acute effects of treatment include transient anorexia, malaise and occasional nausea or dyspepsia.

Tsang RW, Gospodarowicz MK, Pintilie M, et al. Localized mucosa-associated lymphoid tissue lymphoma treated with radiation therapy has excellent clinical outcome. *J Clin Oncol.* 2003;21:4157–4164.

Answer 33

Splenic:
Symptomatic splenomegaly/cytopenia – splenectomy recommended. Chemotherapy/rituximab, or radiation therapy to 30 Gy can also be considered if patient is not a splenectomy candidate.

Nodal:
Involved field radiation therapy to 24–36 Gy.

NCCN Clinical Practice Guidelines in Oncology: Non-Hodgkin's Lymphomas. Fort Washington, PA: National Comprehensive Cancer Network; 2011. http://www.nccn.org/professionals/physician_gls/pdf/nhl.pdf. Accessed October 18, 2011.

Question 34

What is considered part of the routine work-up for mantle cell lymphoma?

Question 35

What are some distinguishing hematologic features between small lymphocytic lymphoma (SLL) and chronic lymphocytic lymphoma (CLL)?

Question 36

Which prospective phase III study investigating consolidative RT for early stage DLBCL did not include bulky stage II disease?

Answer 34

CT chest, abdomen, pelvis with contrast

Peripheral blood smear

Bone marrow biopsy

Colonoscopy

In addition to CT chest, abdomen, pelvis with contrast, peripheral blood smear, and bone marrow biopsy, a colonoscopy is now considered part of the routine staging evaluation, as mantle cell lymphoma may present as lymphomatous polyposis coli, with GI involvement reported as high as 20% of cases.

Chim CS, Hu WH, Loong F, et al. GI manifestations of mantle cell lymphoma. *Gastrointest Endosc*. 2003;58:931–933.

NCCN Clinical Practice Guidelines in Oncology: Non-Hodgkin's Lymphomas. Fort Washington, PA: National Comprehensive Cancer Network; 2011. http://www.nccn.org/professionals/physician_gls/pdf/nhl.pdf. Accessed October 18, 2011.

Answer 35

SLL

peripheral blood lymphocytes $< 5 \times 10^9$/L

$< 30\%$ bone marrow infiltration

lymphadeonpathy, hepatosplenomegaly, or other organ infiltration

CLL

peripheral blood lymphocytes $> 5 \times 10^9$/L

$> 30\%$ bone marrow infiltration

Friedberg JW, Mauch PM, Rimsza LM, et al. Non-Hodgkin's lymphomas. In: DeVita VT, Lawrence TS, Rosenberg SA, eds. *DeVita, Hellman, and Rosenberg's Cancer: Principles & Practice of Oncology*. 8th ed. Philadelphia: Lippincott Williams & Wilkins; 2008:2098–2142.

Answer 36

SWOG 8736

401 pts

Stage I (+/– bulky dz) or II (non-bulky)

intermediate or high grade NHL

Bulky disease was defined as a mediastinal mass with a maximal diameter exceeding one third the maximal chest diameter or any other mass 10 cm or more in maximal diameter.

Mnemonic: "Slim in the Southwest"

Miller TP, Dahlberg S, Cassady JR, et al. Chemotherapy alone compared with chemotherapy plus radiotherapy for localized intermediate- and high-grade non-Hodgkin's lymphoma. *N Engl J Med*. 1998;339:21–26.

Question 37

What major studies investigated consolidative radiation therapy for early stage DLBCL?

Question 38

What are some clinical features of peripheral T-cell lymphoma?

Question 39

What is the most common subtype for testicular lymphoma?

Answer 37

SWOG 8736
    Stage I (+/– bulky dz) or II (non-bulky) intermed/high grade NHL
    CHOP × 8 vs CHOP × 3 + RT
    equivalent PFS and OS after 7, 9 yrs

ECOG 1484
    CHOP × 8; complete responders → IFRT or observation
    6-yr DFS favors RT

GELA LNH-93–4
    CHOP × 4 vs CHOP × 4 + RT; elderly patients
    equivalent 5-yr DFS and OS; controversial methodology

Bonnet C, Fillet G, Mounier N, et al. CHOP alone compared with CHOP plus radiotherapy for localized aggressive lymphoma in elderly patients: a study by the Groupe d'Etude des Lymphomes de l'Adulte. *J Clin Oncol.* 2007;25:787–792.

Horning SJ, Weller E, Kim K, et al. Chemotherapy with or without radiotherapy in limited-stage diffuse aggressive non-Hodgkin's lymphoma: Eastern Cooperative Oncology Group study 1484. *J Clin Oncol.* 2004;22:3032–3038.

Miller TP, Dahlberg S, Cassady JR, et al. Chemotherapy alone compared with chemotherapy plus radiotherapy for localized intermediate- and high-grade non-Hodgkin's lymphoma. *N Engl J Med.* 1998;339:21–26.

Answer 38

Peripheral T-cell lymphoma is an aggressive NHL which commonly presents as stage IV. Worse prognosis than DLBCL with 5-yr OS of 20%. Higher incidence in Asia; median age of diagnosis is 60 years. Conventional chemotherapy offers poor outcomes, and therefore clinical trial participation is encouraged.

Friedberg JW, Mauch PM, Rimsza LM, et al. Non-Hodgkin's lymphomas. In: DeVita VT, Lawrence TS, Rosenberg SA, eds. *DeVita, Hellman, and Rosenberg's Cancer: Principles & Practice of Oncology.* 8th ed. Philadelphia: Lippincott Williams & Wilkins; 2008:2098–2142.

Answer 39

Diffuse large B-cell. Other subtypes, such as peripheral T-cell, lymphoblastic B-cell, are rare.
    Median age of presentation: 60.
    Primary testicular lymphoma is the most common testicular tumor in men over 60.

Vural F, Cagirgan S, Saydam G, et al. Primary testicular lymphoma. *J Natl Med Assoc.* 2007;99:1277–1282.

Question 40

Is orchiectomy sufficient treatment for primary testicular lymphoma?

Question 41

What dose is given to the contralateral testis in the treatment of primary testicular lymphoma?

Question 42

What is an appropriate palliative fractionation for the local palliative treatment of indolent lymphomas?

Question 43

What are the three main subtypes of primary cutaneous B-cell lymphoma?

Which is the most clinically aggressive?

Answer 40

No; in addition to systemic chemotherapy, treatment must include radiation therapy to the involved field, as well as to the contralateral testis. CNS prophylaxis should be administered with high dose methotrexate or intrathecal chemotherapy.

Vitolo U, Chiappella A, Ferreri AJ, et al. First-line treatment for primary testicular diffuse large B-cell lymphoma with rituximab-CHOP, CNS prophylaxis, and contralateral testis irradiation: final results of an international phase II trial. *J Clin Oncol.* 2011;29:2766–2772.

Answer 41

30 Gy

Prophylactic testicular radiation to the contralateral testicle reduces testicular failure from 35% to 8%.

Vitolo U, Chiappella A, Ferreri AJ, et al. First-line treatment for primary testicular diffuse large B-cell lymphoma with rituximab-CHOP, CNS prophylaxis, and contralateral testis irradiation: final results of an international phase II trial. *J Clin Oncol.* 2011;29:2766–2772.

Answer 42

2 Gy × 2 fx, repeating as indicated.

Haas RL, Poortmans P, de Jong D, et al. High response rates and lasting remissions after low-dose involved field radiotherapy in indolent lymphomas. *J Clin Oncol.* 2003;21:2474–2480.

Answer 43

Primary cutaneous follicle center lymphoma (PCFCL)

Primary cutaneous marginal zone lymphoma (PCMZL)

Primary cutaneous large B-cell lymphoma (PCLBCL), leg type

PCLBCL is the most aggressive subtype, with an estimated 5-yr survival of 41%. Estimated 5-yr survival of PCFCL and PCMZL is 95% or greater.

Senff NJ, Hoefnagel JJ, Jansen PM, et al. Reclassification of 300 primary cutaneous B-Cell lymphomas according to the new WHO-EORTC classification for cutaneous lymphomas: comparison with previous classifications and identification of prognostic markers. *J Clin Oncol.* 2007;25:1581–1587.

Question 44

Is bone marrow biopsy required as part of the workup for primary cutaneous diffuse large B-cell lymphoma, leg type?

Question 45

What are two radioimmunotherapies targeting CD20 to treat B-cell non-Hodgkin lymphoma?

Question 46

What are clinically-supported indications to use single-agent radioimmunotherapy in follicular lymphoma (FL)?

Question 47

Which is superior for relapsed or refractory low-grade, follicular B-cell non-Hodgkin lymphoma: Y-90 ibritumomab tiuxetan, or rituximab?

Answer 44

Yes; while optional for the other subtypes of primary cutaneous B-cell lymphoma, bone marrow biopsy is indicated for PCLBCL, leg type.

NCCN Clinical Practice Guidelines in Oncology: Non-Hodgkin's Lymphomas. Fort Washington, PA: National Comprehensive Cancer Network; 2011. http://www.nccn.org/professionals/physician_gls/pdf/nhl.pdf. Accessed October 18, 2011.

Answer 45

Y-90 ibritumomab tiuxetan and I-131 tositumomab.

Side effects of ibritumomab and tositumomab include leukopenia and thrombocytopenia. Tositumomab has also been associated with hypothyroidism in 10–20% of patients. Patients with inadequate bone marrow reserve should not receive radioimmunotherapy.

Witzig TE, White CA, Gordon LI, et al. Safety of yttrium-90 ibritumomab tiuxetan radioimmunotherapy for relapsed low-grade, follicular, or transformed non-Hodgkin's lymphoma. *J Clin Oncol.* 2003;21:1263–1270.

Answer 46

Single agent radioimmunotherapy used for:
  Relapsed/refractory FL
  Selected patients with new, untreated FL
  Consolidation after induction chemotherapy

Witzig TE, Fishkin P, Gordon LI, et al. Treatment recommendations for radioimmunotherapy in follicular lymphoma: a consensus conference report. *Leuk Lymphoma.* 2011;52:1188–1199.

Answer 47

A prospective, randomized, phase III trial demonstrated (90)Y-ibritumomab tiuxetan to have a higher complete response (30% vs 16%; $p = .04$) and overall response rate (80% vs 56%; $p = .002$) when compared to four doses rituxan.

Witzig TE, Gordon LI, Cabanillas F, et al. Randomized controlled trial of yttrium-90-labeled ibritumomab tiuxetan radioimmunotherapy versus rituximab immunotherapy for patients with relapsed or refractory low-grade, follicular, or transformed B-cell non-Hodgkin's lymphoma. *J Clin Oncol.* 2002;20:2453–2463.

Question 48

Does PET SUV intensity distinguish between indolent and aggressive histology for NHL?

Question 49

How does primary CNS lymphoma appear on MRI?

Question 50

In the phase II prospective trial, RTOG 9310, how did the addition of chemotherapy to WBRT improve outcome?

What patients were at greater risk for neurotoxicity?

Question 51

What patients are most appropriate for initial treatment with WBRT for primary CNS lymphoma?

Answer 48

Yes; in a series, SUV > 10 excluded indolent lymphoma with 81% specificity; SUV > 13 with 100% specificity.

Schöder H, Noy A, Gönen M, et al. Intensity of 18fluorodeoxyglucose uptake in positron emission tomography distinguishes between indolent and aggressive non-Hodgkin's lymphoma. *J Clin Oncol.* 2005;23:4643–4651.

Answer 49

Solitary (70%) or multifocal (30%), contrast-enhancing, non-hemorrhagic mass without necrosis, in the deep white matter, adjacent to ventricular surface.

Bühring U, Herrlinger U, Krings T, et al. MRI features of primary central nervous system lymphomas at presentation. *Neurology.* 2001;57:393–396.

Answer 50

Patients received methotrexate (IV and intraventricular), vincristine, and procarbazine. WBRT was planned for 45 Gy (1.8 Gy/fx). WBRT was later modified to 36 Gy (1.2 Gy/fx, BID).

Chemo achieved a 58% CR rate. Median OS for Chemo + WBRT was 36.9 mos; this was an improvement over historical median OS of 12–18 mos for RT alone. Patients > 60 yrs had a significant risk for leukoencephalopathy from combined treatment.

DeAngelis LM, Seiferheld W, Schold SC, et al. Combination chemotherapy and radiotherapy for primary central nervous system lymphoma: Radiation Therapy Oncology Group Study 93-10. *J Clin Oncol.* 2002;20:4643–4648.

Answer 51

Poor performance status patients (KPS < 40) who cannot tolerate high dose systemic chemo

Can be considered following initial chemotherapy for patients < 60 y.o. with good KPS, particularly if there is not a complete response

NCCN Clinical Practice Guidelines in Oncology: Central Nervous System Cancers. Fort Washington, PA: National Comprehensive Cancer Network; 2011. http://www.nccn.org/professionals/physician_gls/pdf/cns.pdf. Accessed October 18, 2011.

Question 52

When can treatment-related leukoencephalopathy occur following methotrexate and WBRT, and how does it clinically manifest?

Question 53

What are appropriate management options to the orbit for primary CNS lymphoma with intraocular involvement?

Question 54

HODGKIN LYMPHOMA

Does PET response following 2 cycles of chemo predict for failure/survival in Hodgkin lymphoma?

Question 55

What is appropriate treatment for stage IA lymphocyte-predominant Hodgkin lymphoma?

Answer 52

Symptoms of neurotoxicity can occur one month after treatment completion. Clinical manifestations include cognitive difficulties, motor disturbances, and gait ataxia. White matter hyperintensity is seen on T2-weighted MRI.

Lai R, Abrey LE, Rosenblum MK, et al. Treatment-induced leukoencephalopathy in primary CNS lymphoma: a clinical and autopsy study. *Neurology.* 2004;62:451–456.

Answer 53

Ocular radiation

Intravitreal chemotherapy

Defer initial ocular treatment and reassess following systemic therapy

Retrospective review demonstrated longer median progression free survival for patients receiving dedicated intraocular therapy but no difference in median overall survival.

Grimm SA, McCannel CA, Omuro AM, et al. Primary CNS lymphoma with intraocular involvement: International PCNSL Collaborative Group Report. *Neurology.* 2008;71:1355–1360.

Answer 54

Yes; conversion to PET negative disease after two cycles predicted for increased complete response (83% vs 58%) and improved 2-yr OS (90% vs 61%).

Hutchings M, Loft A, Hansen M, et al. FDG-PET after two cycles of chemotherapy predicts treatment failure and progression-free survival in Hodgkin lymphoma. *Blood.* 2006;107:52–59.

Answer 55

Involved-Field Radiation Therapy

LPHL has a favorable prognosis and more indolent nature than other subtypes, and radiation therapy alone is acceptable for stage IA–IIA LPHL. Doses of 30–36 Gy are given, with 30 Gy considered sufficient for regions where nodal disease has been excised.

Schlembach PJ, Wilder RB, Jones D, et al. Radiotherapy alone for lymphocyte-predominant Hodgkin's disease. *Cancer J.* 2002;8:377–383.

Question 56

What were the eligibility criteria used for the favorable and unfavorable prognostic groups for the EORTC H7 and H8-F/H8-U phase III trials?

Question 57

EBV positivity is most strongly associated with which subtype of Hodgkin lymphoma?

Question 58

For patients presenting with supradiagphragmatic clinical stage I or II disease, what are four subgroups with a very low (< 10%) probability of subdiaphragmatic involvement?

Answer 56

Favorable prognostic group—all of the following:

 age < 50

 no large mediastinal adenopathy

 ESR of < 50/h and no B symptoms or ESR < 30 mm/hr with B symptoms

 one to three sites of disease (stage I, II2, III3)

 (exception: age < 40, female, stage I, ESR < 50/hr with no B symptoms, and LP/NS histology were not eligible)

Unfavorable prognositc group—any one of the following:

 age ≥ 50

 large mediastinal adenopathy

 four or more sites of involvement (stage II4–II5)

 B symptoms and ESR ≥ 30 mm/hr

 ESR ≥ 50 mm/hr without B symptoms

Eghbali H, Raemaekers J, Carde P. The EORTC strategy in the treatment of Hodgkin's lymphoma. *Eur J Haematol Suppl.* 2005;66:135–140.

Fermé C, Eghbali H, Meerwaldt JH, et al. Chemotherapy plus involved-field radiation in early-stage Hodgkin's disease. *N Engl J Med.* 2007;357:1916–1927.

Answer 57

Mixed cellularity subtype

EBV positivity is associated with the majority of mixed cellularity cases of Hodgkin lymphoma.

Pallesen G, Hamilton-Dutoit SJ, Rowe M, et al. Expression of Epstein–Barr virus latent gene products in tumour cells of Hodgkin's disease. *Lancet.* 1991;337:320–322.

Answer 58

CS I patients with mediastinal-only disease (laparotomy yield: 0%)

Females with CS I disease (lap yield: 6%)

Males with CS I disease and lymphocyte predominance or interfollicular histologies (lap yield: 4%)

Females with CS II, age < 27, and have 3 or fewer sites of clinical involvement (lap yield: 9%)

Mixed cellularity histology and male gender were associated with increased risk for subdiaphragmatic disease.

Leibenhaut MH, Hoppe RT, Efron B, et al. Prognostic indicators of laparotomy findings in clinical stage I-II supradiaphragmatic Hodgkin's disease. *J Clin Oncol.* 1989;7:81–91.

Question 59

What are the chemotherapy agents in Stanford V?

How many cycles of Stanford V are administered for stage I/II favorable disease?

Question 60

In stage I/II unfavorable Hodgkin lymphoma, following 12 weeks of Stanford V, what dose of RT is given to bulky disease (initial sites > 5 cm) and residual PET positive sites?

Question 61

In stage I/II unfavorable Hodgkin lymphoma, following 12 weeks of Stanford V, what dose of RT is given to non-bulky disease for unfavorable patients following 12 weeks of Stanford V?

Answer 59

Adriamycin, Vinblastine, Mechlorethamine, Vincristine, Bleomycin, Etoposide, Prednisone

8 weeks (2 cycles) are administered for stage I/II favorable disease. Following the completion of chemotherapy, complete restaging takes place, and consolidative RT is instituted within 3 weeks.

NCCN Clinical Practice Guidelines in Oncology: Hodgkin Lymphoma. Fort Washington, PA: National Comprehensive Cancer Network; 2011. http://www.nccn.org/professionals/physician_gls/pdf/hodgkins.pdf. Accessed October 18, 2011.

Answer 60

Stage I/II unfavorable patients receive 36 Gy to initial sites > 5 cm and residual PET positive sites after chemotherapy.

NCCN Clinical Practice Guidelines in Oncology: Hodgkin Lymphoma. Fort Washington, PA: National Comprehensive Cancer Network; 2011. http://www.nccn.org/professionals/physician_gls/pdf/hodgkins.pdf. Accessed October 18, 2011.

Answer 61

Patients with unfavorable stage I/II disease based upon B symptoms are treated with Stanford V for 12 wks + 30 Gy IFRT.

Patients with other criteria for unfavorable disease are treated with Stanford V for 8 wks + 30 Gy IFRT.

NCCN Clinical Practice Guidelines in Oncology: Hodgkin Lymphoma. Fort Washington, PA: National Comprehensive Cancer Network; 2011. http://www.nccn.org/professionals/physician_gls/pdf/hodgkins.pdf. Accessed October 18, 2011.

Question 62

EORTC H9U (stage I/II unfavorable Hodgkin lymphoma) found similar 4-year event free and overall survival between three systemic therapy regimens. What were the treatment arms?

Question 63

What is the definition of bulky disease based upon the mediastinal tumor ratio?

Question 64

What is the typical immunohistochemical staining profile for the Reed-Sternberg cells in Classical Hodgkin?

Answer 62

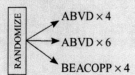

All arms received 30 Gy IFRT. Increased toxicity was found in the BEACOPP arm.

Additionally, EORTC H8U trial for unfavorable stage I/II compared 4 vs 6 cycles of hybrid MOPP/ABV and also showed no difference in 3-yr FFS or OS.

Fermé C, Eghbali H, Meerwaldt JH, et al. Chemotherapy plus involved-field radiation in early-stage Hodgkin's disease. *N Engl J Med.* 2007;357(19):1916–1927.
Noordijk EM, Thomas J, Foerme MB, et al. First results of the EORTC-GELA H9 randomized trials: the H9-F trial (comparing 3 radiation dose levels) and H9-U trial (comparing 3 chemotherapy schemes) in patients with favorable or unfavorable early stage Hodgkin's lymphoma (abstract). *Proc Am Soc Clin Oncol.* 2005;16:6505.

Answer 63

Mediastinal tumor ratio (MMR):
    ratio of the maximum width of the mass and the intrathoracic diameter at the T5–T6 interspace.

Bulky disease = MMR > 0.33

Mauch P, Goodman R, Hellman S. The significance of mediastinal involvement in early stage Hodgkin's disease. *Cancer.* 1978;42:1039–1045.

Answer 64

positive for:
    CD15
    CD30

negative for:
    CD3
    CD45

CD20 detected in < 40% of cases.

Classic Reed-Sternberg cells exhibit multiple nuclear lobes and large, inclusion-like nucleoli. Notably, the nodular lymphocyte predominant subtype does not commonly express the classic Reed-Sternberg cell but has a "lymphocytic and histiocytic" variant.

Diehl V, Re D, Harris NL, et al. Hodgkin lymphoma. In: DeVita VT, Lawrence TS, Rosenberg SA, eds. *DeVita, Hellman, and Rosenberg's Cancer: Principles & Practice of Oncology.* 8th ed. Philadelphia: Lippincott Williams & Wilkins; 2008:2167–2220.

Question 65

What was the largest multi-institutional randomized trial which investigated the efficacy of EFRT versus IFRT in early stage unfavorable Hodgkin lymphoma?

What were the findings?

Question 66

In advanced stage (III/IV) Hodgkin lymphoma patients, what dose of RT is recommended for residual PET-positive sites following 4-cycles of escalated-dose BEACOPP?

Question 67

What are the most common late effects seen with treatment for Hodgkin lymphoma?

Answer 65

HD8 trial from the German Hodgkin Study Group (GHSG):

COPP/ABVD × 4 cycles followed by 30 Gy EFRT + 10 Gy to bulky disease or 30 Gy IFRT + 10 Gy to bulky disease.

No difference in 5-yr Freedom from Treatment Failure (85.8% vs 84.2%, respectively) or 5-yr OS (90.8% vs 92.4%). Higher acute toxicity in the EFRT arm.

Engert A, Schiller P, Josting A, et al. Involved-field radiotherapy is equally effective and less toxic compared with extended-field radiotherapy after four cycles of chemotherapy in patients with early-stage unfavorable Hodgkin's lymphoma: results of the HD8 trial of the German Hodgkin's Lymphoma Study Group. *J Clin Oncol.* 2003;21:3601–3608.

Answer 66

40 Gy

GHSG HD15 is currently investigating the role of consolidative RT for bulky or residual sites for stage III/IV disease.

Kobe C, Dietlein M, Franklin J, et al. Positron emission tomography has a high negative predictive value for progression or early relapse for patients with residual disease after first-line chemotherapy in advanced-stage Hodgkin lymphoma. *Blood.* 2008;112:3989–3994.

Answer 67

Secondary malignancies
(most common: lung, breast)

Cardiovascular Disease
(mediastinal RT and anthracycline-based chemotherapy)

Hypothyroidism
(neck/upper mediastinal RT)

Myelosuppression
(chemotherapy, splenic RT)

Pulmonary toxicity
(bleomycin, pulmonary irradiation)

Diehl V, Re D, Harris NL, et al. Hodgkin lymphoma. In: DeVita VT, Lawrence TS, Rosenberg SA, eds. *DeVita, Hellman, and Rosenberg's Cancer: Principles & Practice of Oncology.* 8th ed. Philadelphia: Lippincott Williams & Wilkins; 2008:2167–2220.

Question 68

What is the age distribution most commonly seen in patients presenting with Hodgkin lymphoma?

Question 69

What are the classical Hodgkin lymphoma histologic subtypes, in order of U.S. frequency, from highest to lowest?

Question 70

What is the histological difference between lymphocyte-predominant Hodgkin lymphoma (LPHL) with a nodular pattern versus a diffuse pattern?

Question 71

What are the chemotherapy agents in BEACOPP?

When would BEACOPP be a more appropriate treatment regimen over Stanford V?

Answer 68

Bimodal age distribution.

Most age common presentation:
    Between 15 and 30 years
    Older than 55 years

Annual incidence in the U.S. is approximately 8800 cases, accounting for 10% of all lymphomas.

Diehl V, Re D, Harris NL, et al. Hodgkin lymphoma. In: DeVita VT, Lawrence TS, Rosenberg SA, eds. *DeVita, Hellman, and Rosenberg's Cancer: Principles & Practice of Oncology*. 8th ed. Philadelphia: Lippincott Williams & Wilkins; 2008:2167–2220.

Answer 69

Nodular sclerosis (70%)

Mixed cellularity (25%)

Lymphocyte rich (5%)

Lymphocyte depleted (< 1%)

Swerdlow SH, Campo E, Harris NL, eds. *World Health Organization Classification of Tumours of Haematopoietic and Lymphoid Tissues*. 4th ed. Lyon, France: IARC Press; 2008.

Answer 70

Nodular subtype – LPHL cells in a background of B-cells

Diffuse subtype – LPHL cells in a background of T-cells

Regula Jr DP, Hoppe RT, Weiss LM. Nodular and diffuse types of lymphocyte predominance Hodgkin's disease. *N Engl J Med*. 1988;318:214–219.

Answer 71

Bleomycin, Etoposide, Doxorubicin, Cyclophosphamide, Vincristine, Procarbazine, and Prednisone

Dose-escalated BEACOPP is preferred over ABVD or Stanford V in advanced disease, when the patient has more than 4 unfavorable factors (IPS ≥ 4).

Diehl V, Franklin J, Pfreundschuh M, et al. Standard and increased-dose BEACOPP chemotherapy compared with COPP-ABVD for advanced Hodgkin's disease. *N Engl J Med*. 2003;348:2386–2395.

Question 72

What is the typical immunohistochemical staining profile for lymphocyte-predominant Hodgkin lymphoma (LPHL)?

Question 73

Which patients should undergo bone marrow biopsy as part of their standard workup for newly diagnosed Hodgkin lymphoma?

Question 74

What were the randomization arms in GHSG HD10?

What were the findings?

Answer 72

positive for:

CD45

CD20

epithelial membrane antigen

negative for:

CD15

rarely express CD30

Diehl V, Re D, Harris NL, et al. Hodgkin lymphoma. In: DeVita VT, Lawrence TS, Rosenberg SA, eds. *DeVita, Hellman, and Rosenberg's Cancer: Principles & Practice of Oncology*. 8th ed. Philadelphia: Lippincott Williams & Wilkins; 2008:2167–2220.

Answer 73

Patients with B symptoms, anemia/leukopenia, or stage III–IV disease.

Bone marrow involvement is 1% for patients with early-stage disease with no B symptoms and no anemia/leukopenia.

Vassilakopoulos TP, Angelopoulou MK, Constantinou N, et al. Development and validation of a clinical prediction rule for bone marrow involvement in patients with Hodgkin lymphoma. *Blood*. 2005;105:1875–1880.

Answer 74

2×2 randomization:

4 cycles ABVD	2 cycles ABVD
30 Gy IFRT	20 Gy IFRT

No significant difference between 2 and 4 cycles ABVD on: 5-yr OS, Freedom from Treatment Failure (FFTF), and PFS.

No significant difference between 30 and 20 Gy on: 5-yr OS, FFTF, and PFS.

Significant differences in WHO grade III/IV toxicity with greater toxicity for 4 cycles (vs 2) and 30 Gy (vs 20).

Engert A, Plütschow A, Eich HT, et al. Reduced treatment intensity in patients with early-stage Hodgkin's lymphoma. *N Engl J Med*. 2010;363:640–652.

Question 75

The Stanford G4 trial compared how many cycles of Stanford V + what dose of IFRT against EFRT?

What was the difference in number of chemo cycles and dose for non-bulky versus bulky stage I–IIA patients?

Question 76

What features comprise the International Prognostic score for advanced stage Hodgkin lymphoma?

Question 77

What are the 5-yr Freedom from Progression (FFP) rates for advanced stage Hodgkin lymphoma based upon International Prognostic Score?

Question 78

What secondary malignancies are encountered following treatment for Hodgkin lymphoma?

Answer 75

Patients with non-bulky stage I/II disease received Stanford V × 8 weeks followed by 30 Gy IFRT.

Patients with bulky stage I/II disease received Stanford V × 12 wks + 36 Gy IFRT.

These regimens were equally effective and less toxic compared to EFRT.

8-yr Freedom From Progression: 96% for non-bulky, 92% for bulky

Advani RH, Hoppe RT, Baer DM, et al. Efficacy of abbreviated Stanford V chemotherapy and involved field radiotherapy in early stage Hodgkin's disease: mature results of the G4 trial. Poster session presented at: American Society of Hematology Annual Meeting and Exposition; 5 December 2009; New Orleans, LA.

Answer 76

Albumin < 4 g/dL

WBC > 15k

Lymphocytes < 600

Stage IV

Hgb < 10.5 g/dL

Age > 45

Male gender

Hasenclever D, Diehl V. A prognostic score for advanced Hodgkin's disease. International Prognostic Factors Project on Advanced Hodgkin's Disease. *N Engl J Med*. 1998;339:1506–1514.

Answer 77

No factors – 84% 5-yr FFP

One factor – 77%

Two factors – 67%

Three factors – 60%

Four factors – 51%

Five factors – 42%

Hasenclever D, Diehl V. A prognostic score for advanced Hodgkin's disease. International Prognostic Factors Project on Advanced Hodgkin's Disease. *N Engl J Med*. 1998;339:1506–1514.

Answer 78

Solid tumors:
    Breast, Lung, Gastrointestinal cancer

Leukemia

Non-Hodgkin Lymphoma

Over half of the second malignancies following treatment for Hodgkin lymphoma are solid tumors.

Women who receive mantle-field RT prior to age 30 are recommended to undergo yearly mammograms beginning 10 years after RT.

Van Leeuwen FE, Klokman WJ, Hagenbeek A, et al. Second cancer risk following Hodgkin's disease: a 20-year follow-up study. *J Clin Oncol*. 1994;12:312–325.

Question 79

What is an estimated rate for secondary malignancy attributable to treatment for Hodgkin lymphoma?

Question 80

What class of chemotherapy agent utilized in lymphoma treatment is associated with cardiotoxicity?

What risk factors correlate with an increased incidence?

Question 81

What class of chemotherapy agents is associated with an increased risk for leukemia?

How long after treatment is the peak incidence seen?

Question 82

When is a unilateral bone marrow biopsy indicated as part of the workup for Hodgkin lymphoma?

Answer 79

0.5–0.7% per year

The risk for leukemia development is highest for patients receiving alkylating chemotherapy. The increased risk for a solid tumor malignancy is attributable to both radiation therapy and chemotherapy. Risk for second malignancy is higher for patients who receive treatment age at 20 or less when compared to older patients.

Henry-Amar M. Second cancer after the treatment for Hodgkin's disease: a report from the International Database on Hodgkin's Disease. *Ann Oncol*. 1992;3(Suppl 4):117–128.

Swerdlow AJ, Douglas AJ, Hudson GV, et al. Risk of second primary cancers after Hodgkin's disease by type of treatment: analysis of 2846 patients in the British National Lymphoma Investigation. *BMJ*. 1992;304:1137–1143.

van Leeuwen FE, Klokman WJ, Veer MB, et al. Long-term risk of second malignancy in survivors of Hodgkin's disease treated during adolescence or young adulthood. *J Clin Oncol*. 2000;18:487–497.

Answer 80

Anthracyclines.

Lifetime cumulative dose, pre-existing heart disease, and cardiac radiation increase the risk.

An estimated cumulative 26% of patients will experience doxorubicin-related CHF at a cumulative dose of 550 mg/m^2

Swain SM, Whaley FS, Ewer MS. Congestive heart failure in patients treated with doxorubicin: a retrospective analysis of three trials. *Cancer*. 2003;97:2869–2879.

Answer 81

Alkylating agents.

Peak incidence is seen between 5–10 years after treatment.

Schonfeld SJ, Gilbert ES, Dores GM, et al. Acute myeloid leukemia following Hodgkin lymphoma: a population-based study of 35,511 patients. *J Natl Cancer Inst*. 2006;98:215–218.

Answer 82

Clinical stage IIB to IV

Presence of B symptoms

Presence of anemia, leukopenia, or thrombocytopenia

Munker R, Hasenclever D, Brosteanu O, et al. Bone marrow involvement in Hodgkin's disease: an analysis of 135 consecutive cases. German Hodgkin's Lymphoma Study Group. *J Clin Oncol*. 1995;13:403–419.

Vassilakopoulos TP, Angelopoulou MK, Constantinou N, et al. Development and validation of a clinical prediction rule for bone marrow involvement in patients with Hodgkin lymphoma. *Blood*. 2005;105:1875–1880.

Question 83

When is radiation therapy indicated following salvage chemotherapy for relapsed Hodgkin lymphoma?

Question 84

What evidence supports IFRT for bulky classical Hodgkin lymphoma, following complete or partial remission to chemotherapy, before or after High Dose Therapy/Autologous Bone Marrow Transplantation?

Question 85

What is the incidence of hypothyroidism as a late-effect following neck or upper mediastinal irradiation for lymphoma?

Question 86

How many cycles of ABVD are given for stage IA to stage IIA favorable disease Hodgkin lymphoma?

What dose is given for IFRT?

Answer 83

Involved field radiation (IFRT) is indicated for localized residual disease.

IFRT also should be considered even if PET is negative after chemotherapy, even in the setting of High-Dose Therapy with Autologous Stem Cell Rescue. RT should be highly considered if the site has not been previously irradiated, or if disease was bulky.

NCCN Clinical Practice Guidelines in Oncology: Non-Hodgkin's Lymphomas. Fort Washington, PA: National Comprehensive Cancer Network; 2011. http://www.nccn.org/professionals/physician_gls/pdf/nhl.pdf. Accessed October 18, 2011.

Answer 84

A prospective study investigated relapsed stage I–III Hodgkin lymphoma, treated with chemotherapy with a subset receiving IFRT as consolidative or cytoreductive therapy before or following HDT/ABMT, median dose 30 Gy. For those not previously irradiated, IFRT demonstrated improved 3-year Freedom From Relapse (100% vs 67%) and a trend for improved survival (85% vs 60%). Benefit was seen in previously irradiated patients as well.

Poen JC, Hoppe RT, Horning SJ. High-dose therapy and autologous bone marrow transplantation for relapsed/refractory Hodgkin's disease: the impact of involved field radiotherapy on patterns of failure and survival. *Int J Radiat Oncol Biol Phys*. 1996;36:3–12.

Answer 85

50%

The same report identified abnormal pulmonary function in up to 30% of long term survivors, and also noted altered fertility even with patients treated with BEACOPP. Infection risk from encapsulated organisms was also higher in patients with functional or anatomical asplenia.

Mauch P, Ng A, Aleman B, et al. Report from the Rockefellar Foundation Sponsored International Workshop on reducing mortality and improving quality of life in long-term survivors of Hodgkin's disease: July 9–16, 2003, Bellagio, Italy. *Eur J Haematol Suppl*. 2005;66:68–76.

Answer 86

2–4 cycles of ABVD are given, followed by 30 Gy IFRT.

If criteria for favorable disease is met (ESR < 50, no extralymphatic involvement, and < 3 nodal regions involved), ABVD × 2 cycles followed by 20 Gy IFRT may be sufficient.

Engert A, Schiller P, Josting A, et al. Involved-field radiotherapy is equally effective and less toxic compared with extended-field radiotherapy after four cycles of chemotherapy in patients with early-stage unfavorable Hodgkin's lymphoma: results of the HD8 trial of the German Hodgkin's Lymphoma Study Group. *J Clin Oncol*. 2003;21:3601–3608.

Question 87

How many weeks of Stanford V are given for stage IA to stage IIA favorable disease Hodgkin lymphoma?

What dose is given for IFRT?

Question 88

How many cycles of ABVD are given for bulky stage I–IIA/B Hodgkin lymphoma?

What dose is given for IFRT?

Question 89

How many weeks of Stanford V are given for bulky stage I–IIA/B Hodgkin lymphoma?

What dose is given for IFRT?

Question 90

Did Intergroup E2496 demonstrate a superior outcome between ABVD and Stanford V for bulky mediastinal stage I–IIA/B and stage III–IV patients?

Answer 87

8 weeks (2 cycles) of Stanford V are given, followed by 30 Gy IFRT.

NCCN Clinical Practice Guidelines in Oncology: Non-Hodgkin's Lymphomas. Fort Washington, PA: National Comprehensive Cancer Network; 2011. http://www.nccn.org/professionals/physician_gls/pdf/nhl.pdf. Accessed October 18, 2011.

Answer 88

6–8 cycles of ABVD are given, followed by 36 Gy IFRT.

ABVD consists of:

Doxorubicin 25 mg/m^2, Bleomycin 10 units/m^2, Vinblastine 6 mg/m^2, Dacarbazine 375 mg/m^2. All agents are given on days 1 and 15.

Cycles are given every 28 days. Dose adjustments of bleomycin are made for renal dysfunction, and doxorubicin and vinblastine for hepatic dysfunction.

Canellos GP, Anderson JR, Propert KJ, et al. Chemotherapy of advanced Hodgkin's disease with MOPP, ABVD, or MOPP alternating with ABVD. *N Engl J Med*. 1992;327:1478–1484.
NCCN Clinical Practice Guidelines in Oncology: Non-Hodgkin's Lymphomas. Fort Washington, PA: National Comprehensive Cancer Network; 2011. http://www.nccn.org/professionals/physician_gls/pdf/hodgkins.pdf. Accessed October 18, 2011.

Answer 89

12 weeks of Stanford V are given, followed by 36 Gy IFRT.

Stanford V consists of:

Doxorubicin 25 mg/m^2 (days 1, 15), Vinblastine 6 mg/m^2 (days 1, 15), Mechlorethamine 6 mg/m^2 (day 1), Vincristine 1.4 mg/m^2 (days 8, 22), Bleomycin 5 units/m^2 (days 8, 22), Etoposide 60 mg/m^2 (days 15, 16), and Prednisone 40 mg/m^2 PO q.o.d. × 9 wks.

Cycles are given every 28 days. Dose adjustments of bleomycin are made for renal dysfunction, and doxorubicin and vinblastine for hepatic dysfunction. Vinblastine and vincristine dose is also reduced during cycle 3 for elderly patients.

Bartlett NL, Rosenberg SA, Hoppe RT, et al. Brief chemotherapy, Stanford V, and adjuvant radiotherapy for bulky or advanced-stage Hodgkin's disease: a preliminary report. *J Clin Oncol*. 1995;13:1080–1088.
Hoppe RT, Advani RH, Ai WZ, et al. Hodgkin lymphoma. *J Natl Compr Canc Netw*. 2011;9:1020–1058.

Answer 90

No. No significant differences were seen between 5-year FFS and OS between the two groups. Toxicity was also similar.

Hoppe RT, Advani RH, Ai WZ, et al. Hodgkin lymphoma. *J Natl Compr Canc Netw*. 2011;9:1020–1058.

Question 91

Can chemotherapy alone be considered for patients with early stage non-bulky Hodgkin lymphoma?

Question 92

What are some of the potential long-term toxicities of ABVD?

Question 93

What considerations would favor the selection of Stanford V over ABVD?

Question 94   **MULTIPLE MYELOMA**

What is an appropriate dose/fractionation for palliative radiation therapy for painful lytic bony lesions from multiple myeloma?

Answer 91

Yes. In trials conducted by the NCIC/ECOG, MSKCC, and Canellos et al., non-bulky stage I/II patients had similar OS with ABVD alone; MSKCC demonstrated no difference in FFP. ABVD alone can be considered for younger patients with stage I–II non-bulky who demonstrate a CR to the first 2 cycles of ABVD.

Canellos GP, Abramson JS, Fisher DC, et al. Treatment of favorable, limited-stage Hodgkin's lymphoma with chemotherapy without consolidation by radiation therapy. *J Clin Oncol.* 2010;28:1611–1615.

Meyer RM, Gospodarowicz MK, Connors JM, et al. Randomized comparison of ABVD chemotherapy with a strategy that includes radiation therapy in patients with limited-stage Hodgkin's lymphoma: National Cancer Institute of Canada Clinical Trials Group and the Eastern Cooperative Oncology Group. *J Clin Oncol.* 2005;23:4634–4642.

Straus DJ, Portlock CS, Qin J, et al. Results of a prospective randomized clinical trial of doxorubicin, bleomycin, vinblastine, and dacarbazine (ABVD) followed by radiation therapy (RT) versus ABVD alone for stages I, II, and IIIA nonbulky Hodgkin disease. *Blood.* 2004;104:3483–3489.

Answer 92

Interstitial pulmonary fibrosis from bleomycin, neuropathy from vinblastine, and cardiomyopathy from doxorubicin.

Diehl V, Re D, Harris NL, et al. Hodgkin lymphoma. In: DeVita VT, Lawrence TS, Rosenberg SA, eds. *DeVita, Hellman, and Rosenberg's Cancer: Principles & Practice of Oncology.* 8th ed. Philadelphia: Lippincott Williams & Wilkins; 2008:2167–2220.

Answer 93

Stanford V may be preferred over ABVD if:

    there are special concerns for potential toxicity from bleomycin or doxorubicin
    the patient is planned to require consolidative RT
    the patient would benefit from a shorter period of treatment

Hoppe RT, Advani RH, Ai WZ, et al. Hodgkin lymphoma. *J Natl Compr Canc Netw.* 2011;9:1020–1058.

Answer 94

20–30 Gy;

Palliative response seen with 150 cGy–200 cGy/fx

Leigh BR, Kurtts TA, Mack CF, et al. Radiation therapy for the palliation of multiple myeloma. *Int J Radiat Oncol Biol Phys.* 1993;25:801–804.

Question 95

What is appropriate management for solitary plasmacytoma of bone?

Question 96

What is the appropriate dose for definitive radiation therapy in the treatment of solitary extramedullary plasmacytoma?

What is the most common location for a solitary extramedullary plasmacytoma?

Question 97

What percent of patients with solitary plasmacytoma of bone progress to develop multiple myeloma?

Question 98

What are the International Myeloma Working Group criteria for the diagnosis of symptomatic multiple myeloma?

Answer 95

Localized radiation therapy to the tumor site.

40–50 Gy using 1.8–2 Gy/fx.

Ozsahin M, Tsang RW, Poortmans P, et al. Outcomes and patterns of failure in solitary plasmacytoma: a multicenter Rare Cancer Network study of 258 patients. *Int J Radiat Oncol Biol Phys.* 2006;64:210–217.

Answer 96

45–50 Gy; 1.8–2 Gy/fx

Extramedullary plasmacytomas most often occur in the head and neck region, but also are found in the GI tract, CNS, bladder, breast, testes, thyroid, skin, parotid gland, and lymph nodes.

Tournier-Rangeard L, Lapeyre M, Graff-Caillaud P, et al. Radiotherapy for solitary extramedullary plasmacytoma in the head-and-neck region: a dose greater than 45 Gy to the target volume improves the local control. *Int J Radiat Oncol Biol Phys.* 2006;64:1013–1017.

Answer 97

50% probability of development of multiple myeloma within 5 years.

Most patients will develop multiple myeloma within 5 years, but progression beyond 5 years is also not uncommon.

Knobel D, Zouhair A, Tsang RW, et al. Prognostic factors in solitary plasmacytoma of the bone: a multicenter Rare Cancer Network study. *BMC Cancer.* 2006;6:118–127.

Answer 98

Presence of an M-protein in serum and/or urine

Presence of 10% or greater clonal bone marrow plasma cells

Presence of related organ or tissue impairment

(Mnemonic: CRAB—increased calcium, renal insufficiency, anemia, or bone lesions)

International Myeloma Working Group. Criteria for the classification of monoclonal gammopathies, multiple myeloma and related disorders: a report of the International Myeloma Working Group. *Br J Haematol.* 2003;121:749–757.

Question 99

What features are used to establish a diagnosis of solitary plasmacytoma of bone?

Question 100

What adjunctive treatment is recommended for all patients receiving therapy for symptomatic multiple myeloma to decrease pain and bone-related complications and preserve quality of life?

Answer 99

No evidence of clonal plasma cells on bone marrow biopsy

No lytic lesions on skeletal survey/MRI

No evidence for multiple myeloma related organ impairment (i.e., hypercalcemia, renal insufficiency, anemia, bone lesions—"CRAB")

Munshi NC, Anderson KC. Plasma cell neoplasms. In: DeVita VT, Lawrence TS, Rosenberg SA, eds. *DeVita, Hellman, and Rosenberg's Cancer: Principles & Practice of Oncology.* 8th ed. Philadelphia: Lippincott Williams & Wilkins; 2008:2305–2342.

Answer 100

Bisphosphonates are recommended for all patients receiving therapy for symptomatic multiple myeloma. Careful monitoring must be undertaken for renal dysfunction and osteonecrosis of the jaw.

Berenson JR, Lichtenstein A, Porter L, et al. Long-term pamidronate treatment of advanced multiple myeloma patients reduces skeletal events. Myeloma Aredia Study Group. *J Clin Oncol.* 1998;16:593–602.

9

PEDIATRIC CANCERS

ERIN MURPHY, SUSAN GUO, AND GAURAV MARWAHA

Question 1

RETINOBLASTOMA

How many cases of retinoblastoma occur in the U.S. each year?

What is the most common presentation of this intraocular tumor?

Question 2

What are some of the key genetic differences between bilateral versus unilateral retinoblastoma?

Question 3

What is the most common secondary tumor associated with retinoblastoma?

Answer 1

Retinoblastoma is the most common intraocular pediatric tumor with approximately 300 new cases per year. It most commonly presents with leukocoria, which is an abnormal white reflection from the retina. The majority of patients present under 2 years of age. Children with bilateral tumors present at a younger age.

Young JL, Smith MA, Roffers SD, et al. Retinoblastoma. In: Ries LA, Smith MA, Gurney JG, eds. *Cancer Incidence and Survival Among Children and Adolescents: United States SEER Program 1975–1995*. Bethesda, MD: National Cancer Institute; 1999. SEER Program, NIH Pub. No. 99–4649; 73.

Answer 2

Bilateral retinoblastoma is always heritable. Bilateral tumors occur more commonly in younger children. Unilateral, multifocal disease is generally heritable. In general, 65–80% of cases are unilateral. The heritable form of retinoblastoma with a germ line mutation can be either familial or sporadic.

Rubenfeld M, Abramson DH, Ellsworth RM, et al. Unilateral vs bilateral retinoblastoma. Correlations between age at diagnosis and stage of ocular disease. *Ophthalmol.* 1986;93:1016–1019.

Answer 3

Osteogenic sarcoma is the most common secondary tumor associated with retinoblastoma. Osteogenic sarcoma accounts for 44% of secondary tumors. The 50-year cumulative incidence of second malignancy is 51% for hereditary and 5% for non-hereditary cases.

Wong FL, Boice JD Jr, Abramson DH, et al. Cancer incidence after retinoblastoma. Radiation dose and sarcoma risk. *JAMA.* 1997;278:1262–1267.

Question 4

What is the pathogenesis of retinoblastoma?

Question 5

What is the estimated 50-year cumulative incidence of second cancers for hereditary and nonhereditary retinoblastoma?

Question 6

What are appropriate treatment approaches for multifocal retinoblastoma, or tumors close to the macula or optic nerve with preservation of vision?

Question 7

When is the focal therapy of photocoagulation appropriate for retinoblastoma?

Answer 4

Both alleles of the Rb gene located on chromosome 13q14 are inactivated, leading to tumorigenesis. The gene acts as a tumor suppressor when it functions normally. The Knudson hypothesis suggests that children with sporadic retinoblastoma are genetically normal at conception and during embryonic development two somatic mutations ("two hits") occur in the cell line leading to the retinal photoreceptors. However, in familial retinoblastoma, the fertilized egg already carries one copy of the mutated allele. In this case if any cell sustains a second hit, retinoblastoma develops.

Friend SH, Bernards R, Rogelj S, et al. A human DNA segment with properties of the gene that predisposes to retinoblastoma and osteosarcoma. *Nature.* 1986;323:643–646.

Fung YK, Murphree AL, T'Ang A, et al. Structural evidence for the authenticity of the human retinoblastoma gene. *Science.* 1987;236:1657–1661.

Knudson AG, Strong LC. Mutation and cancer: a model for Wilms' tumor of the kidney. *J Natl Cancer Inst.* 1972;48:313–324.

Answer 5

The estimated 50-year cumulative incidence of second cancers is 51% for hereditary and 5% for nonhereditary cases. Other radiation-induced second malignant neoplasms include fibrosarcoma and other spindle-cell neoplasms.

Wong FL, Boice JD Jr, Abramson DH, et al. Cancer incidence after retinoblastoma. Radiation dose and sarcoma risk. *JAMA.* 1997;278:1262–1267.

Answer 6

Appropriate treatment options include external beam radiotherapy or the alternative of chemotherapy followed by focal therapy if the target size and location becomes appropriate. The rationale for this approach is to optimize the target volume for radiotherapy and thereby reduce the side effects associated with external beam radiotherapy including second malignancy, and facial hypoplasia.

Fontanessi J, Taub J, Kirkpatrick JP, et al. Retinoblastoma. In: Halperin E, Constine L, Tarbell N, et al., eds. *Pediatric Radiation Oncology.* 5th ed. Philadelphia, PA: Lippincott Williams & Wilkins; 2011:85–107.

Answer 7

Focal photocoagulation, which uses a laser to obliterate the retinal blood vessels feeding the tumor, can be used as primary therapy for tumors ≤ 4.5 mm at the base and ≤ 2.5 mm thick and not close to the macula or optic disc, and without vitreous seeding. It can also be used for a local recurrence postradiation or in conjunction with chemotherapy.

Cassady JR, Sagerman RH, Tretter P, et al. Radiation therapy in retinoblastoma. An analysis of 230 cases. *Radiology.* 1969;93:405–409.

Question 8

When is cryotherapy most appropriate for retinoblastoma?

Question 9

When is plaque radiotherapy appropriate for retinoblastoma?

Question 10   **WILMS**

Which stage of favorable and unfavorable histology Wilms tumor patients requires radiotherapy?

Question 11

What are the stage III indications for radiotherapy for favorable histology Wilms?

Answer 8

Cryotherapy is most appropriate as primary therapy for small tumors anterior to the equator, without vitreous seeding and can be reached by the cryoprobe. It can also be used for a local recurrence post-radiation or in conjunction with chemotherapy.

Murphree AL, Villablanca JG, Deegan WF, et al. Chemotherapy plus local treatment in the management of intraocular retinoblastoma. *Arch Opthalmology*. 1996;114:1348–1356.

Answer 9

Plaque radiotherapy is appropriate as primary treatment for a solitary 2–16 mm basal diameter and < 10 mm thick unilateral lesions located > 3 mm away from optic disc or fovea. It is often used following chemotherapy and some propose a dose reduction of 25–30 Gy to the apex following chemotherapy. The typical dose used is 40 Gy to the tumor apex.

Shields CL, Shields JA, DePotter P, et al. Plaque radiotherapy for retinoblastoma. *Int Opthalmol Clin*. 1993;33:107–118.

Answer 10

Surgery and adjuvant chemotherapy (18–24 wks) are required for all patients. According to COG guidelines: Radiotherapy is used for stage III–IV favorable histology and stage I–IV unfavorable histology (focal and diffuse anaplasia), and all clear cell and rhabdoid tumors (with the exception of stage I CCSK after central review on studies). Radiation therapy should start by postoperative day 9 if possible, but no later than day 14.

Kalapurakal J, Halperin E. Wilms tumor. In: Halperin E, Constine L, Tarbell N, et al., eds. *Pediatric Radiation Oncology*. 5th ed. Philadelphia, PA: Lippincott Williams & Wilkins; 2011:257–289.

Answer 11

SLURPT-B (mnemonic): Spillage (either before or during surgery); **L**ymph nodes (pathologically + in the abdomen or pelvis); **U**nresectable (patient required neoadjuvant chemotherapy); **R**esidual disease (gross or microscopic tumor remains postoperatively or tumor was removed in greater than one piece); **P**eritoneal disease (tumor penetrated peritoneal surface or peritoneal implants); **T**umor thrombus within renal vein (if removed separately from nephrectomy specimen); **B**iopsy prior to removal

Kalapurakal J, Halperin E. Wilms tumor. In: Halperin E, Constine L, Tarbell N, et al., eds. *Pediatric Radiation Oncology*. 5th ed. Philadelphia, PA: Lippincott Williams & Wilkins; 2011:257–289.

Question 12

What are the appropriate Wilms tumor radiation doses for flank irradiation, whole abdominal irradiation, whole lung irradiation, bone metastases, liver irradiation, and residual disease?

Question 13

What are the indications for whole abdominal irradiation?

Question 14

What genetic syndromes are associated with Wilms tumors?

Question 15   **NEUROBLASTOMA**

What is the most common pediatric extracranial malignancy?

What is the median age of diagnosis for this malignancy?

Answer 12

Flank irradiation? 10.8 Gy

Whole abdominal irradiation? 10.5 Gy

Whole lung irradiation? 10.5 Gy (age < 12 mo) or 12 Gy (age ≥ 12 mo)

Bone metastases? 30.6 Gy (or 25.2 Gy if age < 16 yrs)

Liver irradiation? 19.8 Gy to focal metastases

Residual disease? 19.8 Gy

Children's Oncology Group Guidelines as described in the following reference.

Kalapurakal J, Halperin E. Wilms tumor. In: Halperin E, Constine L, Tarbell N, et al., eds. *Pediatric Radiation Oncology*. 5th ed. Philadelphia, PA: Lippincott Williams & Wilkins; 2011:257–289.
Children's Oncology Group Guidelines.

Answer 13

Cytology positive ascites, any preoperative tumor rupture, diffuse surgical spillage, and peritoneal seeding are indications for whole abdominal irradiation. The borders for whole abdominal irradiation are superior: 1 cm above the dome of the diaphragm (must account for respiratory motion), lateral: 1 cm beyond lateral abdominal wall, and inferior: the bottom of the obturator foramens (the femoral heads should be blocked).

Kalapurakal J, Halperin E. Wilms tumor. In: Halperin E, Constine L, Tarbell N, et al., eds. *Pediatric Radiation Oncology*. 5th ed. Philadelphia, PA: Lippincott Williams & Wilkins; 2011:257–289.

Answer 14

WAGR syndrome (Wilms tumor with aniridia, genitourinary malformations, and mental retardation) is associated with a deletion of 11p13 and Beckwith-Wiedemann syndrome (Wilms tumor with macrosomia or hemihypertrophy, macroglossia, omphalocele, abdominal organomegaly, and ear pits is associated with deletion of 11p15).

Bonetta L, Kuetin SE, Huang A, et al. Wilms' tumor locus on 11p13 defined by multiple CpG island-associated transcripts. *Science*. 1990;250:994–997.
Koufos A, Grundy P, Morgan K, et al. Familial Wiedmann-Beckwith syndrome and a second Wilms' tumor locus both map to 11p15.5. *Am J Hum Genet*. 1989;44:711–719.

Answer 15

Neuroblastoma. There are approximately 650 cases of neuroblastoma per year in the U.S. The median age at diagnosis is 22 months.

Goodman MT, Gurney JG, Smith, et al. Sympathetic nervous system tumors. In: Ries LAG, Smith MA, Gurney JG, et al., eds. *Cancer Incidence and Survival Among Children and Adolescents: United States SEER Program 1975–1995*. Bethesda MD: National Cancer Institute; 1999. NIH Pub. No. 99–4649. SEER Program; 65–72.

Question 16

Where does neuroblastoma commonly present?

Question 17

Which biologic features are unfavorable for neuroblastoma?

Question 18

What is the appropriate staging work up for a patient with neuroblastoma?

Question 19

When is radiotherapy used for intermediate risk neuroblastoma patients?

Answer 16

Neuroblastoma most commonly presents in the adrenal gland (35%), followed by the paraspinal ganglia in the thoracic, abdominal, or pelvic chains (30%), the posterior mediastinum (19%), and the cervical sympathetic ganglion (1%). Presenting symptoms may include a palpable abdominal mass, Horner's syndrome, cord compression, respiratory compromise, and gastrointestinal disturbances.

Bernstein ML, Leclerc JM, Bunin G, et al. A population-based study of neuroblastoma incidence, survival, and mortality in North America. *J Clin Oncol.* 1992;10:323–329.

Answer 17

Amplification of MYCN correlates with advanced stage and poor prognosis and occurs in 30–40% of advanced stage neuroblastoma cases. DNA ploidy has shown to be predictive of both progression-free and overall survival, with children with hyperdiploid tumors having a better prognosis. Loss of heterozygosity of 1p and 11q are associated with a poor prognosis.

Attiyeh EF, London WB, Mosse YP, et al. Chromosome 1p and 11 q deletions and outcome in neuroblastoma. *N Engl J Med.* 2005;53:2243–2253.
Bowman LC, Castleberry RP, Cantor A, et al. Genetic staging of unresectable or metastatic neuroblastoma in infants: a Pediatric Oncology Group Study. *J Natl Cancer Inst.* 1997;89:373–380.
Maris JM. The biologic basis for neuroblastoma heterogeneity and risk stratification. *Curr Opin Pediatric.* 2005;17:7–13.

Answer 18

Approximately 60% of patients present with metastatic disease and 80–90% of these patients have bone marrow involvement. Staging work up includes a CT, US, or MRI of the primary site, bilateral iliac bone marrow aspirates and core biopsies, bone radiographs and scintigraphy with or without an MIBG scan, chest radiograph and chest CT, and urinary catecholamines (vanillylmandelic acid and homovanillic acid)

Brodeur GM, Pritchard J, Berthold F, et al. Revisions of the international criteria for neuroblastoma diagnosis, staging, and response to treatment. *J Clin Oncol.* 1993;11:1466–1477.

Answer 19

Intermediate risk patients are expected to have a survival of > 80% after primary tumor resection and chemotherapy. Radiation therapy is reserved for symptomatic palliation (4.5 Gy/3 fx for hepatomegaly), viable residual disease in chemo-refractory pts, or recurrent disease.

Matthay K, Haas-Kogan D, Constine L. Neuroblastoma. In: Halperin E, Constine L, Tarbell N, et al., eds. *Pediatric Radiation Oncology.* 5th ed. Philadelphia, PA: Lippincott Williams & Wilkins; 2011:108–136.

Question 20

What is the 3-year EFS for high-risk disease and what is the appropriate therapy?

Question 21

What is the most common childhood cancer?

Question 22

What is the expected outcome for pediatric ALL and AML?

Question 23

What are good prognostic features of ALL?

Answer 20

The expected 3-year EFS for high-risk neuroblastoma patients is 30–40%. Treatment consists of induction chemotherapy, local control of the primary with surgery and RT (either before or after myeloablative chemotherapy), and myeloablative chemotherapy followed by hematopoietic cell transplant. Radiation therapy is delivered to the post chemo, pre-surgery tumor bed (21.6 Gy at 1.8 Gy/fx for GTR and consider boost to residual for total 36 Gy as per current COG 0532) and any persistent metastatic sites.

Matthay K, Haas-Kogan D, Constine L. Neuroblastoma. In: Halperin E, Constine L, Tarbell N, et al., eds. *Pediatric Radiation Oncology*. 5th ed. Philadelphia, PA: Lippincott Williams & Wilkins; 2011:108–136.

Matthay KK, Reynolds CP, Seeger RC, et al. Long-term results for children with high-risk neuroblastoma treated on a randomized trial of myeloablative therapy followed by 13-cis-retinoic acid: a Children's Oncology Group Study. *J Clin Oncol*. 2009;27:1007–1013.

Answer 21

Acute leukemia (ALL) is the most common childhood malignancy, making up 30% of childhood tumors. There are approximately 3000 children diagnosed with ALL annually in the US. ALL is 5 times more common than AML, with approximately 500 cases of AML annually in the US.

Jemal A, Siegel R, Ward E, et al. Cancer statistics, 2008. *CA Cancer J Clin*. 2008;58:71–96.

Answer 22

The 5-year overall survival for patients with ALL is > 85%. The 5-year EFS for patients with AML is 40–50%, and the 10-year overall survival ranges from 31–43% using dose- and time-intensive induction regimens.

Pui CH, Sandlund JT, Pei D, et al. Improved outcome for children with acute lymphoblastic leukemia: results of total therapy study XIIIB at St Jude children's research hospital. *Blood*. 2004;104:2690–2696.

Smith FO, Alonzo TA, Gerbing RB, et al. Long-term results of children with acute myeloid leukemia: a report of three consecutive Phase III trials by the Children's Cancer Group: CCG 251, CCG213, and CCG 2891. *Leukemia*. 2005;19:2054–2062.

Answer 23

B-precursor ALL, age between 1 and 10 years, and a presenting WBC less than 50×10^9/L, and DNA index > 1.16 or presence of *TEL-AML1* fusion.

Pui CH, Campana D, Pei D, et al. Treatment of childhood acute lymphoblastic leukemia without prophylactic cranial irradiation. *N Engl J Med*. 2009;360:2730–2741.

Smith M, Arthur D, Camitta B, et al. Uniform approach to risk classification and treatment assignment for children with acute lymphoblastic leukemia. *J Clin Oncol*. 1996;14:18–24.

Question 24

What is the role of cranial irradiation for ALL?

Question 25

What are prognostic features of AML?

Question 26   **HODGKIN LYMPHOMA**

What is the age distribution of Hodgkin lymphoma and how common is pediatric Hodgkin lymphoma?

Question 27

How does a child with Hodgkin lymphoma typically present?

Answer 24

Prophylactic cranial irradiation is no longer used for all patients, but is often included in protocols for patients with T cell disease. Most protocols include consolidative cranial irradiation after intensification therapy for children with CNS 3 disease at diagnosis. The standard dose for cranial irradiation is 18 Gy. CNS 3 disease is defined as ≥ 5 WBC/uL and cytologic or biologic evidence of blasts in the CNS.

Kun, L. Leukemias in children. In: Halperin E, Constine L, Tarbell N, et al., eds. *Pediatric Radiation Oncology*. 5th ed. Philadelphia, PA: Lippincott Williams & Wilkins; 2011:12–25.

Answer 25

Favorable AML includes translocation t(8;21), inversion (16) and minimal residual disease < 0.1% after induction, intermediate risk AML includes all others not in favorable/high risk group and the high risk group includes t(6;9), deletions of chromosome 7, 5 and 5q, FAB class M0, M6, or M7 and minimal residual disease > 5% after the first induction or > 1% after second induction. Also, the t(9;22) translocation is a poor prognostic factor.

Campana D. Determination of minimal residual disease in leukaemia patients. *Br J Haemotol*. 2003;121:823–838.
Smith M, Arthur D, Camitta B, et al. Uniform approach to risk classification and treatment assignment for children with acute lymphoblastic leukemia. *J Clin Oncol*. 1996;14:18–24.
Meshinchi S, Arceci RJ. Prognostic factors and risk-based therapy in pediatric acute myeloid leukemia. *Oncologist*. 2007;12:341–355.
Rubitz JE. Childhood acute myeloid leukemia. *Curr Treat Options Oncol*. 2008;9:95–105.

Answer 26

The age specific incidence for Hodgkin lymphoma is bimodal with peaks in the 20s and 50s. Hodgkin lymphoma makes up 6% of childhood cancers, with approximately 900 cases per year in the U.S.

Ries LA, Kosary CL, Hankey BF, et al. eds. *SEER Cancer Statistics Review: 1973–1994*. Bethesda: National Cancer Institute; 1999. SEER Program, NIH Pub. No. 99–4649;35–50.

Answer 27

Most children present with painless cervical adenopathy (80%) and mediastinal involvement occurs in > 70% of adolescents but only 33% in children aged 1–10 years. One-third of patients present with "B" symptoms, consisting of fevers (> 38° C), drenching night sweats, and unexplained weight loss of > 10% of body weight in the preceding 6 months.

Kaplan H. *Hodgkin's Disease*. Cambridge, MA: Harvard University Press; 1980:222.

Question 28

How does nodular lymphocyte predominant Hodgkin lymphoma (NLPHL) differ from the subtypes of classic Hodgkin disease?

Question 29

Which patients are considered to have early or favorable Hodgkin's disease and what is the recommended treatment approach?

Question 30

Which patients are considered to have intermediate risk Hodgkin's disease and what is the recommended treatment approach?

Question 31

Which patients are considered to have unfavorable Hodgkin's disease and what is the recommended treatment approach?

Answer 28

NLPHL has a distinct cell, which is CD20 positive and CD15 negative. Classical Reed-Sternberg cells, which are CD15 and CD30 positive are rare. NLPHL has a long natural history and often presents with a single lymph node involved, often sparing the mediastinum and is more common in young children. Adolescents with early stage NLPHL may be treated with irradiation alone with a dose of 30–36 Gy.

Pellegrino B, Terrier-Lacombe MJ, Oberlin O, et al. Lymphocyte-predominant Hodgkin's lymphoma in children: therapeutic abstention after initial lymph node resection-a study of the French Society of Pediatric Oncology. *J Clin Oncol.* 2003;21:2948–2952.

Schlembach PJ, Wilder RB, Jones D, et al. Radiotherapy alone for lymphocyte-predominant Hodgkin's disease. *Cancer J.* 2002;8:377–383.

Answer 29

Favorable disease includes localized disease (stage IA and IIA) involving less than 4 nodal regions, absence of "B" symptoms, bulk, or extranodal extension. Recommended therapy includes 2–4 cycles of chemotherapy without alkylators plus low-dose, involved field irradiation (15–25 Gy). Alternative approaches include 6 cycles of chemotherapy alone (alternating COPP and ABVD or derivative) or 4 cycles of chemotherapy alone on trial.

Terezakis SA, Hudson MM, Constine LS. Hodgkin lymphoma. In: Halperin E, Constine L, Tarbell N, et al., eds. *Pediatric Radiation Oncology.* 5th ed. Philadelphia, PA: Lippincott Williams & Wilkins; 2011:137–165.

Answer 30

Intermediate risk patients have localized disease involving ≥ 3 nodal regions in the presence of bulky mediastinal adenopathy (stage IA, IIA, IIB) or stage IIIA disease. (Stage IIB is sometimes classified as high risk.) Recommended therapy includes 4–6 cycles of chemotherapy and low-dose, involved field irradiation (15–25 Gy). Alternative approaches include 6–8 cycles of chemotherapy alone.

Terezakis SA, Hudson MM, Constine LS. Hodgkin lymphoma. In: Halperin E, Constine L, Tarbell N, et al., eds. *Pediatric Radiation Oncology.* 5th ed. Philadelphia, PA: Lippincott Williams & Wilkins; 2011:137–165.

Answer 31

Unfavorable patients include stage IIB, IIIB, and IV Hodgkin's disease. Recommended therapy includes 6–8 cycles of advanced chemotherapy with low-dose, involved field irradiation (15–25 Gy). An alternative approach includes 8 cycles of chemotherapy alone.

Terezakis SA, Hudson MM, Constine LS. Hodgkin lymphoma. In: Halperin E, Constine L, Tarbell N, et al., eds. *Pediatric Radiation Oncology.* 5th ed. Philadelphia, PA: Lippincott Williams & Wilkins; 2011:137–165.

Question 32

What are the two important studies that have proven a benefit for IFRT for favorable pediatric Hodgkin's disease?

Question 33   **PEDIATRIC GLIOMAS**

What are the histologic subtypes of low-grade gliomas and what are the expected outcomes after surgical resection?

Question 34

What is the treatment approach for children with low-grade glioma?

Answer 32

The Children's Cancer Group (CCG) trial 5942 randomized children to receive low dose involved field radiotherapy or no radiotherapy after they had obtained a complete response to initial risk-adapted chemotherapy. The 3-year EFS was 93% for those who received radiotherapy compared to 85% for those that did not, which was a statistically significant difference. The German GPOH-HD 95 trial was a prospective study of response-adapted radiotherapy. The children who had a complete response to chemotherapy did not receive radiotherapy and those who obtained a partial response underwent 20–35 Gy IFRT. The 3-year EFS was equivalent for the favorable patients that obtained a CR and PR. However, both the intermediate risk and high risk patients who had a CR and no IFRT had a worse EFS compared to the patients who achieved a PR and received IFRT.

Nachman JB, Sposto R, Herzog P, et al. Children's cancer group. Randomized comparison of low-dose involved-field radiotherapy and no radiotherapy for children with Hodgkin's disease who achieve a complete response to chemotherapy. *J Clin Oncol*. 2002;20:3765–3771.

Ruhl U, Albrecht M, Dieckmann K, et al. Response-adapted radiotherapy in the treatment of pediatric Hodgkin's disease: an interim report at 5 years of the German GPOH-HD 95 trial. *Int J Radiat Oncol Biol Phys*. 2001;51:1209–1218.

Answer 33

WHO grade I includes juvenile pilocytic astrocytoma (JPA), ganglioglioma, subependymal giant cell tumor. The 8 year progression-free survival for a JPA after a gross total resection is 94–95% and after less than a gross total resection is 41–58%. WHO grade II includes diffuse astrocytomas (fibrillary, protoplasmic, and gemistocytic), oligodendroglioma, oligoastrocytoma, pilomyxoid astrocytoma, and pleomorphic xanthoastrocytoma, which are more infiltrative than WHO grade I. The 8-year progression-free survival for non-JPAs after gross total resection is 0–89% depending on the location of the tumor and after less than a gross total resection is 54–56%.

Wisoff JH, Sanford RA, Heier LA, et al. Primary neurosurgery for pediatric low-grade gliomas: a prospective multi-institutional study from the Children's Oncology Group. *Neurosurgery*. 2011;68:1548–1554.

Answer 34

The primary treatment is maximal safe resection. Children are often observed after initial surgery and treatment is offered at time of progression. The timing and sequencing of adjuvant chemotherapy and radiation is controversial. Chemotherapy is often used to delay radiotherapy, particularly in young children.

Kun LE, MacDonald S, Tarbell NJ. Supratentorial brain tumors. In: Halperin E, Constine L, Tarbell N, et al., eds. *Pediatric Radiation Oncology*. 5th ed. Philadelphia, PA: Lippincott Williams & Wilkins; 2011:26–52.

Question 35
What genetic syndrome is associated with optic pathway glioma?

Question 36
What is the risk of a radiation-induced second malignancy for NF-1 patients?

Question 37
What percent of childhood cancers are high-grade glioma and what are the expected outcomes?

Question 38

SOFT TISSUE SARCOMA

How common are pediatric soft tissue sarcomas?

Answer 35

Neurofibromatosis type I results from a mutation of the long arm of chromosome 17 and is characterized by Lisch nodules, café au lait spots, axillary freckling, optic pathway glioma, astrocytoma, and neurofibroma. This tumor impacts children typically less than 15 years of age and may present with visual deficits, proptosis, nystagmus, or optic atrophy. Diagnosis may be based on imaging characteristics alone, a biopsy is not necessary.

Gutmann DH, Aylsworth A, Carey JC, et al. The diagnostic evaluation and multidisciplinary management of neurofibromatosis 1 and neurofibromatosis 2. *JAMA*. 1997;278:51–57.

Answer 36

From a review of 80 NF1 patients with optic pathway gliomas (OPG), the estimated relative risk of second nervous system tumor after radiotherapy was 3.04 (95% CI, 1.29 to 7.15). Fifty-eight patients were assessable for second tumors. Nine (50%) of 18 patients who received radiotherapy for their OPGs developed 12 second tumors in 308 person-years of follow-up after radiotherapy. Eight (20%) of 40 patients who were not treated with radiotherapy developed nine tumors in 721 person-years of follow-up after diagnosis of their OPGs.

Sharif S, Ferner R, Birch JM, et al. Second primary tumors in neurofibromatosis 1 patients treated for optic glioma: substantial risks after radiotherapy. *J Clin Oncol*. 2006;24:2570–2575.

Answer 37

High-grade gliomas account for 6% of childhood cancers. The high-grade gliomas include anaplastic astrocytomas (WHO III) and glioblastoma (WHO grade IV). Children with anaplastic astrocytoma and glioblastoma multiforme after > 90% tumor removal and adjuvant therapy have anticipated 5-year PFS of 43% and 26%, respectively. After less than 90% tumor resection, the 5-year PFS for anaplastic astrocytoma and glioblastoma are 22% and 4%, respectively.

Wisoff JH, Boyett JM, Berger MS, et al. Current neurosurgical management and the impact of the extent of resection in the treatment of malignant gliomas of childhood: a report of the Children's Cancer Group trial no. CCG-945. *J Neurosurg*. 1998;89:52–59.

Answer 38

Pediatric soft tissue sarcomas are rare. They represent 7% of childhood malignancies and more than half are rhabdomyosarcoma. Therefore, non-rhabdomyosarcoma soft tissue sarcomas constitute 3% of childhood tumors, with approximately 250 cases annually in the U.S.

Pappo AS, Parham DM, Rao BN, et al. Soft tissue sarcomas in children. *Semin Surg Oncol*. 1999;16:121–143.

Question 39

What are important prognostic factors for pediatric non-rhabdomyosarcoma soft tissue sarcomas and what is the expected outcome?

Question 40

What is the role for radiotherapy for pediatric soft tissue sarcomas?

Question 41   **LANGERHANS CELL HISTIOCYTOSIS**

What age group and sex predominance is seen in Langerhans cell histiocytosis (LCH)?

Question 42

What is the role of radiation therapy in managing localized bone or soft tissue Langerhans cell histiocytosis (LCH)?

Answer 39

Tumor invasiveness, tumor size, tumor stage, and histologic grade are prognostic for survival. Overall, 66% are expected to have long-term survival. Surgical resection +/− RT achieves local control in over 80% with non-metastatic soft tissue sarcoma. Less than 10% of those presenting with unresectable or metastatic disease survive long-term. 85 of 109 pts with resected disease are long-term survivors.

Spunt SL, Poquette CA, Hurt YS, et al. Prognostic factors for children and adolescents with surgically resected nonrhabdomyosarcoma soft tissue sarcoma: an analysis of 121 patients treated at St Jude Children's Research Hospital. *J Clin Oncol.* 1999;17:3697–3705.

Answer 40

Radiotherapy is used for unresectable soft tissue sarcomas or for resected high-grade soft tissue sarcomas. Krasin et al. reported on 32 pediatric high-grade nonrhabdomyosarcoma soft tissue sarcoma, 27 of whom received adjuvant radiotherapy and 5 received definitive radiotherapy. A 2-cm anatomically constrained margin was used for the study. After a follow up of 32 months, the 3-year cumulative incidence of local failure was 3.7% for patients undergoing surgery and adjuvant radiotherapy.

Krasin MJ, Davidoff AM, Xiong X, et al. Preliminary results from a prospective study using limited margin radiotherapy in pediatric and young adult patients with high-grade nonrhabdomyosarcoma soft-tissue sarcoma. *Int J Radiat Oncol Biol Phys.* 2010;76:874–878.

Answer 41

Male predominance (56–66% of patients). 50% of cases are diagnosed between ages 1–15.

Halperin E. Langerhans cell histiocytosis. In: Halperin E, Constine L, Tarbell N, et al., eds. *Pediatric Radiation Oncology.* 5th ed. Philadelphia, PA: Lippincott Williams & Wilkins; 2011:332–345.

Answer 42

Historically, RT was used as both a diagnostic and therapeutic intervention. However, excellent control rates of 70–90% are seen after surgical excision for localized bone or soft tissue LCH. Radiation in this case is reserved for residual disease or local relapse after surgery.

Halperin E. Langerhans cell histiocytosis. In: Halperin E, Constine L, Tarbell N, et al., eds. *Pediatric Radiation Oncology.* 5th ed. Philadelphia, PA: Lippincott Williams & Wilkins; 2011:332–345.

Question 43

Which patients with Langerhans cell histiocytosis (LCH) may benefit most from radiation therapy?

Question 44

What is the most common complication of CNS involvement in Langerhans cell histiocytosis (LCH)?

Question 45

What common long-term sequelae are seen after treatment of Langerhans cell histiocytosis?

Question 46

LIVER TUMORS IN CHILDREN

What is the breakdown of benign vs malignant liver tumors in children?

Answer 43

Patients with multifocal LCH or with organ dysfunction, painful lesions despite chemotherapy, disfiguring bone or soft tissue lesions, and bones at substantial immediate risk for fracture.

Halperin E. Langerhans cell histiocytosis. In: Halperin E, Constine L, Tarbell N, et al., eds. *Pediatric Radiation Oncology*. 5th ed. Philadelphia, PA: Lippincott Williams & Wilkins; 2011:332–345.

Answer 44

Diabetes insipidus from lesions in the posterior pituitary or pituitary stalk. This is diagnosed by high to normal plasma sodium concentrations, especially if urine osmolality is less than plasma osmolality.

Halperin E. Langerhans cell histiocytosis. In: Halperin E, Constine L, Tarbell N, et al., eds. *Pediatric Radiation Oncology*. 5th ed. Philadelphia, PA: Lippincott Williams & Wilkins; 2011:332–345.
Rose BD, Post TW. Hyperosmolal states- hypernatremia. In: Rose BD, Post TW, eds. *Clinical Physiology of Acid-Base and Electrolyte Disorders*. 5th ed. New York, NY: McGraw-Hill; 2001:748–757, 767–772.

Answer 45

Diabetes insipidus (DI) (18%), GH deficiency and short stature (5%), hypothyroidism (2.5%), deafness (2.5%), and orthopedic sequelae.

French Langerhans Cell Histiocytosis Group. A multicentre retrospective survey of Langerhans' cell histiocytosis. 348 cases observed between 1983 and 1993. *Arch Dis Child*. 1996;75:17–24.

Answer 46

2/3 benign, 1/3 malignant. The most common benign tumor is a benign vascular tumor. Malignant liver tumors account for 1% of all childhood tumors in the United States according to the Surveillance, Epidemiology, and End Results (SEER) cancer registry.

Weinberg AG, Finegold MJ. Primary hepatic tumors of childhood. *Hum Pathol*. 1983;14:512–537.
Finegold MJ, Egler RA, Goss JA, et al. Liver tumors: pediatric population. *Liver Trsnpl*. 2008;14:1545–1546.

Question 47

What are the three most common liver tumors by histopathology in children?

Question 48

What is the typical presentation of children with primary malignant liver tumors?

Question 49

What is the typical demographic for hepatoblastomas?

Question 50

What is the staging system for primary malignant liver tumors according to the Children's Cancer Study Group and Pediatric Oncology Group?

Answer 47

The most common liver tumors by histopathology in children are hepatoblastoma (43%), hepatocellular carcinoma (23%), and benign vascular tumor (13%).

Weinberg AG, Finegold MJ. Primary hepatic tumors of childhood. *Hum Pathol.* 1983;14:512–537.

Answer 48

Abdominal mass or generalized abdominal enlargement, pain localized to right upper quadrant, fever, anorexia, weight loss, jaundice, and vomiting. Rare presentations include: abdominal crisis caused by tumor rupture and hemoperitoneum, paraneoplastic syndrome (e.g., precocious sexual development), anemia, and thrombocytopenia.

Chen B, Tsai S, Cheng SH, et al. Liver tumors in children. In: Halperin E, Constine L, Tarbell N, et al., eds. *Pediatric Radiation Oncology.* 5th ed. Philadelphia, PA: Lippincott Williams & Wilkins; 2011:290–301.

Answer 49

Median age of diagnosis 16–19 months, only 5% occur in children greater than 4 years.
Male predominance.

Chen B, Tsai S, Cheng SH, et al. Liver tumors in children. In: Halperin E, Constine L, Tarbell N, et al., eds. *Pediatric Radiation Oncology.* 5th ed. Philadelphia, PA: Lippincott Williams & Wilkins; 2011:290–301.

Answer 50

Both use same staging:

i. Complete resection of the tumor
ii. Microscopic residual tumor
iii. Macroscopic residual tumor
iv. Distant metastatic tumor

Bellani FF, Massimino M. Liver tumors in childhood: epidemiology and clinics. *J Surg Oncol Suppl.* 1993;3:119–121.
Bowman LC, Riely CA. Management of pediatric liver tumors. *Surg Oncol Clin N Am.* 1996;5:451–459.
Cohen MD, Bugaieski EM, Haliloglu M, et al. Visual presentation of the staging of pediatric solid tumors. *Radiographics.* 1996;16:523–545.
Schnater JM, Kohler SE, Lamers WH, et al. Where do we stand with hepatoblastoma? A review. *Cancer.* 2003;98:668–678.

Question 51

What is the treatment paradigm for hemangioblastoma of the liver?

Question 52

What doses should be used for neoadjuvant radiation for hepatoblastoma and hepatocellular carcinoma?

Question 53

What doses should be used for adjuvant radiation for hepatoblastoma and hepatocellular carcinoma?

Question 54   EWING SARCOMA

How common is Ewing's sarcoma relative to other primary childhood bone tumors?

Answer 51

American Intergroup Studies favor primary surgery and adjuvant chemotherapy, except for clearly unresectable tumors.

SIOP prefers biopsy, neoadjuvant chemotherapy to reduce tumor burden, and definitive surgery. May also consider radiotherapy to improve resectability if not possible after neoadjuvant chemotherapy.

Chen B, Tsai S, Cheng SH, et al. Liver tumors in children. In: Halperin E, Constine L, Tarbell N, et al., eds. *Pediatric Radiation Oncology*. 5th ed. Philadelphia, PA: Lippincott Williams & Wilkins; 2011:290–301.

Answer 52

50–60 Gy to the GTV plus margin, if normal liver can be spared. Respiratory motion needs to be accounted for within the treatment plan. The normal liver should be restricted to a maximum dose of 30 Gy.

Chen B, Tsai S, Cheng SH, et al. Liver tumors in children. In: Halperin E, Constine L, Tarbell N, et al., eds. *Pediatric Radiation Oncology*. 5th ed. Philadelphia, PA: Lippincott Williams & Wilkins; 2011:290–301.

Answer 53

45 Gy to limited area for microscopic disease, 50–60 Gy for bulkier residual disease.

Chen B, Tsai S, Cheng SH, et al. Liver tumors in children. In: Halperin E, Constine L, Tarbell N, et al., eds. *Pediatric Radiation Oncology*. 5th ed. Philadelphia, PA: Lippincott Williams & Wilkins; 2011:290–301.

Answer 54

Second most common primary childhood bone tumor, represents 3% of pediatric cancers. Approximately 200 cases are diagnosed each year in the U.S.

Marcus K, Yock T, Tarbell NJ. Ewing sarcoma. In: Halperin E, Constine L, Tarbell N, et al., eds. *Pediatric Radiation Oncology*. 5th ed. Philadelphia, PA: Lippincott Williams & Wilkins; 2011:172–183.

Question 55

What is the cellular morphology seen in Ewing's sarcoma?

Question 56

What are the most important prognostic factors in Ewing's sarcoma?

Question 57

What are the classical radiographic findings of Ewing's sarcoma, and how does this differ from those found in osteosarcoma?

Question 58

What is the overall treatment approach for Ewing's sarcoma?

Answer 55

Small round malignant cells with hyperchromatic nuclei, periodic acid-Schiff (PAS) positive, uniformly vimentin positive and often cytokeratin positive.

Marcus K, Yock T, Tarbell NJ. Ewing sarcoma. In: Halperin E, Constine L, Tarbell N, et al., eds. *Pediatric Radiation Oncology*. 5th ed. Philadelphia, PA: Lippincott Williams & Wilkins; 2011:172–183.

Answer 56

The key prognostic factor is the presence or absence of metastases. In patients with no metastases at diagnosis, other poor prognostic factors include tumor volume (> 100 cc), axial site, and age ≥ 15.

Cotterill SJ, Ahrens S, Paulussen M. Prognostic factors in Ewing's tumor of bone: analysis of 975 patients from the European intergroup cooperative Ewing's sarcoma study group. *J Clin Oncol*. 2000;18:3108–3114.

Answer 57

Ewing's sarcoma typically shows an "onion skin" and "moth-eaten" reaction on plain films, whereas osteosarcoma is associated with a "sunburst" appearance. Areas of new subperiosteal bone formation, "Codman triangle," can be seen in both tumor types.

Conrad III, EU. Ewing's sarcoma of the hand. In: Conrad EU, ed. *Orthopaedic Oncology: Diagnosis and Treatment*. New York, NY: Thieme; 2008:75–80.

Answer 58

Induction chemotherapy, local therapy (surgery +/− adjuvant RT or definitive RT), and adjuvant chemotherapy. Whole lung irradiation is indicated for lung metastases. The indications for postoperative RT include marginal and intralesional resection or poor response to initial chemotherapy (> 10% viable tumor cells in resected tumor). The dose for whole lung is 18–21 Gy.

Dunst J, Paulussen M, Jergens H. Lung irradiation for Ewing's sarcoma with pulmonary metastases at diagnosis: results of the CESS-studies. *Strahlenther Onkol*. 1993;169:1514–1524.

Marcus K, Yock T, Tarbell NJ. Ewing sarcoma. In: Halperin E, Constine L, Tarbell N, et al., eds. *Pediatric Radiation Oncology*. 5th ed. Philadelphia, PA: Lippincott Williams & Wilkins; 2011:172–183.

Schuck A, Ahrens S, von Schorlemer I. Radiotherapy in Ewing tumors of the vertebrae: treatment results and local relapse analysis of the CESS 81/86 and EICESS 92 trials. *Int J Radiat Oncol Biol Phys*. 2005;63:1562–1567.

Question 59

What was examined in the phase III INT-0091 study and what were the major findings?

Question 60

What is the expected 5-year relapse-free survival for local vs metastatic Ewing's sarcoma?

Question 61

What is the rate of secondary malignancies after Ewing's sarcoma, and which factor increases the risk?

Question 62   **RHABDOMYOSARCOMA**

What is the incidence and age distribution of rhabdomyosarcoma?

Answer 59

INT-0091 was a phase III study of patients with localized and metastatic Ewing's, PNET of bone, and primitive sarcoma of bone. Patients were randomized to vincristine, dactinomycin, cyclophosphamide, adriamycin (VACAdr) or VACAdr alternating with ifosfamide and etoposide (IE). For patients with localized disease, induction VACAdr alternating with IE improved 5 year overall survival (72% vs 61%) and reduced 5 year local recurrence (5% vs 15%). There was no survival advantage for the addition of IE for patients with metastatic disease at presentation.

Grier HE, Krailo MD, Tarbell NJ, et al. Addition of ifosfamide and etoposide to standard chemotherapy for Ewing's sarcoma and primitive neuroectodermal tumor of bone. *N Engl J Med*. 2003;348:694–701.

Answer 60

From the European Intergroup experience, the 5-year relapse-free survival rates for patients with localized and metastatic disease at presentation were 55% and 21%, respectively.

Cotterill SJ, Ahrens S, Paulussen M. Prognostic factors in Ewing's tumor of bone: analysis of 975 patients from the European intergroup cooperative Ewing's sarcoma study group. *J Clin Oncol*. 2000;18:3108–3114.

Answer 61

Per St. Jude's experience, the estimated cumulative incidence rate at 20 years was 9.2% for any second malignancy and 6.5% for sarcoma. No secondary sarcomas developed among patients who received less than 48 Gy. The absolute risk of secondary sarcoma was 130 cases per 10,000 person-years of observation among patients who had received ≥ 60 Gy.

Kuttesch JF Jr, Wexler LH, Marcus RB, et al. Second malignancies after Ewing's sarcoma: radiation dose-dependency of secondary sarcomas. *J Clin Oncol*. 1996;14:2818–2825.

Answer 62

Rhabdomyosarcoma is the most common soft tissue sarcoma in children, accounting for 3–4% of all cases of childhood cancer, with approximately 350 new cases per year in the U.S. This tumor is more common in males, and 60% occur in patients under the age of 10 years.

Pappo AS, Russell HV, Komguth DG, et al. Cancers of childhood. In: DeVita V, Hellman S, Rosenberg SA, eds. *Cancer: Principles and Practice of Oncology*. 8th ed. Philadelphia, PA: Wolters Kluwe Health Lippincott Williams & Wilkins; 2008:2043–2083.

Question 63

What are the most common sites, and which are favorable for rhabdomyosarcoma?

Question 64

What is the grouping system for rhabdomyosarcoma?

Question 65

What is the staging system for rhabdomyosarcoma?

Answer 63

The most common sites are head and neck (40%: subdivided into parameningeal 25%, orbit 9%, and non-parameningeal 6%), genitourinary 30%, extremity 15%, and trunk 15%. Favorable sites include the orbit, head and neck (excluding parameningeal), genitourinary (non-bladder and non-prostate), and biliary tract.

Pappo AS, Russell HV, Komguth DG, et al. Cancers of childhood. In: DeVita V, Hellman S, Rosenberg SA, eds. *Cancer: Principles and Practice of Oncology.* 8th ed. Philadelphia, PA: Wolters Kluwe Health Lippincott Williams & Wilkins; 2008:2043–2083.

Answer 64

Clinical grouping is a surgical-pathologic staging system that depends on the surgical resectability of the disease and the presence or absence of metastases:

· Group I: R0 resection, localized disease
· Group II: R1 resection and/or resected with positive lymph nodes
· Group III: R2 (both primary and positive lymph nodes) or biopsy only
· Group IV: Distant mets

The grouping and staging systems, in addition to histologic subtype, should be used to stage patients with pediatric rhabdomyosarcoma because therapy and outcome closely depend on the variables outlined by each system.

Pappo AS, Russell HV, Komguth DG, et al. Cancers of childhood. In: DeVita V, Hellman S, Rosenberg SA, eds. *Cancer: Principles and Practice of Oncology.* 8th ed. Philadelphia, PA: Wolters Kluwe Health Lippincott Williams & Wilkins; 2008:2043–2083.

Answer 65

The pretreatment TNM staging system stratifies patients into four different categories based on the site of the primary tumor, tumor size, presence or absence of nodal and distant disease, and invasiveness.

· T1: Confined to anatomic site of origin
  T1a: ≤ 5 cm
  T1b: > 5 cm
· T2: Extension or fixed to adjacent tissue
  T2a: ≤ 5 cm
  T2b: > 5 cm
· N1: regional node involvement
· M1: distant mets
· Stage I: Favorable site (any T, any N)
· Stage II: Unfavorable site, T1a–T2a (< 5 cm), N0
· Stage III: Unfavorable site, T1b–T2b (> 5 cm), and/or N1
· Stage IV: Any M1

The grouping and staging systems, in addition to histologic subtype, should be used to stage patients with pediatric rhabdomyosarcoma because therapy and outcome closely depend on the variables outlined by each system.

Pappo AS, Russell HV, Komguth DG, et al. Cancers of childhood. In: DeVita V, Hellman S, Rosenberg SA, eds. *Cancer: Principles and Practice of Oncology.* 8th ed. Philadelphia, PA: Wolters Kluwe Health Lippincott Williams & Wilkins; 2008:2043–2083.

Question 66

What factors define the risk groups and what is the expected outcome for each risk group for rhabdomyosarcoma?

Question 67

What is the benefit of RT for unfavorable histology in rhabdomyosarcoma?

Question 68

How should orbital rhabdomyosarcoma be treated?

Question 69

GERM CELL TUMORS (NON-CNS)

What is the most common histological subtype of germ cell tumors in children?

Answer 66

Low risk (5 year OS 90–95%): nonmetastatic, embryonal, *and*
- Favorable site (group I–III) or
- Unfavorable site groups I–II

Intermediate risk
- Nonmetastatic, group III embryonal, unfavorable site (5-year OS 70–85%) or
- Nonmetastatic unfavorable histology, any site (5-year OS 55–60%)
- Metastatic embryonal (stage IV group IV), age 2–10 (as per current COG study)

High risk (5-year OS 25–35%): all other metastatic disease

Pappo AS, Russell HV, Komguth DG, et al. Cancers of childhood. In: DeVita V, Hellman S, Rosenberg SA, eds. *Cancer: Principles and Practice of Oncology*. 8th ed. Philadelphia, PA: Wolters Kluwe Health Lippincott Williams & Wilkins; 2008:2043–2083.

Answer 67

Based on IRS I-III, patients in clinical group 1 with unfavorable histology who received RT had improved failure-free survival and overall survival. In IRS-1 and II, patients with alveolar or undifferentiated histologies who received RT compared to those who did not receive RT had improved 10-year failure-free survival rates (73% vs 44%, $p = .03$) and overall survival rates (82% vs 52%, $p = .02$). In IRS-III, these patients also experienced improved 10-year FFS (95% vs 69%, $p = .01$) and overall survival (95% vs 86%, $p = .23$).

Wolden SL, Anderson JR, Crist WM, et al. Indications for radiotherapy and chemotherapy after complete resection in rhabdomyosarcoma: A report from the Intergroup Rhabdomyosarcoma Studies I to III. *J Clin Oncol*. 1999;17:3468–3475.

Answer 68

Primary surgery is not recommended for the orbit, and treatment should consist of chemotherapy and radiation. The radiation dose is 45 Gy to the tumor volume plus margin taking into consideration doses delivered to the lens, lacrimal gland, cornea, retina, optic nerve, bony structures, and brain. The volume does not need to include the entire orbit if the tumor is small. Treatment with the eye open to avoid bolus effect of the lids, unless the lids are involved, may be preferred.

MacDonald SM, Friedmann AM, Tarbell NJ, et al. Rhabdomyosarcoma. In: Halperin E, Constine L, Tarbell N, et al., eds. *Pediatric Radiation Oncology*. 5th ed. Philadelphia, PA: Lippincott Williams & Wilkins; 2011:204–229.

Answer 69

Mature teratoma is the most common histologic subtype. Other subtypes include germinomas, embryonal carcinoma, yolk sac tumor, malignant mixed germ cell tumors, and immature teratomas.

Carrie C, Halperin EC. Germ and stromal tumors of the gonads and extragonadal germ cell tumors. In: Halperin E, Constine L, Tarbell N, et al., eds. *Pediatric Radiation Oncology*. 5th ed. Philadelphia, PA: Lippincott Williams & Wilkins; 2011: 303–310.

Question 70

What are the most common anatomical sites for extragonadal germ cell tumors?

Question 71

What are the common tumor markers associated with yolk sac tumors?

Germinomas?

Choriocarcinomas?

Question 72

How are children with mature teratomas managed?

Question 73

What is the optimal surgical procedure to evaluate a suspected testicular malignancy in a young boy?

Is a retroperitoneal dissection of lymph nodes indicated for staging in young boys?

Answer 70

The most common sites are the midline sites, consistent with embryonic patterns of migration. The midline sites include sacrococcygeal, presacral, and buttock regions. Additional sites of extragonadal germ cell tumors include the mediastinal, vaginal, uterine, and prostatic regions.

Carrie C, Halperin EC. Germ and stromal tumors of the gonads and extragonadal germ cell tumors. In: Halperin E, Constine L, Tarbell N, et al., eds. *Pediatric Radiation Oncology*. 5th ed. Philadelphia, PA: Lippincott Williams & Wilkins; 2011: 303–310.

Answer 71

a. Yolk sac: alpha feto proteins (AFP)
b. Germinomas: beta hCG < 100ng/mL (pure germinomas do not secrete AFP)
c. Choriocarcinomas: beta hCG > 100ng/mL

The half-life for AFP is 5–7 days and for beta hCG is 24–36 hours.

Carrie C, Halperin EC. Germ and stromal tumors of the gonads and extragonadal germ cell tumors. In: Halperin E, Constine L, Tarbell N, et al., eds. *Pediatric Radiation Oncology*. 5th ed. Philadelphia, PA: Lippincott Williams & Wilkins; 2011: 303–310.

Answer 72

Surgery and observation can be done with excellent prognosis. In a review of 153 children with nontesticular mature teratoma, the 6-year relapse-free survival for completely resected disease was 96% versus 55% for incomplete resection.

Göbel U, Calaminus G, Engert J, et al. Teratomas in infancy and childhood. *Med Pediatr Oncol*. 1998;31:8–15.

Answer 73

Radical inguinal orchiectomy with initial high ligation of the spermatic cord is the procedure of choice. Transscrotal biopsy can risk inguinal node metastasis. Retroperitoneal dissection of lymph nodes is not beneficial in the staging of testicular GCTs in young boys.

Rescorla FJ. Pediatric germ cell tumors. *Semin Surg Oncol*. 1999;16:144–158.
Schlatter M, Rescorla F, Giller R, et al. Excellent outcome in patients with stage I germ cell tumors of the testes: a study of the Children's Cancer Group/Pediatric Oncology Group. *J Pediatr Surg*. 2003;38:319–324.

Question 74

What is the standard chemotherapy for both children and adults with malignant nonseminomatous GCTs?

Question 75

What is the role of RT in extragonadal germ cell tumors?

Question 76   MEDULLOBLASTOMA

What percentage of pediatric CNS tumors do medulloblastomas comprise?

What genetic syndromes are associated with this diagnosis?

Question 77

What are poor prognostic factors for medulloblastoma?

Answer 74

Bleomycin, etoposide, cisplatin (BEP). Typically, 4–6 cycles are given.

Cushing B, Giller R, Cullen JW, et al. Randomized comparison of combination chemotherapy with etoposide, bleomycin, and either high-dose or standard-dose cisplatin in children and adolescents with high-risk malignant germ cell tumors: a pediatric intergroup study-Pediatric Oncology Group 9049 and Children's Cancer Group 8882. *J Clin Oncol.* 2004;22:2691–2700.

Answer 75

Radiotherapy is not necessary for children who have a documented complete response to surgery and chemotherapy, with low local recurrence rates in this patient population. When only a partial response to chemotherapy and surgery is achieved in localized disease, the chance of irradiation in achieving local control is modest, although the radiotherapy literature in this patient population is based on older forms of chemotherapy. Doses of 45–50 Gy are recommended, as limited by the tolerance of surrounding normal tissue.

Carrie C, Halperin EC. Germ and stromal tumors of the gonads and extragonadal germ cell tumors. In: Halperin E, Constine L, Tarbell N, et al., eds. *Pediatric Radiation Oncology.* 5th ed. Philadelphia, PA: Lippincott Williams & Wilkins; 2011:303–310.
Ablin AR, Krailo MD, Ramsay NK, et al. Results of treatment of malignant germ cell tumors in 93 children: a report from the Children's Cancer Study Group. *J Clin Oncol.* 1991;9:1782–1792.

Answer 76

20%. This makes it the 2nd most common pediatric CNS tumor behind low-grade glioma (35–50%). The U.S. incidence is 500 cases per year. Gorlin syndrome (nevoid basal cell carcinoma syndrome) and desmoplastic medulloblastoma are associated through the Sonic Hedgehog Pathway. Turcot syndrome, which is associated with the APC gene, is associated with medulloblastoma that develop via the WNT pathway. Li-Fraumeni syndrome, which results from p53 mutations, accounts for a small percentage of medulloblastoma.

McNeil DE, Coté TR, Clegg L, et al. Incidence and trends in pediatric malignancies medulloblastoma/primitive neuroectodermal tumor: a SEER update. Surveillance epidemiology and end results. *Med Pediatr Oncol.* 2002;39:554–557.
Garrè ML, Cama A, Bagnasco F, et al. Medulloblastoma variants: age-dependent occurrence and relation to Gorlin syndrome-a new clinical perspective. *Clin Cancer Res.* 2009;15:2463–2471.

Answer 77

Male gender, age < 5 years old, < GTR and M+ disease

Kun LE, MacDonald S, Tarbell NJ. Medulloblastoma. In: Halperin E, Constine L, Tarbell N, et al., eds. *Pediatric Radiation Oncology.* 5th ed. Philadelphia, PA: Lippincott Williams & Wilkins; 2011:53–63.

Question 78

What are the T and M stages in the modified Chang staging system for medulloblastoma?

Question 79

Which patients are considered standard risk medulloblastoma and how should they be treated?

Question 80

What are the borders for the spinal and cranial fields in traditional, prone technique craniospinal irradiation (CSI)?

Answer 78

Extent of Tumor

T1	≤ 3 cm
T2	> 3 cm
T3a	> 3 cm with extension into the aqueduct of Sylvius and/or the foramen of Luschka
T3b	> 3 cm with unequivocal extension into the brainstem (can be defined by intraoperative demonstration of tumor extension into the brainstem in the absence of radiographic evidence)
T4	> 3 cm with extension up past the aqueduct of Sylvius and/or down past the foramen magnum

Degree of Metastasis

M0	No evidence of gross subarachnoid or hematogenous metastasis
M1	Microscopic tumor cells found in the cerebrospinal fluid
M2	Gross nodular seeding demonstrated in the cerebellar/cerebral subarachnoid space or in the third or lateral ventricles
M3	Gross nodular seeding in the spinal subarachnoid space
M4	Metastasis outside the cerebrospinal axis

Chang CH, Housepain EM, Herbert C. An operative staging system and a megavoltage radiotherapeutic technique for cerebellar medulloblastomas. *Radiology.* 1969;93:1351–1359.

Kun LE, MacDonald S, Tarbell NJ. Medulloblastoma. In: Halperin E, Constine L, Tarbell N, et al., eds. *Pediatric Radiation Oncology.* 5th ed. Philadelphia, PA: Lippincott Williams & Wilkins; 2011:53–63.

Answer 79

Standard risk is defined as age ≥ 3 years old, GTR/STR (with < 1.5 cm of residual disease), and M0. Treatment: Surgical resection → CSI 23.4 Gy (1.8 Gy/fx) with posterior fossa boost to 54 Gy with concurrent weekly vincristine → PCV (procarbazine, CCNU, vincristine). The Children's Oncology Group ACNS0331 is currently evaluating the role of posterior fossa boost versus resection cavity boost on a randomized trial.

Packer RJ, Gajjar A, Vezina G, et al. Phase III study of craniospinal radiation therapy followed by adjuvant chemotherapy for newly diagnosed average-risk medulloblastoma. *J Clin Oncol.* 2006;24:4202–4208.

Answer 80

	Spinal (Simulate First)	Cranial (Parallel/Opposed Laterals)
Superior	As low as possible along the cervical spine. (slight neck hyper-extension, to minimize exit through mouth)	Flash scalp
Inferior	1–2 cm margin on lowest level of thecal sac on sagittal spine MRI (usually bottom of S2)	As low as possible along the cervical spine, 0.5–1 cm on cribriform plate 1 cm on middle cranial fossa
Lateral	1 cm from lateral edge of pedicles (increase by 1–2 cm in sacrum)	
Anterior		Ensure coverage on cribriform plate, middle cranial fossa and spinal cord

Kun LE, MacDonald S, Tarbell NJ. Medulloblastoma. In: Halperin E, Constine L, Tarbell N, et al., eds. *Pediatric Radiation Oncology.* 5th ed. Philadelphia, PA: Lippincott Williams & Wilkins; 2011:53–63.

Question 81

What is the appropriate management for medulloblastoma patients < 3 years old?

Question 82

What did the CCG 921 high-risk medulloblastoma trial investigate?

Question 83   **BRAINSTEM GLIOMA**

How common are brainstem gliomas in children and adolescents, and what histologies are most frequently seen?

Question 84

What is the prognosis in terms of median overall survival in children with brainstem gliomas?

What factors bode for worse prognosis overall in brainstem gliomas?

Answer 81

Maximal safe resection → chemo until patient reaches age 3 (at which point can consider CSI → more chemo). In a Children's Cancer Group study, patients were treated with one of two 4-drug combination chemotherapy regimens, and RT was withheld unless there was evidence of tumor progression. At 5 years, 10 of 38 children who had M0 disease were alive and event-free without having received RT.

Geyer JR, Sposto R, Jennings M, et al; Children's Cancer Group. Multiagent chemotherapy and deferred radiotherapy in infants with malignant brain tumors: a report from the Children's Cancer Group. *J Clin Oncol.* 2005;23:7621–7631.

Answer 82

In CCG 921, high-risk patients (classified as age 1.5–21, or M1-4, or T3-4, or residual > 1.5 cm^2) were randomized to CSI 36 Gy/PF 54 Gy/spinal mets 50.4–54 Gy (age < 3 received CSI 23.4 Gy/PF 45 Gy) + concurrent vincristine → Vincristine, lomustine, and prednisone (VCP). x8 versus "8 in 1" (vincristine, prednisone, lomustine, hydroxyurea, procarbazine, cisplatin, cyclophosphamide, cytarabine) chemotherapy x2 → RT → "8 in 1" chemo x8. Better 5-year PFS with VCP arm (65% vs 45%, $p = .006$).

Zeltzer PM, Boyett JM, Finlay JL, et al. Metastasis stage, adjuvant treatment, and residual tumor are prognostic factors for medulloblastoma in children: conclusions from the Children's Cancer Group 921 randomized phase III study. *J Clin Oncol.* 1999;17:832–845.

Answer 83

Brainstem gliomas comprise roughly 10% of all intracranial tumors in children. The incidence peaks between ages 5–9, and is seen more often in males than females. Diffusely infiltrating brainstem gliomas are most common, comprising 75–85% of brainstem neoplasms in children and adolescents (15–25% are focal or "exophytic"). High-grade astrocytomas comprise 70–80%.

Kun LE, MacDonald S, Tarbell NJ. Brainstem glioma. In: Halperin E, Constine L, Tarbell N, et al., eds. *Pediatric Radiation Oncology.* 5th ed. Philadelphia, PA: Lippincott Williams & Wilkins; 2011:72–77.

Answer 84

The prognosis is very poor with a 1-year average median survival. The disease is fatal in > 90% of patients. Diffuse infiltrating, high-grade, and younger age bode for worse prognosis. Patients with focal disease have a 10-year OS of 50–70%. Dorsally exophytic and tectal lesion locations are considered more favorable.

Kun LE, MacDonald S, Tarbell NJ. Brainstem glioma. In: Halperin E, Constine L, Tarbell N, et al., eds. *Pediatric Radiation Oncology.* 5th ed. Philadelphia, PA: Lippincott Williams & Wilkins; 2011:72–77.

Question 85

What is the typical treatment sequence for children with a diffusely infiltrating pontine glioma?

What is the role for chemotherapy?

Question 86

Are there roles for dose escalation or hyperfractionation in brainstem gliomas?

Question 87

What kind of impact does radiation therapy have on disease progression of brainstem glioma?

Question 88   EPENDYMOMA

What are the expected outcomes for children with ependymoma treated with surgical resection and adjuvant conformal radiotherapy?

Answer 85

Steroids/shunt (if necessary), followed by radiation (54–59 Gy in 1.8–2 Gy fractions). Chemotherapy has not shown to be effective in the treatment of diffuse pontine gliomas. Most recently, temozolomide was tested in a COG phase II trial and found to be ineffective.

Cohen KJ, Heideman RL, Zhou T, et al. Temozolomide in the treatment of children with newly diagnosed diffuse intrinsic pontine gliomas: a report from the Children's Oncology Group. *Neuro-Oncology.* 2011;13:410–416.

Answer 86

No. In various trials (POG, CHOP/NYU, CCG, UCSF), dose escalation to anywhere from 66–78 Gy showed no benefit in disease control or survival. For example, POG 9239 compared conventional fractionation of 54 Gy at 1.8 Gy per fraction versus a twice daily regimen of 1.17 Gy for a total dose of 70.2 Gy. Cisplatin was used as a radiation sensitizer. There was no difference in median time to progression (6 months in the standard arm versus 5 months in the hyperfractionated arm) and median overall survival (8.5 months in the standard arm versus 8 months in the hyperfractionated arm).

Freeman CR, Krischer JP, Sanford RA, et al. Final results of a study of escalating doses of hyperfractionated radiotherapy in brain stem tumors in children: a Pediatric Oncology Group study. *Int J Radiat Oncol Biol Phys.* 1993;27:197–206.
Mandell LR, Kadota R, Freeman C, et al. There is no role for hyperfractionated radiotherapy in the management of children with newly diagnosed diffuse intrinsic brainstem tumors: results of a Pediatric Oncology Group phase III trial comparing conventional vs hyperfractionated radiotherapy. *Int J Radiat Oncol Biol Phys.* 1999;43:959–964.
Prados MD, Wara WM, Edwards MS, et al. The treatment of brain stem and thalamic gliomas with 78 Gy of hyperfractionated radiation therapy. *Int J Radiat Oncol Biol Phys.* 1995;32:85–91.

Answer 87

60–70% of those with classic pontine glioma show improvement of functional status. Ultimately, radiotherapy can delay median time to progression by 6–8 months.

Kun LE, MacDonald S, Tarbell NJ. Brainstem glioma. In: Halperin E, Constine L, Tarbell N, et al., eds. *Pediatric Radiation Oncology.* 5th ed. Philadelphia, PA: Lippincott Williams & Wilkins; 2011:72–77.

Answer 88

There is an overall survival benefit to postoperative radiation therapy as published by the St. Jude's experience. In a study of 153 patients (median age 2.9 years) treated with conformal radiotherapy after definitive surgery (59.4 Gy or 54 Gy), after a median follow-up of 5.3 years, 10 year OS was 75%, LC was 87%, and EFS was 69%.

Merchant TE, Li C, Xiong X, et al. Conformal radiotherapy after surgery for paediatric ependymoma: a prospective study. *Lancet Oncol.* 2009;10:258–266.

Question 89

What are poor prognostic factors for an intracranial ependymoma?

Question 90

What is the most common location for pediatric ependymomas?

Where else can they be found?

Question 91

What are the histological subtypes of ependymoma?

What is the classic pathological feature?

Question 92

Can patients < 3 years of age be given high-dose radiation therapy after surgical resection?

Answer 89

Less than GTR (most important factor), age < 4 years old, supratentorial location, and overexpression of erbB-2/erbB-4.

Kun LE, MacDonald S, Tarbell NJ. Ependymomas (infants, children, and adolescents). In: Halperin E, Constine L, Tarbell N, et al., eds. *Pediatric Radiation Oncology*. 5th ed. Philadelphia, PA: Lippincott Williams & Wilkins; 2011:66–72.

Answer 90

Posterior fossa (2/3 of all pediatric ependymomas) is the most common location. Greater than 90% of pediatric ependymomas are intracranial, representing 5–8% of intracranial neoplasms in children. Ependymomas are also found in the spine, representing 25% of pediatric spinal tumors. In adults, the majority of ependymomas are located in the spine.

Kun LE, MacDonald S, Tarbell NJ. Ependymomas (infants, children, and adolescents). In: Halperin E, Constine L, Tarbell N, et al., eds. *Pediatric Radiation Oncology*. 5th ed. Philadelphia, PA: Lippincott Williams & Wilkins; 2011:66–72.

Answer 91

Grade 1: Myxopapillary (spinal) and subependymoma
Grade 2: Classic ependymoma (cellular, papillary, clear cell, tanycytic, giant cell, epitheliod)
Grade 3: Anaplastic
Grade 4: Ependymoblastoma

The classical pathologic feature is perivascular pseudorosettes.

Kun LE, MacDonald S, Tarbell NJ. Ependymomas (infants, children, and adolescents). In: Halperin E, Constine L, Tarbell N, et al., eds. *Pediatric Radiation Oncology*. 5th ed. Philadelphia, PA: Lippincott Williams & Wilkins; 2011:66–72.

Answer 92

Yes. St. Jude's experience suggests (prospective study including 78% of patients < 3 years of age) that RT can be given safely and effectively in these patients. Young age should not prevent patients from receiving standard 54 to 59.4 Gy adjuvant radiation therapy unless they are infants < 1 year old.

Merchant TE, Li C, Xiong X, et al. Conformal radiotherapy after surgery for paediatric ependymoma: a prospective study. *Lancet Oncol*. 2009;10:258–266.

Question 93 OSTEOSARCOMA

How common is osteosarcoma, and who is primarily affected?

Question 94

What are the most common sites for osteosarcoma?

Question 95

What is the T-N-M staging for osteosarcomas?

Question 96

What is the role of chemotherapy in the treatment of osteosarcoma?

Answer 93

Osteosarcoma is the most common primary bone tumor in the pediatric population. It typically affects male children in the second decade of life. There is a strong genetic correlation with the inactivation of the retinoblastoma (Rb) gene.

Woo S, Halperin E. Osteosarcoma, chordoma, and chondrosarcoma. In: Halperin E, Constine L, Tarbell N, et al., eds. *Pediatric Radiation Oncology.* 5th ed. Philadelphia, PA: Lippincott Williams & Wilkins; 2011:184–202.

Answer 94

Osteosarcomas affect the metaphyses of long bones, especially the knee joint. Bony distribution based on a large group of patients treated on Neoadjuvant German-Austrian-Swiss Cooperative Osteosarcoma Study Group (COSS): Femur (50%), tibia (26%), humerus (15%), fibula (6%), and pelvis (5%).

Bielack S, Kempf-Bielack B, Delling G, et al. Prognostic factors in high-grade osteosarcoma of the extremities or trunk: an analysis of 1,702 patients treated on neoadjuvant Cooperative Osteosarcoma Study Group protocols. *J Clin Oncol.* 2002;20:776–790.

Answer 95

The staging system is consistent with that of bone tumors.

- Tx: Primary tumor cannot be assessed
- T0: No evidence of primary tumor
- T1: Tumor ≤ 8 cm in greatest dimension
- T2: Tumor > 8 cm in greatest dimension
- T3: Discontinuous tumors in the primary bone site
- Nx: Regional lymph nodes cannot be assessed
- N0: No regional lymph node metastases
- N1: Regional lymph node metastases
- M0: No distant metastases
- M1a: Lung metastasis
- M1b: Other distant metastasis besides lung

Edge SB, Byrd DR, Compton CC, et al., eds. Bone. *AJCC Cancer Staging Handbook: from the AJCC Cancer Staging Manual.* 7th ed. New York, NY: Springer; 2010:284.

Answer 96

Randomized trials have established that both neoadjuvant and adjuvant chemotherapy should be incorporated with surgical resection (for localized, resectable primary tumors) in order to prevent relapse and recurrence.

Eilber F, Giuliano A, Eckardt J, et al. Adjuvant chemotherapy for osteosarcoma: a randomized prospective trial. *J Clin Oncol.* 1987;5:21–26.

Link MP, Goorin AM, Miser AW, et al. The effect of adjuvant chemotherapy on relapse-free survival in patients with osteosarcoma of the extremity. *N Engl J Med.* 1986;314:1600–1606.

Question 97

What is the 5-year survival for nonmetastatic and metastatic osteosarcoma?

Question 98

What is the recommended radiation dose for definitive management of unresectable osteosarcoma?

Question 99   **CRANIOPHARYNGIOMA**

What is the main histology for craniopharyngioma in children, and what are its characteristics? How does this differ from the histology seen in adults?

Question 100

What endocrine abnormalities are most commonly seen at time of diagnosis of craniopharyngiomas?

Answer 97

In the setting of treatment with chemotherapy and surgery for nonmetastatic osteosarcoma, the 5-year overall survival is 60–70%. Metastatic osteosarcoma 5 year overall survival is approximately 20%. Histologic response predicts for survival in non-metastatic patients. Primary site, number of metastases, and location of metastases predict for EFS for patients with metastatic disease.

Kager L, Zoubek A, Potschger U, et al.; Cooperative German-Austrian-Swiss Osteosarcoma Study Group. Primary metastatic osteosarcoma: presentation and outcome of patients treated on neoadjuvant Cooperative Osteosarcoma Study Group Protocols. *J Clin Oncol.* 2003;21:2011–2018.

Woo S, Halperin E. Osteosarcoma, chordoma, and chondrosarcoma. In: Halperin E, Constine L, Tarbell N, et al., eds. *Pediatric Radiation Oncology.* 5th ed. Philadelphia, PA: Lippincott Williams & Wilkins; 2011:184–202.

Answer 98

Older studies suggest radiation doses up to 60–75 Gy (or as high as normal tissue tolerance allows), with shrinking fields for definitive management of unresectable osteosarcoma. In a more recent retrospective review, the recommended radiation dosage is at least 55 Gy. This review suggested that doses > 55 Gy were associated with improved local control rates. The local control rate was 71% +/− 9% for 32 patients receiving doses ≥ 55 Gy vs 53.6% +/− 20.1% for 9 patients receiving < 55 Gy.

DeLaney TF, Park L, Goldberg SI, et al. Radiotherapy for local control of osteosarcoma. *Int J Radiat Oncol Biol Phys.* 2005;61:492–498.

Answer 99

The major histology seen in childhood craniopharyngioma is adamantinomatous. These tumors are typically calcified, comprised of solid components and large complex cysts filled with lipid-laden fluid described as "crankcase oil." Squamous cell histology is seen almost exclusively in adults. These tumors tend to be solid, without cystic components.

Kun LE, MacDonald S, Tarbell NJ. Craniopharyngioma. In: Halperin E, Constine L, Tarbell N, et al., eds. *Pediatric Radiation Oncology.* 5th ed. Philadelphia, PA: Lippincott Williams & Wilkins; 2011:40–44.

Answer 100

At diagnosis, 50–90% of pediatric patients will present with endocrine abnormalities, with growth hormone deficiency being the most common, though diabetes insipidus (DI) can be seen in 10–20% of cases as well. Sexual dysfunction is the most frequently seen endocrine abnormality in adults.

Kun LE, MacDonald S, Tarbell NJ. Craniopharyngioma. In: Halperin E, Constine L, Tarbell N, et al., eds. *Pediatric Radiation Oncology.* 5th ed. Philadelphia, PA: Lippincott Williams & Wilkins; 2011:40–44.

Question 101

What is the role for radiosurgery (SRS), and what is the recommended dose in the management of craniopharyngioma?

Question 102

What is the consensus on initial primary management of craniopharyngioma?

Question 103

What is the overall expected survival and the prognostic features for patients with craniopharyngioma?

Answer 101

The role for SRS in craniopharyngioma is primarily for postoperative residual disease, or in the setting of recurrent disease, where tumors should be at least 5 mm away from the optic apparatus and hypothalamus. Dose for SRS is 12–14 Gy.

Plowman PN, Wraith C, Royle N, et al. Stereotactic radiosurgery. IX. Craniopharyngioma: durable complete imaging responses and indications for treatment. *Br J Neurosurg*. 1999;13:352–358.

Answer 102

The two primary approaches for craniopharyngioma management include GTR or maximal safe resection followed by adjuvant radiotherapy (54–55 Gy with 1.8 Gy/fx). In a recent study, the 10-year local control with surgery (GTR or STR) alone versus surgery and radiation was found to be 42% vs 84%, respectively. Additionally, St. Jude data (2002) revealed that the IQ deficit for aggressive surgical management was 8.8 points compared to limited surgery with radiation group where average IQ loss was 1.25 points.

Merchant TE, Kiehna EN, Sanford RA, et al. Craniopharyngioma: the St. Jude Children's Research Hospital experience 1984–2001. *Int J Radiat Oncol Biol Phys*. 2002;53:533–542.

Stripp DC, Maity A, Janss AJ, et al. Surgery with or without radiation therapy in the management of craniopharyngiomas in children and young adults. *Int J Radiat Oncol Biol Phys*. 2004;58:714–720.

Answer 103

Overall, the prognosis is very good, with 5 and 10 year overall survival rates of 89–96% and 85–91%, respectively, and local control rates of 63% and 53–75%. Poor prognostic factors include: age ≤ 5 years, severe hydrocephalus, ≥ 3.5 cm tumor height in midline, presence of signs of hypothalamic disturbance, intraoperative complications, and removal of tumor observed to be adherent to hypothalamus.

De Vile CJ, Grant DB, Kendall BE, et al. Management of childhood craniopharyngioma: can the morbidity of radical surgery be predicted? *J Neurosurg*. 1996;85:73–81.

Scott RM, Hetelekidis S, Barnes PD, et al. Surgery, radiation, and combination therapy in the treatment of childhood craniopharyngioma–a 20-year experience. *Pediatr Neurosurg*. 1994;21(suppl 1):75–81.

Stripp DC, Maity A, Janss AJ, et al. Surgery with or without radiation therapy in the management of craniopharyngiomas in children and young adults. *Int J Radiat Oncol Biol Phys*. 2004;58:714–720.

INDEX